Physics Applied to Anaesthesia

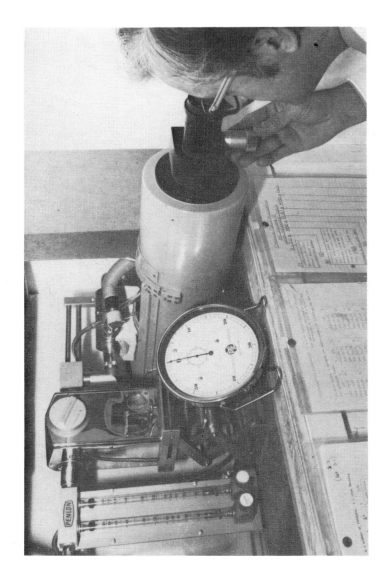

A Carl Zeiss interferometer in the thoroughly ventilated, air conditioned calibration room of Penlon Ltd, being used to test a vaporizer. (By courtesy of Penlon Ltd)

Physics Applied to Anaesthesia

Fourth Edition

D. W. Hill M.Sc., Ph.D., D.Sc., F.Inst.P., F.I.E.E.

Regional Scientific Officer
North East Thames Regional Health Authority

Butterworths
London – Boston
Sydney – Wellington – Durban – Toronto

United Kingdom London	Butterworth & Co (Publishers) Ltd 88 Kingsway, WC2B 6AB
Australia Sydney	Butterworths Pty Ltd 586 Pacific Highway, Chatswood, SW 2067 Also at Melbourne, Brisbane, Adelaide and Perth
Canada Toronto	Butterworth & Co (Canada) Ltd 2265 Midland Avenue, Scarborough, Ontario, M1P 4S1
New Zealand Wellington	Butterworths of New Zealand Ltd T & W Young Building, 77–85 Customhouse Quay, 1, CPO Box 472
South Africa Durban	Butterworth & Co (South Africa) (Pty) Ltd 152–154 Gale Street
USA Boston	Butterworths (Publishers) Inc 10, Tower Office Park, Woburn, Massachusetts 01801

First published 1967
Second edition 1972
Third edition 1976
Reprinted 1978
Fourth edition 1980

© Butterworth & Co (Publishers) Ltd 1980

ISBN 0 407 00188 3

British Library Cataloguing in Publication Data

Hill, Dennis Walter
    Physics applied to anaesthesia. - 4th ed.
    1. Anesthesia
    2, Medical physics
    I. Title
    530′ .02′4617   RD82   80-4011

    ISBN 0-407-001883

Typeset by Scribe Design, Medway, Kent
Printed by W & J Mackay Ltd., Chatham

Foreword to the first edition

Shortly after the Research Department of Anaesthetics was founded in the Royal College of Surgeons in 1957 under the chairmanship of the late Professor R.F. Woolmer, Dr. Hill was appointed lecturer in Physics. His book *Physics Applied to Anaesthesia* not only reflects the range and depth of Dr. Hill's experience since his appointment but also confirms the fundamental soundness of Professor Woolmer's approach to the developing needs of Anaesthesia. As Professor Woolmer's successor I am greatly honoured that his pupil should have asked me to introduce his work.

Of recent years much has been written about the inadequacies of medical education and the controversy has not been confined to the undergraduate curriculum. Differences have arisen in the postgraduate field and nowhere has this been more apparent than in the specialty of Anaesthesia. The great technical advances of the last decade have altered the pattern of the anaesthetist's duties and increased the range of his responsibilities so much that there has been a widespread demand for a radical change in training programmes. In particular the curriculum for the Fellowship examination in anaesthetics has been widely criticized and indeed the need for revision has been fairly generally accepted for some time. But there has also been an understandable reluctance to upset an order which appeared both solid and incontrovertible. However, the need for reform has finally prevailed and a decision to revise the curriculum and the pattern of the examination has now been taken. Shortly, Anatomy will lose its predominant position in the primary examination to be replaced by Physics, Clinical Measurement and Clinical Chemistry, subjects more closely related to the needs of modern Anaesthesia. This decision is undoubtedly the right one and marks a significant step in the emancipation of the anaesthetist from a curriculum ordained more by tradition and historical association than by present day requirements. Many will agree that the reformers' case must have been greatly strengthened by the substantial contributions made to anaesthetics teaching and research by those physicists who have chosen to work within the speciality.

Thus, Dr. Hill's book is opportune. Based on the series of lectures on medical physics presented to the postgraduate students in the Royal College of Surgeons he has expanded his material to ensure that all aspects of his subject of interest to anaesthetists have been covered. Dr. Hill combines an ease of expression with a wealth of practical experience from which a substantial amount of this material is derived. Scrutiny of his text reveals Dr. Hill's close association with colleagues trained in many different scientific disciplines and emphasizes once again the advantages of a multi-discipline approach to research problems. The nature and extent of these cooperative efforts augur well for the future of research in Anaesthesia. Professor Woolmer's foresight in appointing a physicist to his staff and encouraging him to become involved in the general research activities of his department has been amply justified.

Research Department of Anaesthetics
Royal College of Surgeons of England   **J.P. Payne**

Preface

Whatever else might be said of *Physics Applied to Anaesthesia* it has stood the test of time in the thirteen years that have passed since the first edition appeared.

Throughout this period there has been a steadily increasing appreciation of the physical foundations of much of anaesthetic practice and equipment and this applies equally to intensive care. Successive editions at roughly four year intervals have provided the opportunities to thoroughly revise the text and to incorporate new material where appropriate. The SI system of units is now adopted in the United Kingdom and these units appear throughout the book, although the equivalents in earlier units are provided since older equipment will still be scaled in non-SI units.

General purpose computers are now generally available and are widely used for statistical treatment of data. Many anaesthetists will be familiar with at least one high-level computing language. On the other hand, the increasing incorporation of microcomputers into devices such as blood-gas analysers will place much more computing power in the hands of the user of 'intelligent' instruments.

When a book reaches its fourth edition, it is apparent that it must be supplying a genuine need and the author will have the advantage of perusing a number of reviews of his work. Several helpful suggestions made by reviewers have been incorporated into this edition. From the start, the book was never conceived as an elementary primer on physics for the anaesthetist. Rather it was written as a source book of information, both for F.F.A.R.C.S. students and for anaesthetists and physicists requiring a textbook to assist in their understanding of specific physics topics likely to be required in their practice or research. The former will need to be selective in their reading under the guidance of a tutor in order that they can concentrate on the main principles and leave the details until later.

Students working for the F.F.A.R.C.S. come from diverse backgrounds and many find physics a difficult subject. In addition to reading a textbook, it is helpful – in the author's experience at the University of London Institute of Basic Medical Sciences – to have an alternative audio-visual approach as a back-up. With the cooperation of the Audio-Visual Centre of London University and my colleague Dr. I.R. Perry, it has been possible to make a series of videotapes covering: Logarithms and Exponentials for the Anaesthetist (2 tapes); Statistics (2 tapes); SI Units; Laminar and Turbulent Flow; Electrical Safety; Blood-gas Analysis; Vaporizers; Automatic Lung Ventilators; The Gas Laws. The tapes are available in most formats and can be obtained from the University of London Audio-Visual Centre, 11 Bedford Square, London WC1.

The preparation of this book owed much to the constructive suggestions of students on the Primary F.F.A.R.C.S. courses held at a number of teaching hospitals and the technical information provided by a number of manufacturers of equipment.

The staff of the Medical Division of Butterworths have taken a keen interest in the preparation of another edition and I am most grateful for their loyal support and encouragement.

D.W. Hill

Abbreviations and conversion factors

Metre	m	Pound-force (similarly for kilogram-force etc.)	lbf
Micrometre	μm	Bar (10^6 dyn cm^{-2})	bar
Nanometre	nm	Millibar	mb
Inch	in	Atmosphere, standard	atm
Foot	ft	Atmosphere, absolute	ata
Square metre (similarly for square centimetre, etc.)	m^2	Atmosphere, gauge	atg
Square inch (similarly for square foot, etc.)	in^2	Millimetre of mercury	mmHg
Cubic metre (similarly for cubic centimetre, etc.)	m^3	Joule	J
		Erg	erg
Cubic inch (similarly for cubic foot, etc.)	in^3	Kilowatt hour	kWh
Litre	l	Foot-pound-force	ft lbf
Gallon	gal	Calorie	cal
		Kilocalorie	kcal
Second (time)	s	Watt	W
Minute (time)	min	Decibel	dB
Hour	h	Degree Celsius	°C
Day	d	Degree Kelvin	K
		Degree Fahrenheit	°F
Degree:minute:second (angle)	° ′ ″	Candela	cd
		Lumen	lm
Radian	rad	Lux	lx
Radian per second	rad s^{-1}		
Cycle per second (hertz)	Hz	Hydrogen ion exponent	pH
Revolution per minute	rev min^{-1}	Coulomb	C
		Ampere	A
Gram	g	Volt	V
Kilogram	kg	Ohm	Ω
Pound	lb	Farad	F
Dyne	dyn	Henry	H
Newton	N		
Stokes	St	Curie	Ci
Poise	P	Becquerel	Bq
		Gray	Gy
		Sievert	Sv

Prefixes

Prefixes denoting decimal multiples or submultiples

Indicating submultiples			*Indicating multiples*		
$\times 10^{-2}$	: centi	c	$\times 10^{12}$	: tera	T
$\times 10^{-3}$	: milli	m	$\times 10^{9}$	: giga	G
$\times 10^{-6}$	: micro	μ	$\times 10^{6}$	: mega	M
$\times 10^{-9}$	: nano	n	$\times 10^{3}$	: kilo	k
$\times 10^{-12}$	: pico	p			

The symbols listed above are in accordance with British Standard
Specification 1991 : Part 6:1963

Conversion table

To Convert	*Multiply by*
Calories to joules	4.186
Cubic inches to cubic centimetres	16.39
Cubic feet to cubic metres	0.0283
Cubic feet to litres	28.32
Gallons (Imperial) to gallons (U.S.A.)	1.201
Gallons (Imperial) to fluid ounces	160.0
Gallons (Imperial) to cubic feet	0.161
Gallons (Imperial) to litres	4.546
Pounds weight to newtons	4.448
Foot pounds to joules	1.356
Horse power to watts	746
Horse power to foot pounds per second	550
Inches to centimetres	2.540
Pounds to grams	453.6
Square inches to square centimetres	6.452
Pounds per square inch to kiloponds per square centimetre	0.070
Pounds per square inch to newtons per square metre	6895
Pounds per square inch to bars	0.069
Millimetres of mercury to newtons per square metre	133
Centimetres of water to newtons per square metre	0.98
Metre-kiloponds to joules	9.086
Kiloponds per square centimetre to pounds per square inch	14.22
Dynes per square centimetre to newtons per square metre	0.10

Contents

1 Some mathematical concepts

Physics is traditionally a mathematical subject, and in applying the concepts of physics, and modern physical techniques, to anaesthesia it is helpful to have at least some background of elementary mathematics. Many anaesthetists instinctively recoil from anything mathematical, but on reflection most will agree with these sentiments, particularly those with research interests. It is the purpose of this introductory chapter to provide a revision of some of the more frequently encountered topics.

Trigonometry

The trigonometrical ratios

Consider the right-angled triangle OXP in *Figure 1.1*. For angle $\angle$POX, the following trigonometrical ratios apply: the sine of $\angle$POX is given by the ratio of the sides PX to PO, i.e. $\sin \angle POX = PX/PO$. The cosine of $\angle$POX is given by the ratio of the sides OX to OP, i.e. $\cos \angle POX = OX/OP$, and the tangent of $\angle$POX is given by $\tan \angle POX = XP/XO$. It

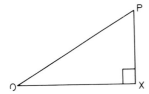

Figure 1.1

is worth remembering that $\sin 30° = \frac{1}{2}$, $\cos 30° = (\sqrt{3})/2$, $\sin 45° = (\sqrt{2})/2$, $\cos 45° = (\sqrt{2})/2$, $\tan 45° = 1$, $\sin 60° = (\sqrt{3})/2$, $\cos 60° = \frac{1}{2}$, $\sin 90° = 1$, $\cos 90° = 0$, and $\tan 90° = \infty$.

The inverse functions

Suppose that $\angle POX = 30°$, then this fact can also be written as $\angle POX = \sin^{-1}(\frac{1}{2})$, this notation simply means that $\angle POX$ is the angle whose sine has a value of $\frac{1}{2}$. It has nothing to do with the reciprocal of a sine. Similarly, $\angle POX = \cos^{-1}(\sqrt{3}/2)$ and $\angle POX = \tan^{-1}(\sqrt{3}/3)$. To avoid the possibility of confusion, the inverse ratios are sometimes written as arcsin, arccos and arctan. The mathematical compilers of digital computers usually contain a routine for calculating the angle for a given value of the tangent, i.e. an arctan routine. Some pocket calculators also have an arc key. This is used in conjunction with the sin, cos or tan keys. For example, to find the angle in degrees whose sine is 0.44444, enter 0.44444 into the calculator, press the arc key followed by the sin key and the answer displayed is 26.38 degrees. Entering the angle in degrees and pressing the sin, cos or tan keys will give the appropriate trigonometrical ratio. Long gone are the days of trigonometrical tables!

Very small angles

For small angles, $\sin \theta$ and $\tan \theta$ are approximately equal to the value of θ in radians. The smaller the angle, the more accurate is this approximation. The error is less than 2 per cent for angles up to $20°$ for sines and up to $13°$ for tangents.

Triangles

It will be recalled that from Pythagoras' theorem, $OP^2 = OX^2 + XP^2$ (*Figure 1.1*). Thus if the lengths of the sides of the triangle are in the ratio of 5:12:13 or 3:4:5, the triangle must be right-angled. The sum of the internal angles of any triangle equals $180°$. For any angle $\angle POX$, $\sin^2 \angle POX + \cos^2 \angle POX = 1$.

Similar triangles

Consider the triangles ABC and ADE in *Figure 1.2*. ADE is clearly an extension of ABC and the triangles are said to be similar in shape. It is

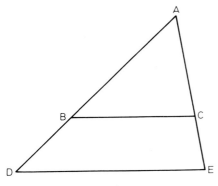

Figure 1.2

a property of similar triangles that AB/AD=AC/AE. Since BC is parallel to DE, the angles of the two triangles will correspond.

Circular measure

In *Figure 1.3* let OX and OP be radii of a circle, centre O. If OP rotates to the position OX, the angle ∠POX is swept out. If OX turns through one complete revolution to return to its initial position ∠POX=360°.

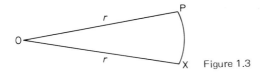

Figure 1.3

Angle ∠POX can also be expressed in *circular measure,* that is in radians. The number of radians in the angle is given by the ratio of its arc to its radius, i.e. PX/XO (*Figure 1.3*). If XO=r, then the circumference of the circle has a length of $2\pi r$, and the angle in radians equivalent to one complete revolution is given by $2\pi r/r=2\pi$ radians. It is seen that $90°=\pi/2$ radians and $180°=\pi$ radians.

In *Figure 1.4* let OP represent a crank which revolves at a rate of f revolutions per second. The angular velocity ω of the crank will be equal to $2\pi f$ radians per second. At time $t=0$, the crank starts from position OS. After a further t seconds, the crank will have turned through an angle (ωt) radians. If the crank is connected to a piston U in a gas-filled cylinder by a long connecting rod, the volume of gas v swept out by the piston at any instant will be given by the equation

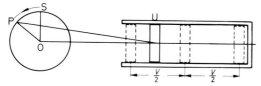

Figure 1.4

$v=\frac{1}{2}V \sin(\omega t)$, where V is the volume of the cylinder. Measuring from the mid-point of the stroke, the variation of the volume swept out with time is shown in *Figure 1.5*. In one complete movement of the piston, the swept volume is V. Taking a rotation of $360°$ to give one complete cycle, and remembering that $\sin 0°=0$, $\sin 90°=1$ etc., it is seen that the curve of *Figure 1.5* is a sine waveform.

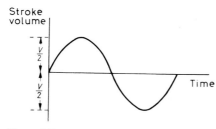

Figure 1.5

Sine waveform pumps give an easily reproducible waveform and are widely specified for the testing of items such as anaesthetic vaporizers and demand-type anaesthetic machines. *Figure 1.6* shows a sine-wave respiratory waveform simulator due to Hill, Hook and Bell (1961) which employs an electronic speed control system. It can be shown that the maximum velocity of the pump's piston, and hence of the gas leaving the cylinder, is equal to π times the minute volume pumped (Cooper, 1961). Thus this type of pump can be used to provide known gas flow rates without the need to actually measure the flow. A typical application occurs in the calibration of a pneumotachograph and also in the testing of demand regulators designed for use with pre-mixed nitrous oxide and oxygen.

The plotting of graphs with linear axes

In *Figure 1.7* the position of a point P can be defined in respect of two axes OX and OY at right-angles to each other. These are traditionally

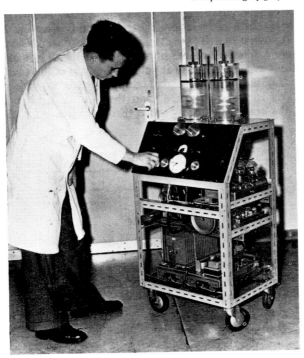

Figure 1.6. Servo-controlled respiratory waveform simulator

called the X and Y axes. Point O is called the *origin*. Let OQ have a length equal to x units, and QP equal to y units. Any point in the two-dimensional plane containing the X and Y axes can be now defined in terms of its x and y co-ordinates. These are also known as *cartesian* co-ordinates. The x co-ordinate is called the *abscissa* and the y co-ordinate is known as the *ordinate* of the point in question.

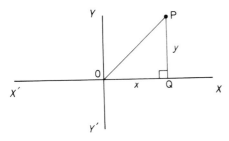

Figure 1.7

OX and OY are taken as positive and OX' and OY' are taken as negative, tan $\angle POQ = y/x$, hence $y = x$ tan $\angle POQ$. Let tan $\angle POQ = m$, then any point which lies on the straight line OP is defined by the equation $y = mx$. The term m is known as the *slope* or *gradient* of the line. The line $y = mx$ passes through the origin ($x = 0, y = 0$). In *Figure 1.8* the line makes an intercept of length c on the Y axis, and the equation to this line is $y = mx + c$, in *Figure 1.8* and $y = mx - c$ in *Figure 1.9*. This idea of

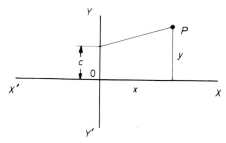

Figure 1.8

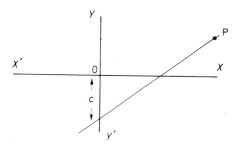

Figure 1.9

the 'slope' of a line becomes important when it is necessary to consider the physical concept of a differential coefficient in the calculus notation. With this simple straight-line relationship, y is linearly related to x. Such a linear function is often assumed to be the natural order of things. For example, it can be easily taken for granted that the expansion of the mercury thread in a thermometer is linear, i.e. that the calibration will be the same at both high and low temperatures, which of course it is not. It is also very tempting to draw a straight line through a series of scattered points on a graph, when in fact a curved relationship may exist. It is a fact that non-linear relationships are often encountered in anaesthetic practice. During streamline or laminar flow conditions, the volume flow of a gas through a tube is linearly related to the pressure drop existing across the tube. However, when turbulence is produced, a power relationship occurs between the volume flow and the pressure drop. This fact can be readily evaluated by means of a semi-logarithmic, rather than a linear plot. The need to plot semi-logarithmic graphs also occurs in estimating the rate of decay of the activity of a radio-iodinated human serum albumin solution used in plasma-volume studies, and in dealing with the uptake or elimination of volatile anaesthetic agents from various body compartments.

Indices

Any number X multiplied by itself n times is said to be raised to the power n, and this is written as X^n. In digital computing, 2 to the power n is frequently encountered, e.g. $2^4=16$. The numbers n and 4 are called indices.

$X^n \times X^m = X^{(n+m)}$. Thus to multiply together powers of the same number, the indices are added. $X^n \times X^o = X^{(n+0)} = X^n$ so that $X^o = 1$. Any number raised to the power zero equals unity.

$(X^n)^m = X^{nm}$, i.e. when a power is itself raised to a power, the two indices are multiplied together.

$(XY)^n = X^n \times Y^n$, i.e. when the product of two numbers is raised to a power, the result is equal to the product of the two numbers each raised to that power.

$$X^{-n} = 1/X^n \text{ and } X^{(1/n)} = \sqrt[n]{X}, \text{i.e., the } n\text{th root of } X.$$

In particular, $\sqrt{XY} = \sqrt{X} \times \sqrt{Y}$ and

$$\sqrt{\frac{X}{Y}} = \frac{\sqrt{X}}{\sqrt{Y}}$$

Surds

A square root that cannot be further reduced is known as a surd, e.g. $\sqrt{2}, \sqrt{3}, \sqrt{5}$.

Rationalization

The evaluation of an expression such as $1/\sqrt{2}$ can be speeded by multiplying the numerator and denominator by $\sqrt{2}$; this will leave the value of the expression unaltered. Thus

$$\frac{1}{\sqrt{2}} = \frac{1}{\sqrt{2}} \times \frac{\sqrt{2}}{\sqrt{2}} = \frac{\sqrt{2}}{2} = \frac{1.414}{2} = 0.707$$

Logarithms

When dealing with very large or very small numbers, calculations are greatly simplified by working in terms of indices. Thus one million equals 1 000 000 which is 10 to the power 6, i.e. 10^6. One thousandth equals 10^{-3} and so on. In electronics one is frequently concerned with currents of the order of 10^{-10} A and resistances of the order of $10^{12}\,\Omega$.

It is possible to express any number in terms of the appropriate power of 10. The power to which a fixed number (the base) must be raised to produce a given number is called the logarithm (Greek *logos*, reckoning, *arithmos*, number) of that number to that particular base. Thus 6 is the logarithm to the base 10 of 1 000 000, written as $\log_{10}$ (1 000 000)=6, and 2 is the logarithm to the base 10 of 100. Since $10^{(a+b)}=10^a \times 10^b$, the logarithm of the product of two numbers is equal to the sum of the logarithms of the individual numbers. The logarithm of the quotient of the two numbers is equal to the difference of the logarithms of the individual numbers, thus $\log_{10}(ab)=\log_{10} a + \log_{10} b$ and $\log_{10}(a/b)=\log_{10} a - \log_{10} b$. These rules apply whatever the value of the base. The usual *common logarithms* are to the base 10, but tables are also available of *natural* or *Naperian logarithms* which are to the base e.

The *exponential* e has a value of 2.7183 and is an important quantity in mathematics. Exponential functions govern a number of relationships encountered in anaesthesia. The value of e can be calculated from the infinite series

$$e = 1 + \frac{1}{1} + \frac{1}{2 \times 1} + \frac{1}{3 \times 2 \times 1} + \frac{1}{4 \times 3 \times 2 \times 1} \cdots$$

This is a form of the general expression

$$e^x = 1 + x + \frac{x^2}{2 \times 1} + \frac{x^3}{3 \times 2 \times 1} + \ldots \qquad \text{with } x = 1.$$

The usefulness of the series is that it enables any number raised to a power to be expressed in terms of a series. Thus, using this series, logarithms could be calculated.

Natural logarithms are often denoted by ln, for example, ln x. Digital computers calculate the natural logarithms of numbers and these must then often be converted into common logarithms by means of a conversion factor.

$\log_e N = \log_{10} N / \log_{10} e$; but $\log_{10} 2.718 = 0.4343$

Thus

$\log_e N = \log_{10} N / 0.4343$,

i.e.

$\log_e N = 2.30261 \log_{10} N$

and

$\log_{10} N = 0.4343 \log_e N$

The whole concept of pH is based upon the use of logarithms. For simplicity we can say that the pH value of a solution is equal to -1 multiplied by the power to which 10 must be raised to give the hydrogen ion concentration of the solution. Thus a pH of 7 indicates a hydrogen ion concentration of 10^{-7} moles per litre. Because the scale is logarithmic and not linear, the average of pH 6, pH 7 and pH 8 is not simply pH 7. The average hydrogen ion concentration of the three solutions is $(3.7) \times 10^{-7}$ giving an average pH value of 7.57.

Linear, semi-logarithmic and logarithmic plots

Most graphs are plotted on simple linear graph paper, where equal increments of length on the axes now represent equal additions of the variables. *Figure 1.10* illustrates a simple linear scale starting from zero, and *Figure 1.11* shows a logarithmic scale. These never start from zero. This follows since 10^0 is not 0 but 1. For a logarithmic scale, equal increments represent multiplication by a constant factor, in this case by a factor of ten. Some organs such as the eye and the ear have a logarithmic response, and can handle a wide range of input intensities without overloading. For this reason, sound intensity is expressed in terms of a logarithmic unit, the decibel.

Organs in which a subjective sensation increases with the logarithm of the objective influence obey the Weber—Fechner law. The retina is able to accept light intensity variations over a range of 10^8 at least, the

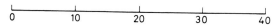

Figure 1.10

corresponding pupil area changing only by a factor of about 5. Over a range of light intensity from about 3×10^{-6} to 3 candelas m^{-2}, there is a linear decrease in the pupil area from some 35 to 10 mm^2. The process follows an equation of the type $A = A_0 - K \log I$. A plot of A

| 1 | 10 | 100 | 1000 | 10 000 |
| 10^0 | 10^1 | 10^2 | 10^3 | 10^4 |

Figure 1.11

against $\log I$ will give a straight line of slope $-K$. The wide range of stimuli that can be handled by an organ is also illustrated in the case of the ear where the sound pressure ratio is $10^{5.5}:1$ between the threshold of pain and the auditory threshold.

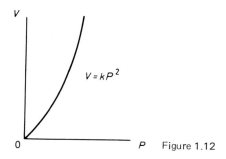

$V = kP^2$

0   P   Figure 1.12

If a turbulent gas flow occurs when a pressure difference P exists across a pipe, it can be shown that the minute volume of gas flow is given by an equation of the form $V = kP^n$. If $n = 2$, the graph plotted on linear axes would have the form of *Figure 1.12*. Taking the logarithms of both sides, we have $\log_{10} V = n \log_{10} P + \log_{10} k$. This is similar in form to $y = mx + c$ and represents a straight line. The slope of the line is equal to the value of the constant n. This is now a logarithmic plot, since log V is plotted against log P. This type of plot has been used by Cooper (1961) to evaluate the performance of breathing apparatus.

In a semi-logarithmic plot, one axis is linear and the other logarithmic. The linear axis may often represent time. Both logarithmic and semi-logarithmic graph papers are available. Semi-logarithmic plots are widely used for the stripping (separating) of the components of multi-exponential curves and for the re-plotting of dye dilution cardiac output curves.

In plotting either linear or logarithmic graphs using cartesian co-ordinates, each point on the graph is plotted with respect to its x and y co-ordinates. The x and y values are known as variables, since their magnitudes are not fixed, but change throughout the period of the observations for which the graph is plotted. However, for each individual graph point some relationship will exist between the corresponding x and y value. It is usually convenient to decide on some particular values of x and then to find the corresponding values of y and plot them. In this case x is called the independent variable and y the dependent variable. Conventionally, the independent variable is plotted as the abscissa and the dependent variable as the ordinate. For example, the stroke volume of a patient might be plotted against time, with time as the independent variable.

Decibels
In a complex electronic system containing a large number of circuits each contributing a gain or a loss, calculation of the overall transmission gain or loss may be tedious. The calculation is simplified by expressing individual power ratios in terms of decibels (abbreviation dB). The power loss or gain of a circuit expressed in decibels is given by $D = 10 \log_{10} (P_2/P_1)$ where P_2 is the output power and P_1 is the input power. If (P_2/P_1) is less than unity, then $10 \log_{10} (P_2/P_1)$ will be negative. Thus a negative sign indicates a power loss while a positive sign indicates a power gain. If the input power to an amplifier is 2 mW and the output power is 2 watts, the power gain is 1000. Since $\log_{10} 1000$ is 3, this represents a power gain of 30 dB. The decibel is fundamentally a unit of power ratio and not of absolute power. However, if some power level is taken as a standard, then any absolute power can be expressed in terms of so many dB above or below this standard. The standard level usually adopted is one milliwatt. Thus one watt is +30 dB with respect of 1 mW. This is often contracted to 30 dBm.

When it is required to compare the powers developed in two *equal* resistors, it is sufficient to measure just the two currents or the two voltages. The power ratio in decibels is given by $D=20 \log_{10} (V_2/V_1)$ or $20 \log_{10} (I_1/I_2)$. The factor 20 instead of 10 arises from the fact that the power developed in a resistor is proportional to the square of the voltage or current.

Generally speaking, the frequency response of an amplifier will be reasonably flat over quite a wide range of frequencies, but will fall off at the upper and lower ends of the frequency spectrum. It is conventional to define the upper and lower limits of the frequency response in terms of the half-power points. A fall in power of 50 per cent is equivalent to -3 dB, so that these points are also known as the 3 dB points. At the half-power points the output voltage of the device will have fallen to $(1/\sqrt{2})$ i.e. 0.707 of its original value at 0 dB. Hence the frequency response of pen galvanometers is often specified in terms of the 3 dB frequency, i.e. the upper frequency at which the pen amplitude has fallen to 70 per cent of its value when on the flat portion of the frequency response curve. The input signal is of course kept constant. When discussing the frequency response of pressure transducer—catheter systems the 3 dB frequency may be too coarse a measure and it may be preferable to talk in terms of that frequency at which the signal amplitude has fallen by 5 per cent.

The circle

On the basis of a knowledge of the pairs of x and y co-ordinates for each point, it is possible to plot graphs showing the relationship of x and y on a variety of scales for the axes. In a number of cases, particular shapes of graphs can be associated with an equation, so that substitution of pairs of x and y values will give rise to a set of points which can then be joined up to describe the graphical relationship existing between x and y. A simple example is the equation to a straight line $y = mx + c$. Another simple equation is that to a circle, *Figure 1.13*. Let O be the origin ($x = 0$, $y = 0$) and also the centre of the circle. Let $OP = r$ be any radius. Then by Pythagoras' theorem, $x^2 + y^2 = r^2$ which is the equation defining a circle with its centre at O and radius r. If another circle has its centre not now at the origin but at some point C ($x = a, y = b$) as shown in *Figure 1.14*, then the equation to that circle is $(x - a)^2 + (y - b)^2 = r^2$.

A knowledge of the principles of co-ordinate geometry and the use of equations to define curves is essential in order to be able to write a computer program which can instruct a digital graph plotter to trace

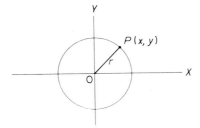

Figure 1.13

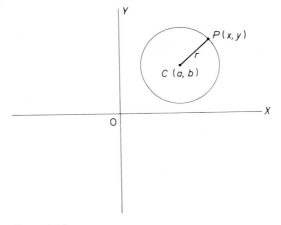

Figure 1.14

out particular shapes, for example, a family of oxygen dissociation curves corresponding to various carbon dioxide tensions in arterial blood.

Conic sections

When a right circular cone is sliced by a plane, the cut surface can be either a parabola, an ellipse or a hyperbola (or a circle, of course) depending upon the angle between the plane and the axis of the cone.

Hence, the parabola, ellipse and hyperbola are called conic sections. The parabola and the hyperbola occur in a number of relationships found in physiology and anaesthesia.

An alternative definition of a conic section is that it is the locus of a point which moves in a plane so that its distance from a fixed point in the plane is in a constant ratio to its distance from a fixed straight line in the plane. The fixed point is known as the *focus*, the fixed line is the *directrix* and the constant ratio is the *eccentricity* of the curve.

The standard equation of the parabola

Referring to *Figure 1.15*, O is the origin of the parabola ($x = 0, y = 0$), S is the focus ($x = a$, $y = 0$) and the directrix passes through the point ($x = -a$, $y = 0$) at right-angles to OX the axis of the parabola. For a parabola, the eccentricity has a value of unity, so that if any point P on the parabola has co-ordinates (x, y) then PS = PM i.e. $PS^2 = PM^2$ so

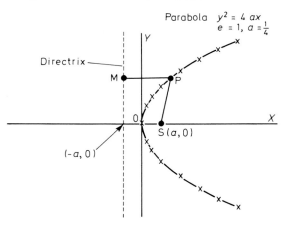

Figure 1.15

that $(x - a)^2 + y^2 = (x + a)^2$ giving $y^2 = 4ax$ which is the standard equation of a parabola. Because of the y^2 term, for all values of y, x will be positive, so that no part of the curve can lie to the left of the origin.

If a source of light or heat radiation is placed at the focus of the parabola, then after reflection at the parabolic surface all the rays from the focus will emerge as a beam parallel to the axis. Thus, parabolic reflectors are commonly encountered in optical systems, searchlights and electric radiant fires. The velocity profile of a fluid flowing down a pipe with a streamline motion is also parabolic. When the flow pattern through the pipe is fully turbulent, the parabolic relationship $P = kF^2$ obtains, where P is the pressure drop across the pipe, F is the volume flow rate and k is a constant.

The standard equation of the ellipse

Figure 1.16 shows an ellipse which is symmetrical about the origin O. Because of the symmetry there are now two foci S and S', and two directrices DD' and $D_1D'_1$. For an ellipse, the eccentricity is less than unity. The equation of this ellipse is

$$\frac{x^2}{a^2} + \frac{y^2}{b^2} = 1$$

where the length of the major axis AA' is equal to $2a$, the length of the minor axis BB' is equal to $2b$, the focal distances OS and OS' are

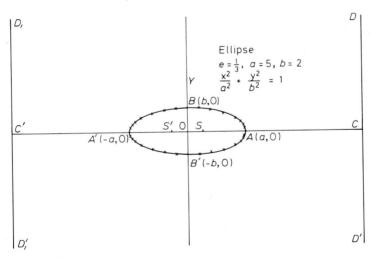

Figure 1.16

respectively $+ae$ and $-ae$, OC $= +a/e$ and OC' $= -a/e$. If the inner surface of an elliptical cavity is silvered to act as a reflector and a source of light is situated at one focus, then light from it will be brought to a focus at the second focal point. This arrangement is employed in ruby lasers which have been built into opthalmoscopes and used for welding detached retinas back into place, although this is no longer the technique of choice. A powerful xenon flash tube is located at one focus and the ruby rod at the other. When the flash tube is discharged, its light emission irradiates the ruby rod and causes a flash of ruby laser light to be emitted.

The standard equation of the hyperbola

For the third conic section, the hyperbola, the eccentricity is greater than unity. *Figure 1.17* shows the two portions of a symmetrical hyperbola whose equation is

$$\frac{x^2}{a^2} - \frac{y^2}{b^2} = 1.$$

The point O is the origin $(0, 0)$, S and S' are the foci where $OS = +ae$ and $OS' = -ae$. DD' and $D_1 D'_1$ are the directrices where $OC = +a/e$ and $OC' = -a/e$. The equation for a hyperbola can be re-written as

$$y = \pm \frac{bx}{a} \sqrt{\left(1 - \frac{a^2}{x^2}\right)}$$

so that when x becomes very large, y tends towards a value $(b/a)x$. The lines $y = +(b/a)x$ and $y = -(b/a)x$ are shown in *Figure 1.17* and are known as the asymptotes of the hyperbola. When x has a value of plus or minus infinity they will be tangents to the hyperbola. The transverse axis of the hyperbola has a length of $2a$. The conjugate axis lies along the y-axis and has a length of $2b$.

The rectangular hyperbola

A hyperbola is said to be rectangular when its transverse and conjugate axes are equal in length, thus $a = b$ and the equation for a rectangular hyperbola referred to its axes as the axes of co-ordinates becomes $x^2 - y^2 = a^2$. If the asymptotes are taken as the axes of co-ordinates this simplifies to $xy =$ a constant, the curve now having the form of *Figure 1.18*. This is the familiar equation of Boyle's law for a perfect gas which states that for a given mass of gas at a constant temperature, the product of its pressure and volume is a constant. For the given mass of gas, a family of rectangular hyperbolas will exist, each corresponding to a different temperature. The curve can be shifted up or down the y-axis by the addition of a second constant term 'b', i.e. $y = (k/x) + b$. This is

Hyperbola $\quad e = \frac{4}{3} \qquad a = 1 \qquad b = 0.78$

$$\frac{x^2}{a^2} - \frac{y^2}{b^2} = 1$$

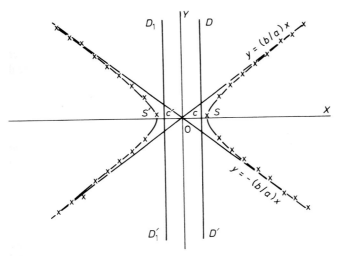

Figure 1.17

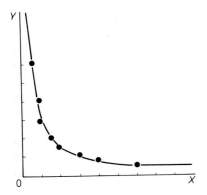

Figure 1.18

well illustrated in *Figure 1.19* which shows the empirical strength–duration curve for the electrical excitation of muscle or nerve. The threshold strength of the stimulating current required to just excite the tissue depends on the duration of the current flow, the greater the current the less the time for which it need be applied. Here '*b*'

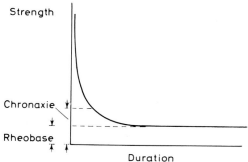

Figure 1.19

represents the minimum value of current which will just excite the tissue whatever the duration of current flow. This critical minimum value of the current is called the rheobase. The minimum time needed to excite a tissue at a current equal to twice the rheobase is known as the chronaxie.

Calculus

Differentiation

It can be most useful to have even an elementary notion of the elements of the differential and integral calculus. The idea of a differential coefficient can be gathered from *Figure 1.20*. The slope of the

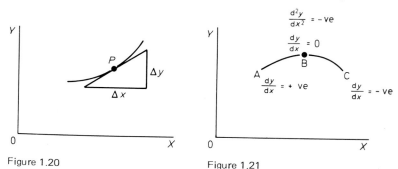

Figure 1.20

Figure 1.21

curve at point P is given by the slope of the tangent drawn at point P. Numerically, this is equal to $\Delta y/\Delta x$, where Δy, Δx are small increments of y and x respectively. Using the conventional calculus notation, if Δy and Δx are made vanishingly small they are written as dy and dx. The differential coefficient dy/dx represents the instantaneous rate of change of y with x at a particular point.

Suppose that y varies with x, we say that y is a function of x. This is written as $y=f(x)$. On the other hand, if y depends on time, then $y=f(t)$. By using the standard techniques of the differential calculus, it is possible to determine the differential coefficient of any function (Thompson, 1957). In the case of the curve $y=kx^2$ (similar to that of *Figure 1.12*), the slope (differential coefficient of y with respect to x) increases rapidly with increasing x. It can be shown that for this curve, $dy/dx=2kx$ and the value of the slope at any point can be found by substituting for the appropriate values of y and x. The fact that the slope of an ECG waveform has its largest negative value on the down-slope of each R-wave is a useful criterion which can be used together with an amplitude criterion to identify valid R-waves. This approach was adopted by Sandman *et al.* (1973) in the design of an analogue pre-processor for the determination of R-R intervals and R-wave widths on-line from an ECG recording. In *Figure 1.21* is shown a graph which has a maximum at B. At a maximum, the slope changes sign. Thus over the portion AB, the slope has a positive value since y increases with increasing x. Over the portion BC, it has a negative value,

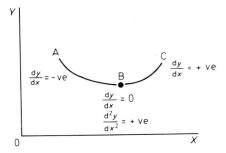

Figure 1.22

since y now decreases with increasing x. At point B the value of the slope is zero. As y passes through a maximum, dy/dx changes from +ve to −ve, it is therefore decreasing as x increases. Thus the differential coefficient of dy/dx is negative at a maximum. The second differential coefficient, written as d^2y/dx^2, represents the rate of change of the slope of the curve. Thus the two conditions which must be satisfied for a maximum are $dy/dx = 0$ and d^2y/dx^2 is negative. In *Figure 1.22* at the minimum, dy/dx is again zero, but d^2y/dx^2 is now positive. These conditions become of importance when it is desired to determine from the equation to a curve the period of time which must elapse before the curve reaches a maximum; for example, the time which will elapse after an injection before a particular drug will attain its maximum concentration in the blood.

Integration

It is possible to take the equation to a curve, and differentiate it to obtain the differential coefficient. The reverse process is known as integration. By integrating a differential coefficient the original equation can be regained. For example, the differential coefficient of y with respect to x when $y=x^2$ is $2x$. In fact the integral of $dy/dx=2x$ must be written as $y=x^2 +C$ where C is a constant of integration. Since C is just a constant term and does not contain x, its differential coefficient would be zero and would not appear in the differentiating process. The value of a constant of integration can be determined if the value of y for some definite value of x is known. Thus if $y = 2$ when $x = 1$, then $C = 1$. The value of C will also correspond with the initial condition for y, i.e. when $x = 0, y = C = 1$.

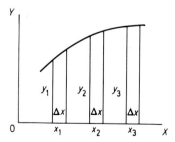

Figure 1.23

The action of integrating the equation to a curve is to determine the area under the curve between specified limits. In *Figure 1.23*, let the area under the curve between the values of $x=x_1$ and $x=x_3$ be divided up into a series of strips each of width Δx. The areas of the individual strips will be given by $y_1\Delta x$, $y_2\Delta x$, $y_3\Delta x$, etc. The whole of the area under the curve between the limits of x_1 and x_3 is simply equal to the sum of the areas of the strips. If Δx is made vanishingly small, then the total area A is given by

$$A = \int_{x=x_1}^{x=x_3} y dx.$$

The sign $\int$ simply means the continuous summation of the individual strip areas ($y dx$) between the limits of $x=x_1$ and $x=x_3$. This is called a *definite integral* because the process of integration is only performed between the definite limits of x_1 and x_3. Digital computer programs often use this method of summating the areas of thin strips to calculate the area under a dye dilution curve for cardiac output determination.

Exponential equations

If C is the concentration of an anaesthetic agent in the blood at a particular body site at any instant, then dC/dt represents the rate of change of the concentration with time. Equations containing differential coefficients are known as *differential equations*. A simple example would be the differential equation $dy/dx=2kx$, derived by differentiation of both sides of the original equation $y = kx^2$. The equation $dy/dx = (2k)x$ shows that the slope dy/dx of the original equation is directly proportional to the corresponding value of x. In physical terms the slope of $y = kx^2$ becomes progressively more steep as x increases.

Differential equations are commonly encountered in calculations concerning the uptake and elimination of volatile anaesthetic agents, the metabolism of drugs or the ventilation of the lungs. The decay with time of radioactive isotopes used for tracer studies can be expressed by a differential equation following an exponential law and this topic provides a convenient introduction to the subject.

Consider a quantity of a radioactive isotope which is decaying and changing into another form and during the process emits radioactivity. Suppose that a scintillation counter is used to count a constant fraction of the number of atoms disintegrating per second. At time $t=0$, at the start of the counting experiment, let there be a total of N_0 atoms still ready to decay. After an interval of t seconds, suppose that N_0 has fallen to N. Experiments reveal that the value of the time rate of decay (dN/dt) at any instant is proportional to the number of atoms left unchanged at that instant. That is to say, there is a simple linear relationship existing between the decay rate and the number of unchanged atoms. This can be expressed by writing $dN/dt = -kN$. The two related values dN/dt and N are linked by the factor k which is known as a *constant of proportionality*. The equation can be written in the form $dN/N = -k dt$, and both sides can now be integrated.

Standard textbooks on calculus show that the integral of $dN/N = \log_e N$. The integral of dt is simply t. By integrating, the equation $\log_e N = -kt + A$ is obtained, where A is a constant of integration. If A is a constant, then so will be $\log_e A$. In practice, it is more convenient to write the constant in this form. Thus $\log_e N = -kt + \log_e A$. Let $N = N_0$ at $t=0$. Then at $t=0$, $\log_e A = \log_e N_0$. Thus $\log_e N/N_0 = -kt$. This is the logarithmic form of $N = N_0 e^{-kt} = N_0 \exp(-kt)$. Because of the exponential term this is known as an *exponential equation*. The graph

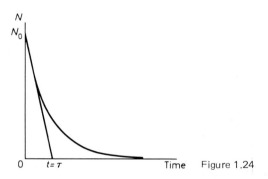

Figure 1.24

of this equation is given in *Figure 1.24*. Since the slope (dN/dt) is proportional to N, it falls off rapidly at first, and then more slowly. The equation has only one exponential term and is known as a simple exponential equation.

Time constant and half-life

The time constant of a simple exponential curve is defined as the time taken for the ordinate to fall to $1/e$ of its initial value. In the case of the radioactivity decay curve it is the time taken to fall to N_0/e, i.e. to 37 per cent of N_0. After an interval equal to two time constants, N will have fallen to 13.5 per cent of N_0 and to 5 per cent of N_0 after three time constants. As an approximation, a process is often said to be complete after the passage of four time constants since it will then be 1.8 per cent away from completion. If the line of the initial slope is projected as shown, it will strike the time axis at a value equal to one time constant. The half-life of the isotope is defined as the time taken for the initial level of the activity to fall to one half, i.e. at $t_{1/2}$, $N=N_0/2$. It can be shown that the half-life has a value equal to 69.3 per cent of the time constant. The physical half-life of radioactive krypton-85 used in cerebral blood flow studies is 10.6 years and that of radioactive iodine-131 used in blood volume determinations and thyroid and renal function tests is 8.04 days. It may not always be possible to count samples of blood and urine until a few days later and the count N can be back-corrected to its original value N_0 using the equation $N_0=N$ exp $(+kt)$ where t is the time interval which has elapsed prior to counting. The decay equation can also be written in the form $N=N_0$ exp $(-t/\tau)$ where τ is the time constant. Taking logarithms of both sides of the equation gives $\log_e N = -kt + \log_e N_0$. This can be re-written in the form $\log N = -C_1 t + C_2$. Thus for a simple exponential equation, a plot of $\log_e N$ against t will yield a straight line. This will also apply for $\log_{10} N$ since this is a semi-log plot. The availability of a semi-log plot is extremely useful in the dispensing of solutions of radioactive isotopes. The x-axis of the graph paper is scaled in days and a point marked at $t = 0$ with a y-value of unity. A y-value of 0.5 is marked at a time corresponding to the half-life and the two points joined with a straight line. Solutions of radiopharmaceuticals are normally supplied containing a known activity, say 1 millicurie in a volume of 1 ml, at 12 noon on a stated date. On receipt, the original 1 ml is usually diluted to 10 ml by the addition of 9 ml of sterile saline. Thus at 12 noon on the day in question each 1 ml will contain an activity of 100 microcuries. After the elapse of a time equal to the half-life, each 1 ml will now only contain 50 microcuries. Thus to obtain a dose of 100 microcuries, 2 ml will have to be injected. The reciprocal of the fraction left at any given day will give the number of millilitres which must be injected to provide the activity originally contained in a volume of 1 ml. If a y-value of 2 is plotted at the half-time and joined by a straight line to the y-value of one at $t = 0$, then the multiplying factors for the original volume of 1 ml can be read off directly from the graph. It is convenient to have a set of such graphs available for each of the commonly used radiopharmaceuticals.

Another example occurs in the measurement of cardiac output by the dye dilution technique. For a normal heart, the down-slope of the dye dilution curve is very close to a straight line plot prior to the recirculation peak when plotted on semi-log paper.

Multi-component exponential wash-out curves are frequently

encountered when the substance is cleared from several body compartments, as for example, in a nitrogen wash-out curve, or when counting over the heart following an injection of [131] I-labelled Hippuran in order to measure the effective renal plasma flow (Lavender, 1970; Rosen *et al.*, 1967). The nitrogen curve can be resolved into three components and the Hippuran curve can be resolved into two distinct components. In the case of the nitrogen curve, the fast component corresponds to a well-ventilated lung compartment and the slow component to a relatively poorly ventilated compartment. Another well known example is with the inert gas wash-out technique for the measurement of cerebral blood flow or renal blood flow (Thorburn *et al.*, 1963).

The exponential decay of a dye dilution curve

Let the volume of blood in the heart and pulmonary vessels be V litres and the cardiac output assumed to be a steady $\dot{Q}$ litres/minute.

At time $t=0$, M_0 milligrams of dye are injected as a bolus into the right heart and continuous mixing is assumed to occur when the

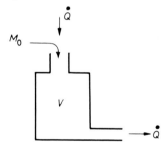

injection is complete. Then the rate at which dye leaves the heart equals the rate at which it passes through the aorta (*Figure 1.25*). The rate of decline of the mass of dye in the heart is $-\mathrm{d}M/\mathrm{d}t$ and the average concentration of dye at any instant is M/V where M is the mass present t seconds after the injection.

Then

$$\frac{-\mathrm{d}M}{\mathrm{d}t} = \frac{M}{V}\,\dot{Q};$$

re-arranging,

$$\frac{-\mathrm{d}M}{M} = \frac{\dot{Q}}{V}\,\mathrm{d}t$$

Integrating from $t=0$ to $t=t$

$$-\int_{M_0}^{M} \frac{dM}{M} = \int_{t=0}^{t=t} \frac{\dot{Q}}{V}\, dt$$

i.e.

$$\log_e (M/M_0) = -(\dot{Q}/V)t$$

so that

$$M = M_0 \exp(-\dot{Q}/V)t$$

This equation shows that the mass of dye remaining in the heart is diminishing with time in a simple exponential fashion and so therefore will the mass leaving the heart per unit time and, since the cardiac output is assumed to be steady, so will the concentration of dye expressed in mg per 100 ml of blood flowing into the aorta.

Thus the wash-out curve for the dye should follow a simple exponential law if the assumptions made are valid. Analysing 256 consecutive dye curves; the Sanborn Company (Medical Division of Hewlett Packard Ltd) found that over 95 per cent were exponential in form when the dye concentration was in the range 40–60 per cent of the peak value for the curve. Deviations from an exponential down slope are likely to occur with very low cardiac outputs and in patients with a marked degree of regurgitation due to aortic valve incompetence.

Elimination of a substance from more than one body compartment

The graph of the concentration of a volatile anaesthetic agent in the expired air against time may resemble the simple exponential curve of *Figure 1.24*, but in practice it will consist of a series of exponential terms, e.g. $C = C_1 \exp(-k_1 t) + C_2 \exp(-k_2 t)$. In this case the data will not yield a single straight line when plotted on semi-logarithmic paper. A number of digital computer programs have been written to strip out the pairs of constants and exponents which define each term. It is possible to recover three terms if the constants are separated by a ratio of at least 3:1 and the exponents separated by a ratio of at least 5:1 for successive terms. References to suitable digital computer programs are those of Gardner *et al.* (1959) and Borman, Shahn and Weiss (1962).

For those without access to such programs, it is necessary to resort to the technique of *backward projection*. The final portion of the semi-log plot of the original multi-component curve which is considered to be a single exponential is projected backwards to cut the *C* axis, and the values for the ordinates at suitable time intervals of the projected line are subtracted in turn from the corresponding ordinates of the original curve (*Figure 1.26*). If the plot of these differences against time is now a straight line, then the original curve can be considered as containing only two components. If however, the second plot is still curved then the backwards projection method is continued until only a straight line does remain. Usually, no more than three components can be isolated by backwards projection owing to lack of accuracy in the original data. The slopes and intercepts found will not be exact because of the difficulties in fitting the straight lines by eye. With the computer programs this is done by a least squares fit. Van Liew (1962) points out that many physiological processes, such as the wash-out of nitrogen from the lungs, can be considered as occurring from a great many compartments with time constants which are distributed continuously, rather than from the conventional two or three compartments. He

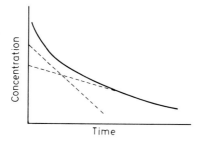

Figure 1.26. Isolation of two exponential terms from a compound exponential curve by the backwards projection technique

found that the backward projection technique gave misleading results when applied to systems in which the processes are distributed so that the standard deviation of half-times is large compared with the mean half-time. Examples of the backward projection technique are given by Matthews (1957).

Figure 1.27, taken from Whelpton (1969), shows the primary nitrogen wash-out curve from a patient. Broken down into its three constituent components, the expired nitrogen concentration measured with a gas-discharge nitrogen meter is plotted against breath number.

Curve 1 describes the regions of the lungs which are relatively well ventilated, curve 2 describes the poorly ventilated regions of the lungs and curve 3 represents the nitrogen returning to the lungs from the tissues to a first approximation. Whelpton found that the largest discrepancy between the composite curve and the clinical curve was about 5 per cent of the clinical values, and for most of the curve the

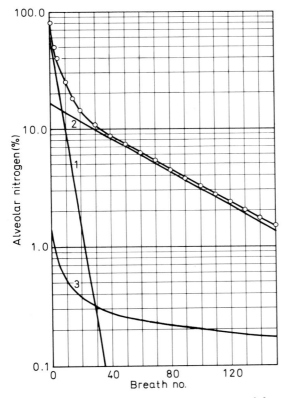

Figure 1.27. Analysis of a nitrogen wash-out curve (after Whelpton, 1969)

discrepany was less than 3 per cent of the clinical values. Let I_2 be the intercept made by curve 2 with the vertical axis. Following the analysis of Briscoe *et al.* (1960), the regional ventilation of the second less-well ventilated compartment is given by $\dot{V}_{A2} = \dot{V}_A I_2$ per cent where 80 per cent nitrogen represents the initial expired nitrogen value (in this case the patient had been breathing air and then changed over to oxygen). For this patient the alveolar ventilation $\dot{V}_A$ was 5 litres per minute and from *Figure 1.27*, $I_2 = 16$ per cent so that $\dot{V}_{A_2} = 1$ litre per minute. Since the total ventilation was 5 litres per minute, then $\dot{V}_{A_1} = 4$ litres per minute. Whelpton reports that the oxygen consumption for this patient was 343 ml per minute (STPD) so that $\dot{V}_A / \dot{V}_{O_2} = 5.0/0.343 = 14.6/1$, $\dot{V}_{A_2} / \dot{V}_{O_2} = 1.0/0.343 = 2.92/1$ and $\dot{V}_{A_1} / \dot{V}_{O_2} = 1.0/5.0 = 0.2/1$. The analysis of Briscoe *et al.* (1960) also allows the perfusion of each region to be determined. In this case the blood flow (assuming a constant haematocrit) to the lungs divides between regions 1 and 2 in the ratio 1.33:1 and ventilation in the ratio 4.0:1. The ratio of the volume of region 1 to that of region 2 is 0.35:1.

Applications of exponential equations

Mushin, Rendell-Baker and Thompson (1959) and Mapleson (1962) discuss the application of exponential curves to the inflation of the lungs; for example, they show that both the volume and the pressure in the lungs rise exponentially when a constant-pressure type of ventilator is used for inflation. Bergman (1963) proposed a two-compartment exponential equation for the clearance of thiopentone from dogs. For convenience, Bergman works to the power of 10 rather than to the power of e, and his equation is $C = (20.3) \, 10^{-0.037\,t} + (29.0) \, 10^{-0.00152\,t}$, where C is the concentration of thiopentone in the plasma in $mg\,l^{-1}$, and t is the time in minutes from the injection. Fink (1966) is in favour of equations to the base 10 for anaesthetics applications. It should be remembered that the decimal time constant for the process to decay to one tenth of its initial value is 2.3 times the conventional exponential time constant (time to decay to $1/e$ of the original value). Bowes (1964) discusses the exponential uptake and elimination of anaesthetic gases. Severinghaus (1963), Mapleson (1962) and Waters and Mapleson (1964) discuss in detail the application of exponential functions to anaesthesia. Defares, Sneddon and Wise (1973) consider a number of interesting pharmacological and physiological applications of exponential functions. These include the variation with time of the concentration of a drug in the body as a function of the number of doses administered, the increase with time of the concentration of carbon dioxide in a lung with breath holding, and the concentration-time curve of drugs in the blood stream when injected intramuscularly, subcutaneously or intraperitoneally.

So far, the exponential equations mentioned have all contained at least one negative exponential term. The equations are all self-limiting, tending either towards zero, or towards a maximum value as in the case of an uptake equation $C=C_s [1-\exp(-kt)]$. The concentration C at any time t will tend towards the saturation value C_s as time progresses.

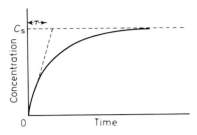

Figure 1.28. Uptake curve of the concentration of a volatile anaesthetic in a single body compartment plotted against time

(*Figure 1.28*). In theory, saturation will be reached after an infinite time. The time constant τ of the uptake process is defined as the time taken for C to attain a value equal to 63 per cent of C_s. The equation can also be written $C=C_s [1-\exp(-t/\tau)]$. This limiting does not occur in an equation having a positive exponential term.

Consider the case of the growth equation for a colony of bacteria, where the rate of increase of the colony population is linearly proportional to the number present at that time. The growth equation has the form $N_t = N_0 \exp(+kt)$ where N_0 is the initial number of bacteria at the start of the observation period when $t=0$, and N_t is the number present after a further time interval t. The slope of the curve increases rapidly upwards with time. This is the population explosion curve, the positive value of k implying a net excess of births over deaths.

Suppose that for a particular colony of insects on day 0 the number of both newly hatched and dead insects is counted and the difference is found to be 125. Putting $t = 0$ in the equation $N_t = N_0 \exp(+kt)$ gives $N_0 = 125$ since $e^0 = 1$. At the start of the next day, $t = 1$, and the net increase in the colony's numbers is found to be 200. This is determined from the numbers of newly hatched and dead insects. Hence $200 = 125 \exp(k \times 1)$ so that $k = \log_e(200/125) = 0.47$ giving $N_t = 125 \exp(+0.47t)$ where t is the time in days since the start of the observations. The increase in the numbers on any one day is given by

$$N_t - N_{t-1} = 125(e^{0.47t} - e^{0.47(t-1)}) = 125e^{0.47t}(1 - e^{0.47})$$

$$= 125e^{(0.47t)} \times 0.375 = 46.87 \exp(0.47t)$$

The colony's rate of growth is:

Day	Increase in numbers
1	75
2	120
3	192
4	307
5	491
6	786
7	1258
8	2013
9	3220
10	5153

This is clearly an explosive situation which is likely to be limited by other factors, e.g. a limit on the available supply of food.

References

BERGMAN, N.A. (1963). Effect of haemorrhage on rate of fall of plasma thiopental concentration. *Anesthiology* **24**, 123

BORMAN, M., SHAHN, E. and WEISS, M.F. (1962). The routine fitting of kinetic data to models: A mathematical formulation for digital computers. *Biophysical. J.* **2**, 275

BOWES, J.B. (1964). Changes in blood gases at the end of anaesthesia. *Anaesthesia* **35**, 684

BRISCOE, W.W., CREA, E.M., FILLER, J., HOUSSAY, H.E.J. and COURNAND, A. (1960). Lung volume, alveolar ventilation, and perfusion inter-relationships in chronic pulmonary emphysema *J. appl. Physiol.* **15**, 785

COOPER, E.A. (1961). Behaviour of respiratory apparatus. *Med. Res. Memo. natn. Coal Bd. med. Serv.*, **2**, 11

DEFARES, J.G., SNEDDON, I.N. and WISE, M.E, (1973). *An Introduction to the Mathematics of Medicine and Biology*. 2nd edn. Amsterdam; North Holland

FINK, B.R. (1966). Time constants in anesthesiology. *Anesthesiology* **27**, 838

GARDNER, D.G., GARDNER, J.C., LAUSCH, G. and MEINKE, W.W. (1959). Method for the analysis of multicomponent exponential decay curves. *J. chem. Phys.* **31**, 978

HILL, D.W., HOOK, J.R. and BELL, E.G. (1961). A servo-operated respiratory waveform simulator. *J. scient. Instrum.* **38**, 100

LAVENDER, S. (1970). Estimation of glomerular filtration rate and effective renal plasma flow by isotopic methods. *Br. J. Urol.* **41**, Suppl. 76

MAPLESON, W.W. (1962). The effect of lung characteristics on the functioning of automatic ventilators. *Anaesthesia* **17**, 300

MAPLESON, W.W. (1963). An electrical analogue for uptake and exchange of inert gases. *J. appl. Physiol.* **18**, 197

MATTHEWS, C.M.E. (1957). The theory of tracer experiments with I-131 labelled plasma proteins. *Physics Med. Biol.* **1**, 36

MUSHIN, W.W., RENDEL-BAKER, L. and THOMPSON, P.W. (1959). *Automatic Ventilation of the Lungs.* Oxford; Blackwell

ROSEN, S.M., TRUNIGER, B.P., KRIEK, H.R., MURRAY, J.E. and MERRILL, J.P. (1967). Intrarenal distribution of blood flow in the transplanted dog kidney: effect of denervation and rejection. *J. clin. Invest.* **46**, 1239

SANDMAN, A., HILL, D.W. and WILCOCK, A.H. (1973). Analogue preprocessor for the measurement by a digital computer of R-R intervals and R-wave widths. *Med. Biol. Eng.* **11**, 191

SEVERINGHAUS, J.W. (1963). Role of lung factors. In *Uptake and Distribution of Anaesthetic Agents* (Ed. by E.M. Papper and R.J. Kitz). New York; McGraw-Hill

THOMPSON, S.P. (1957). *Calculus Made Easy.* London; Macmillan

THORBURN, G.D., KOPALD, H.H., HERD, A., HOLLENBERG, M., O'MARCHOE, C.C.C. and BARGER, A.C. (1963). Intrarenal distribution of nutrient blood flow determined with 85-Krypton in the unanaesthetized dog. *Circ. Res.* **13**, 290

VAN LIEW, H.D. (1962). Semilogarithmic plots of data which reflect a continuity of exponential processes. *Science, N.Y.* **138**, 682

WATERS, D.J. and MAPLESON, W.W. (1964). Exponentials and the anaesthetist. *Anaesthesia* **19**, 274

WHELPTON, D. (1969). The use of an analogue computer in the study of the uptake of inhalational anaesthetics in fit and diseased patients. Sheffield University, PhD Thesis

2 Computer techniques

Digital computers

Anaesthetists are coming increasingly into contact with computers, particularly digital computers. A digital computer is a machine designed to perform operations upon data represented in digital or number form. For simplicity digital computers use the binary number system, that is, only the numbers 0 and 1. It performs these operations in a series of discrete steps. This is in contrast with an analogue computer which operates continuously upon the analogue signals which are fed into it. A digital computer can be considered in terms of a large calculating machine which is capable of making its own decisions in regard to the processing of its calculation, but operating under the control of a stored set of instructions, known as a computer *program*. The individual steps are simple such as adding or subtracting two numbers, multiplying or dividing, but they can be performed very rapidly, each taking perhaps only a few microseconds. The computer can also repeat an instruction or group of instructions until a desired result is attained. This facility is invaluable in approximation methods and in curve fitting where the process can be continued until the result converges to within a specified limit. Simple decision tests can be applied by the program to compare two numbers. By this means a program can be made to take various of its branches depending upon the conditions obtaining with the particular data provided as the program is running.

Input of data

A block diagram of a simple digital computer is shown in *Figure 2.1*. The basic input to the system could be via punched paper tape readers.

The punched paper tape is prepared by means of a teleprinter. This is rather like an electric typewriter, but each time a key is pressed a pattern of up to eight holes in a line is punched out of a reel of one-inch-wide paper tape driven from the teleprinter. Both the instructions for the computer program and the numerical data to be used are punched up in this way. When a tape has to be fed into the computer it is threaded into the tape reader. An electric motor in the reader then pulls the tape through at a steady rate over a line of eight miniature photocells. The tape is illuminated by a bulb and the pattern of holes passing over the photocells is converted into a corresponding pattern of electrical signals which can be interpreted by the computer. The presence of a hole corresponds to a binary 'one' and a space to a binary

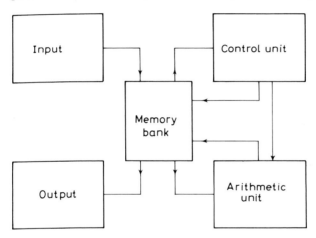

Figure 2.1. Block diagram of a simple digital computer (in practice the links are organized into a 'data highway')

'nought'. A common arrangement is for the computer to work on *even parity,* that is to say, that the number of holes in the pattern for each character read in should add up to an even number. The computer checks for this as it reads in each number. If a fault has arisen in the teleprinter, resulting in the mispunching of a character, there is usually one hole too many or one too few and the parity check fails. The computer then gives an *error message* to draw attention to the dubious character.

Punched paper tape is still widely used as an input medium for scientific minicomputers and it is a compact medium which is relatively cheap to produce. It does mean, however, that a whole reel of tape has to be repunched in order to alter a single character when the characters are such that the particular character concerned cannot be altered on its own by the use of a hand punch. Digital tape cassettes are often employed as the input device for programs run on small laboratory computers. Punched cards are widely employed as an input medium, particularly for large batch processing computer systems. Since each statement is punched on an individual card, only that card need be changed in order to alter a statement.

Central processing unit (CPU)

Referring to *Figure 2.1,* the computer is organized on the *'data highway'* principle. Each unit in the computer can, under the direction of the control unit, send information to, or accept information from, a main highway linking all the units. The central processing unit of the computer contains three main sub-units. The control unit interprets the instructions of the program and initiates the steps involved in obeying them. The arithmetic unit performs the various arithmetic and logic operations required, under the command of the control unit. The central memory stores the program instructions and some of the data.

Before the computer can perform any calculations, it clearly must be fed with the instructions telling it what to do. These will be stored in the memory or store of the computer for subsequent use. The manufacturer of the computer arranges that the store already contains a small number of wired-in *initial instructions* which are sufficient to enable it to read in further programs as required by the user. As the instructions are read in, each is allocated a specific location or address in the store. This is normally in the central memory of the computer. It can be thought of as a nest of pigeon holes, small machines containing perhaps 4k, 8k or 16k locations (k represents the 'binary kilo', that is, 2^{10} or 1024). Each consists of a number of small rings of ferrite material which can be magnetized or not depending on whether it represents a binary one or nought. Alternatively a semiconductor memory may be used.

When the program is run, each instruction is normally used in sequence. At the appropriate time, numerical data is read in and either stored for later use or taken straight to the arithmetic unit. This contains a number of *registers*—units for storing numbers and results. The main register in which the results of arithmetic operations appear is called the *accumulator*. A possible sequence might be for the control unit following the program instructions to place one number already held in store into the accumulator, read in a second number from a data tape and add this to the number in the accumulator. Finally, the sum of the two which is now in the accumulator is stored back in a new location in the store.

Computer languages

The basic instructions with which a computer operates are written in a coding system known as *machine code* which is specific for a particular computer. This is a low-level language, i.e. one in which each instruction has a single corresponding machine code equivalent. Although tedious to write, a machine code program is the most direct and hence the fastest to execute.

The next level up in complexity is the assembly language which is again specific for a particular computer. Whereas the machine code program instructions consist of numerals, the assembly language uses mneumonics and the assembly language program once written is operated upon by an assembly program to convert it into machine code instructions. Assembly language or 'code' procedures are often introduced in high-level language programs where repetitive tasks such as analogue-to-digital conversion have to be performed at high speed. The code procedure is considerably faster to run than its equivalent version in a high-level language.

A popular language for high-level working in scientific applications is Fortran (*For*mula *tran*slator). The original 'source' program consists of English-like statements and this is input into the computer with the Fortran compiler program in store. The translator part of the compiler translates the high-level source program into an object program of machine code statements. A compiler is distinguished from an assembly program by the fact that the compiler usually generates more than one machine code instruction for each source statement, whereas an assembly language is one-for-one with machine code. In a two-pass compiler the object program from the translator is run through the compiler to pick up any necessary procedures such as a plotter package. When this has been done the complete machine code version of the source program is in the computer's memory and is ready to run. Once any errors have been removed from the object program by editing, it can be stored on paper tape, disc or magnetic tape so that compilation is then not required each time the program is required to run.

Another popular high-level language, particularly for interactive multiterminal computer systems is Basic (*B*eginners' *A*ll-purpose *S*ymbolic *I*nstruction *C*ode). Although it is a high-level language Basic differs from Fortran in that it is an interpretive language. The original source program is acted on line by line by an interpretive program for Basic held in the computer's store. Each line is translated into machine code and executed immediately, no intermediate object program being introduced.

The object code approach is effective in batch processing, but the execution line-by-line approach is convenient with an interactive system where the computer terminal operator may wish to change the course of the program as it is running.

Large batch operation computers are encountered in university computer centres and commercial computer bureaux, but many scientific and medical departments now have their own powerful mini-computer with a large fast store which may be at least 100k words, two or more discs, printer, plotter, visual display terminals and analogue-to-digital and digital-to-analogue converters. It is common for anaesthetists to write their own programs in a high-level language.

The core store of the computer is very fast in operation (particularly if semiconductor rather than magnetic core elements are used), but limited in size. A fast, random access, store is not required for all the data or instructions in use, so that almost all systems augment the central processor unit's store with one or more forms of larger, but slower, backing store. Magnetic tapes are still used, particularly for archival purposes. However, fixed head discs, exchangeable discs and floppy discs are most commonly employed. With magnetic tapes or discs, data or programs are stored in the form of discrete blocks. Each block is allocated a label to identify it. Thus it is subsequently possible to search a particular *file* on tape or disc and locate a specified block which is transferred into the main store for further operations. Typical uses of the backing store would be to hold a sequence of programs which have already been compiled and tested, or to hold a cumulative record of patients' data. This can then be systematically searched to reveal any trends developing in a patient's condition.

The central processor unit contains the fast store, arithmetic and control units and various registers. Associated with it are the peripheral devices for input and output (e.g. paper tape reader, analogue-to-digital converter, visual display units; line printer, graph plotter, magnetic discs, magnetic tape, digital-to-analogue converter).

In addition to providing for the input of numerical data to the computer in the form of punched paper tape or keyboard entry from a teleprinter or visual display unit, provision may be made to feed in analogue electrical signals via an analogue-to-digital converter (ADC). This device samples the continuous analogue signal at a predetermined rate, typically 300 or 500 samples per minute for an ECG and 100 per second for an EEG. The output of the ADC for each sample is a digital value corresponding with the amplitude of the signal at the moment of sampling and the sequence of these values is placed into the computer's store. If the signal is rapidly varying during the time of sampling it may be necessary to precede the ADC with a sample-and-hold circuit which captures the instantaneous value of the signal for subsequent reading by the ADC.

The sampling rate needs to be chosen with care and in general, it should be at least twice the frequency of the highest frequency component present in the analogue signal.

Output of data

The output from the computer can be printed-up directly on the control teleprinter, or more rapidly, on a line-printer which prints a complete line of text at a time, or it may be displayed on a cathode-ray tube visual display unit or plotted in graphical form on a digital graph plotter driven from the computer. If it is not wanted to be seen immediately, the data can be stored in a backing store.

It is possible for computer installations to be operated in a number of possible modes. In off-line operation, human intervention is required for the transfer of control commands and data between two units of the system. A typical off-line operation occurs with batch processing where batches of data obtained on previous occasions are subsequently processed by the computer at some convenient time. This is in contrast with on-line operation where control commands and data can be passed automatically between two units of the system. For example, in suitable patients the computer might check that the 15 minute urine volume was satisfactory. If it was not, the computer could command a pump to infuse a diuretic agent. In real-time operation, the computer will process the incoming data at such a speed that it keeps up with the input rate. An example occurs in the computer detection of ventricular ectopic beats in an ECG.

The heart of a real-time digital computer system is the *operating system* program which schedules the various programs to be used such that they come into operation as required by a predetermined plan. For example the sampling of an ECG may be interlaced with the taking of blood pressure and tidal volume samples. In the case of minicomputers, sophisticated operating systems will occupy typically 32k of core-store. They are capable of foreground and background operation, i.e. when the computer is free from running foreground tasks such as sampling physiological signals, it can be doing background tasks such as compiling programs or checking them for errors. This facility enables routine development work to be slotted in with dedicated real-time operation.

It is usual to refer to the digital computer and its peripherals as *hardware*, while the computer programs are known as *software*. An active computer installation performing real-time operations will call extensively upon computer engineers for maintenance and the design of interfaces whilst resident programmers will be engaged in modifying and up-dating the software.

Uses of digital computers

A clear introduction to the use of digital computers for medical applications is given by both Payne (1966) and Coles (1973). Digital computers are being widely exploited in anaesthetic research studies where a large number of tedious routine calculations have to be made. Kelman (1966) describes a sub-program for the conversion of oxygen tension into oxygen saturation, and also for the conversion of Pco_2 into blood CO_2 content (Kelman, 1967). Respiratory investigations provide a useful outlet for computer assistance. Borgstedt, Goodson and Gillies (1966) give a Fortran program for the reduction of gas volumes to the conditions of 0 °C and 760 mmHg. Bleich (1969) has described a computer evaluation of acid-base disorders, as have Valbona, Penny and McMath (1971). Menin, Barnett and Schmechel (1973) have used a computer program in the care of patients with acute respiratory failure. The use of such conversational-type programs run on a silent terminal in a ward or unit office will undoubtedly help in the clinical training of junior staff by drawing their attention to a logical presentation of symptoms and extending the range of possible diagnoses. Useful formulae for computing total peripheral resistance and left ventricular work are given by Mostert, Moore and Murphy (1969).

Digital computers are playing a growing part in patient monitoring schemes. Jensen *et al.* (1966) give a detailed account of a two-bedded monitoring system in which the computer records the systolic, diastolic, pulse and mean arterial pressures together with the central venous pressure. Normally, the blood pressure program is gated from the ECG. Heart rate is obtained from both the ECG and blood-pressure signals, any difference giving an indication of a pulse deficit. Respiration rate is obtained from the pressure swings on the central venous pressure. In patients suffering from shock, temperature is measured rectally and at a number of peripheral sites. Following an injection of dye, the computer calculates not only the cardiac output, but also the cardiac work and peripheral resistance. Other accounts of computer patient-monitoring systems are those of Osborn *et al.* (1969) and Warner (1972). The advantage offered by the computer over conventional patient monitors lies in its ability to recall readings taken over several hours and to provide an analysis of them, and also to draw attention to subtle changes occurring in more than one parameter (Hope *et al.*, 1973).

The development of reliable analogue and digital telephone data links means that now the computer need not be situated close to the clinical area. Using a simple frequency modulation system it is feasible to transmit electrocardiograms over distances of more than 100 miles (Colbeck *et al.*, 1968). In practice, three channels each 100 Hz wide can be made available on a single telephone line (Hill and Payne, 1972). The output from the computer can be sent back over a digital telephone data link to a visual display unit situated at the bedside or in the operating room. A number of computer programs have been developed for analysing conventional 12-lead electrocardiograms off-line, the ECGs being recorded on analogue magnetic tape and sent in batches over a telephone link to the central computer (Caceres *et al.*, 1964). A number of computer programs are now available for the interpretation of conventional 12-lead ECGs (Pordy *et al.*, 1968; Bonner *et al.*, 1972). Bailey *et al.* (1974) report that their group of cardiologists found essential agreement with the results from the program of Bonner *et al.* in 76 per cent of 1150 unselected tracings. Clinically significant disagreements based strictly on the application of different criteria occurred in 20 per cent of the tracings, whereas disagreements based on program errors occurred in only 4 per cent of the ECGs. With the increasing desire by anaesthetists for all patients having a general anaesthetic to have had an ECG recorded beforehand, it is likely that in some countries anaesthetists will come into contact with ECG interpretation computer systems. The present diagnostic accuracy is of the order of 75 per cent and this means that the ECGs must also be checked by a clinician.

Computers have also been applied to the analysis of EEG recordings. This can be a major task if all 16 channels have to be analysed (Brazier, 1961; Dummermüth and Flühler, 1967). However, the situation is simplified if a power spectral analysis is performed on-line for a single channel for monitoring purposes during anaesthesia. Myers *et al.* (1973) have described the use of a three-dimensional display of the frequency spectra of successive EEG epochs on a cathode ray tube during anaesthesia.

Apart from pattern recognition procedures, a digital computer can easily be programmed to analyse data obtained from anaesthetic record cards. Galla, Schwarzbach and Buccigrossi (1969) describe the design of an anaesthetic record card with computer processing in mind. Hill and Bodman (1968) discuss the use of a computer program for sorting anaesthetic record cards from a series of prostatectomy patients in teaching and non-teaching hospitals. Computers have also been employed for the scheduling of anaesthetic staff (Ernst and Matlak, 1974; Ernst *et al.*, 1973).

Other applications of interest to anaesthetists include the quality control of blood acid–base results (Solberg, 1973), the interpretation of ventilatory studies (Hoffer *et al.*, 1973), the continuous monitoring of cardiac output in the operating room (Wesseling *et al.*, 1976) and intensive therapy unit monitoring (Blackburn, 1976; Taylor, 1976).

An outstanding contribution to medical and scientific instrumentation has occurred with the increasing incorporation of microprocessors into instruments such as centrifuges, gas chromatographs, arterial blood pressure recorders, spectral analysers for use with Doppler shift blood flow meters, spectrophotometers and blood-gas analysers (Mergler and Primiano, 1978). The actual microprocessor is fabricated on a single chip by large scale integration techniques and other components such as a real-time clock, analogue-to-digital converter and memories (e.g. PROM – programmed read-only memory for holding computer program instructions which do not need to be changed or RAM – random access memory for holding data) are added inside a single multi-pin package to form a complete microprocessor. The development of 'intelligent' instruments leads to more sophisticated calibration and baseline checks and processing facilities for the original raw data. Repeated operation under identical conditions is also possible.

Kenny and Davis (1979) describe the use of a microcomputer programmed in Basic for the teaching of anaesthetists, with the microcomputer driving a visual display and operating a slide projector.

Analogue computer elements

The use of operational amplifiers

Operational amplifiers form the basis of analogue computers. The availability of compact integrated-circuit operational amplifiers for a few pence has revolutionized medical electronics. Operational amplifiers are high-gain, direct-coupled transistor circuits whose gain and frequency characteristics can be set by the addition of external passive components. Operational amplifiers can be adapted to perform various mathematical functions such as summation, inversion, integration and differentiation. They can provide a high input impedance and a low output impedance if this is required. Modern versions are internally compensated against instability and are protected against accidental short-circuiting of the input and output.

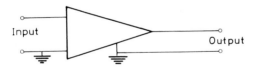

Figure 2.2

Continuously varying analogue signals are commonly encountered in anaesthetic practice since they are the primary output from transducers which transform a physical variable such as the arterial blood pressure or body temperature into a corresponding electrical signal. Once an analogue signal has been converted into a series of discrete values by means of an analogue-to-digital converter and is in digital form it can be operated upon by a digital computer. However, in order to save computer time, it is convenient to perform various manipulations such as peak-picking, integration or differentiation and filtering while the signal is still in analogue form by means of hard-wired circuitry using operational amplifiers. This is known as pre-processing. The more complicated analogue pre-processing is now being taken over by microcomputer.

Assume that the basic amplifier has an infinite gain (in practice of

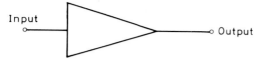

Figure 2.3

the order of 100 000), produces a negative output for a positive input, and draws a negligible input current. Such an amplifier might be illustrated in diagrammatic form as in *Figure 2.2*, but since all signals in analogue computing are usually measured with reference to earth, (ground), the earth lines do not need to be drawn each time and are usually omitted as in *Figure 2.3*.

Summation

In *Figure 2.4*, a feedback resistor R_F (1MΩ) is connected from the output to the input of the amplifier. R_1 is a resistor connected from point A which is the circuit input to the amplifier input B. Suppose that the maximum voltage output obtainable from the amplifier is 10 V. With a gain of 100 000 the input voltage at point B cannot exceed 10/100 000 V=0.01 mV. Thus point B can be taken as being sensibly at a level of 0 V, although it is not directly connected to earth.

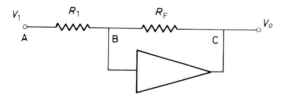

Figure 2.4

Hence it is known as a virtual earth point. The input current to the circuit is V_1/R_1 where V_1 is the applied voltage. The amplifier is designed to have a high value of input impedance, so that it does not draw any significant current. Resistors R_1 and R_F thus carry equal currents since the amount lost into the amplifier can be neglected. Therefore, numerically,

$$i = \frac{V_1}{R_1} = \frac{V_0}{R_F}$$ where V_0 is the output voltage.

And

$$V_o = -V_1 \frac{R_F}{R_1}$$

If $R_F=R_1$ then $V_o=V_1$. The effective circuit gain is unity under these conditions. If there are several inputs V_1, V_2, and V_3 and $R_1=R_2=R_3=R_F$ then $V_o = -(V_1 + V_2 + V_3)$. Hence the output voltage is equal to the sum of the input voltages (*Figure 2.5*).

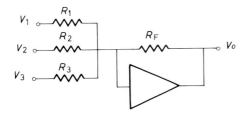

Figure 2.5

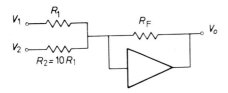

Figure 2.6

In *Figure 2.6* if $R_2 = 10R_1$

then

$$V_o = V_1 + \frac{V_2}{10}$$

Integration
Making the same assumptions about the amplifier as before, but now using capacitive feedback (*Figure 2.7*),

$$V_1 = i_R R, \qquad i_R = \frac{V_1}{R}$$

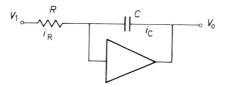

Figure 2.7

and

$$i_C = \frac{\mathrm{d}V_o}{\mathrm{d}t}\, C$$

Since

$$i_C = i_R, \quad \frac{V_1}{R} = \frac{\mathrm{d}V_o}{\mathrm{d}t}\, C$$

thus

$$\mathrm{d}V_o = \frac{V_1}{RC}\, \mathrm{d}t$$

Integrating,

$$\int_0^{V_o} \mathrm{d}V_o = \frac{1}{RC} \int_0^t V_1 \, \mathrm{d}t$$

The output voltage of the circuit is now proportional to the integral with respect to time of the input voltage.

Applications of integrating circuits

Figure 2.8 shows the record from a pneumotachograph obtained with a sine wave pump (Hill *et al.*, 1961). This is a plot of gas flow rate against time (in practice it is usually respiratory flow rate). The ripple

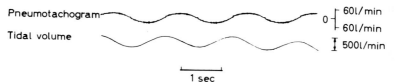

Figure 2.8

on the flow tracing arises from friction between the piston and cylinder. The electrical output from the pressure transducer of the pneumotachograph is the electrical analogue signal of this waveform. If this is fed into an integrating circuit (Hill, 1959; Whelpton and Watson, 1966) then the output of the integrating circuit over one complete cycle is the analogue of

$$\int_{t=t_1}^{t=t_2} f\mathrm{d}t \quad \text{and} \quad \int_{t=t_2}^{t=t_3} f\mathrm{d}t$$

where f is the instantaneous value of the flow rate in litres per minute (*Figure 2.9*). The product of (litres per minute $\times$ minutes) is equal to a

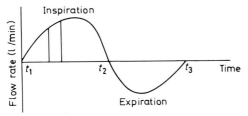

Figure 2.9

volume in litres. The output of the integrating circuit is shown in the tidal volume tracing of *Figure 2.8*, the height of the trace being proportional to the tidal volume. It is seen that the tidal volume tracing is a cosine wave which is 90°, or a quarter of a cycle, out of phase with the sine wave tracing of the flow pattern. This follows since mathematically the integral of a sine wave can be shown to be a cosine wave. Integrating circuits are also used to obtain a mean value from a blood pressure waveform. Essentially, integration is a form of low-pass filtering and varying degrees of integration can be used for removing cardiac pulsations from, for example, an oesophageal pressure tracing.

Differentiation

in *Figure 2.10*, resistive feedback is used with a capacitive input.

$$V_o = i_R R,$$

therefore

$$i_R = \frac{V_o}{R}$$

and

$$i_C = C \frac{dV_1}{dt}$$

since

$$i_R = i_C$$

$$\frac{V_o}{R} = C \frac{dV_1}{dt}$$

so that

$$V_o = RC \frac{dV_1}{dt}$$

The output voltage is now proportional to the time rate of change (differential) of the input voltage. In practice, this is not an easy

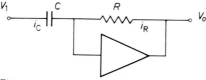

Figure 2.10

technique to use, since rapidly varying noise signals are preferentially amplified relative to the more slowly varying signal.

Applications of differentiating circuits

Much of the instrumentation associated with surgery and anaesthesia is concerned with the production of electrical signals which are analogues of physiological processes. Typical examples are the electrical output signals from a blood pressure transducer or a blood flow probe. It is often necessary to be able to observe the time rate of change of such signals, and this can be accomplished by feeding the signal into a differentiating circuit. An elegant example of the use of a differentiating circuit is given by Angelakos (1964). By placing a semiconductor micropressure transducer at the tip of a cardiac catheter, he was able to accurately record intraventricular pressure. This was then differentiated once to give velocity and twice to give acceleration (acceleration is the rate of change of velocity). dP/dt is taken as one index of myocardial contractility. Shinozaki *et al.* (1966) describe means for the linear calibration of pressure derivatives. Differentiating circuitry is essential for the non-invasive electrical impedance method of cardiac output measurement described by Kubicek *et al.* (1966) and is commonly used in the detection of the R-waves of an electro-cardiogram. The downslope of the ECG usually has the greatest negative value of slope and this fact together with an amplitude criterion was employed by Sandman, Hill and Wilcock (1973) to distinguish valid R-waves in an ECG having ventricular ectopic beats.

Inversion

A signal is inverted on passing through an operational amplifier having $R_F = R_1$. The gain is simply unity, but the output signal is inverted with respect to the input.

Multiplication by a constant

A multi-turn potentiometer (*Figure 2.11*) is employed to produce an output voltage V_0 where $V_0 = KV_1$ ($0 < K < 1$). The potentiometer

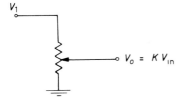

Figure 2.11

simply taps off $1/K$ of the input. The factor K should be set up using an accurate voltmeter, with the potentiometer connected to its load resistance at the time.

Analogue cardiac output computers

The more usual types of cardiac output computer are designed to accept an input signal provided by the optical densitometer associated with the dye dilution technique. From a venous catheter, a bolus of suitable dye is injected as nearly as possible into the right heart. By means of a constant speed drive syringe, a sample of arterial blood is drawn through the cuvette of the densitometer. When the bolus of dye reaches the cuvette, the increasing optical density of the blood causes the chart recorder attached to the densitometer to trace out the well known 'dilution curve' of *Figure 2.12*. As the bolus passes through the cuvette, the recorder pen starts to return to its original baseline, this part of the curve having a high probability of being an exponential. A second, smaller peak is then traced out due to the arrival of dye which has made a second transit of the circulation. The primary peak of

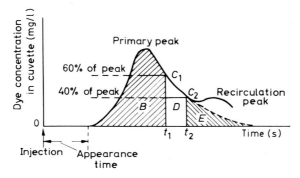

Figure 2.12

Figure 2.12 is shown extrapolated as though recirculation did not exist. If C is the concentration of dye at time t minutes after the injection of M_0 milligrams of dye, then the cardiac output in litres per minute

$$\dot{Q} = \frac{M_0 \times 60}{\displaystyle\int_0^\infty C\mathrm{d}t}$$

Now $\int_0^\infty C\mathrm{d}t$ is the total area A under the curve (in mg/litre $\times$ seconds) where $A = B + D + E$ (*Figure 2.12*). If a substantial number of cardiac outputs have to be determined, it becomes tedious to measure each area by counting squares on a graph or by the use of a planimeter.

The cardiac output computer automatically calculates a value for the area under each dye curve without recirculation. The computer is first calibrated by passing known concentrations of dye in blood through the cuvette of the densitometer and adjusting the sensitivity of the computer to a pre-set value. The output meter of the computer can then indicate the value of the cardiac output in litres per minute.

In the majority of cases, the down slope of the dilution curve is a simple exponential function. In *Figure 2.12*, let C_1 and C_2 be the dye concentrations at times t_1 and t_2 on the exponential portion of the curve. Then the area under the curve from $t=t_1$ to $t=$infinity is equal to

$$\int_{t_1}^{\infty} C_1 \exp(-kt)dt = \left(\frac{-C_1}{k} \exp(-k \times \infty) - (-1) \times \frac{C_1}{k} \exp(-kt_1) \right)$$

$$= \frac{+C_1}{k} \exp(-kt_1)$$

$$= \frac{C_1}{K}$$

$$= \text{area (D+E)}$$

Similarly, the area under the curve from $t=t_2$ to $t=\infty$ is equal to

$$\int_{t_2}^{\infty} C_1 \exp(-kt)dt = \frac{1}{k} C_1 \exp(-kt_2) = \frac{C_2}{K}$$

Suppose that the concentrations C_1 and C_2 are in the ratio $x : 1$,

i.e. $C_2 = \dfrac{C_1}{x}$, then area $E = \dfrac{C_2}{K} = \dfrac{C_1}{Kx}$

Area $D = \dfrac{C_1}{K} - \dfrac{C_1}{Kx} = \dfrac{C_1}{K}\left(1 - \dfrac{1}{x}\right) = \dfrac{C_1}{K}\dfrac{(x-1)}{x}$

so that area $(D + E) = \dfrac{x}{(x-1)}$ area D

The procedure for finding the total area A under the dye curve is as follows.

The computer integrates the dye concentration (proportional to the densitometer output signal) from $t=0$ to $t=t_1$. The integration sensitivity is then multiplied by a factor $x/(x-1)$ and integration continued at the enhanced rate for time interval (t_2-t_1). At time $t=t_2$, the output from the integrator is proportional to the wanted area A.

As will be explained later, the fact that area $(D+E) = x/(x-1) \times$ area D is used in a number of digital computer programs for dye dilution calculations.

In one commercial cardiac output computer, $C_1 = 60$ per cent of the peak concentration and $C_2 = 40$ per cent of the peak concentration, so that $C_2 = C_1/1.5$ giving $(x-1)/x = \frac{1}{3}$. Thus area A=(B+D+E)

=B+3D. The rate of integration is automatically increased three-fold from $t=t_1$ to $t=t_2$. At $t=t_1$ the computer generates a voltage equal to C_1/x and compares this continuously with the diminishing value of C, at the same time increasing the rate of integrating threefold. When C becomes equal to the pre-set value of C_1/x, integration is stopped and the output of the integrator shown on a set of digital display tubes. This figure is proportional to the area under the dye curve without recirculation. The cardiac output $\dot{Q}$ in litres per minute is given by

$$\dot{Q} = \frac{M_o \times 60}{A}$$

where A is the area under the curve expressed in terms of (mg/litre $\times$ seconds) and M_o is the mass of dye in mg injected. By pulling a known concentration of dye in blood for a known time through the cuvette it is possible to produce a known area and thus to obtain a factor to convert the computer reading directly into cardiac output. Another commercial cardiac output computer using a fibre optic cardiac catheter takes C_1 as 75 per cent of the peak concentration and C_2 as 55 per cent of the peak concentration. For sampling close to the aortic valve or in the cardiac chambers, current practice is to employ a fibre optic densitometer. With this device no blood has to be drawn from the circulation to an external cuvette. The response is sufficiently fast that the dye curve has returned to the baseline before the recirculation peak has arrived and simple integration is adequate for determining the area under the dye curve. This mode is employed when a recirculation peak is present. This will occur when the site of sampling is peripheral. When the sampling site is located close to the left ventricle, the recirculation peak may be absent. Under these circumstances provision has been made to alter the mode of operation of the computer so that the area under the dye curve is determined by integration until the amplitude of the curve has fallen to 10 per cent of the peak concentration. The remaining portion of the area under the curve is found by means of a correction factor.

The use of room-temperature isotonic saline solution as the indicator substance, rather than dye, simplifies the design of the associated analogue computer since with this method the recirculation peak is negligible. Good accounts of analogue computers designed for cardiac output determinations by the cool saline technique in intensive care units are those of Cowell and Bray (1970) and Braithwaite and Bradley (1968).

Typically, 10 ml of cool saline is used. Assuming that the injectate mixes thoroughly with the blood, and that negligible net heat flow occurs through the vessel walls during the passage of the saline between the points of system and measurement, then the heat injected can be equated to the heat detected. If the volume of saline injected is small compared to the volume of blood with which it mixes, then to a good approximation,

$$V D_i S_i (T_i - T_b) = \dot{Q} D_b S_b \int \Delta T \mathrm{d}t$$

where $\dot{Q}$ is the blood volume flow, V is the volume of saline injected, T is the body temperature, D is density, S is the specific heat, ΔT is the temperature difference between the blood and the injected saline and the suffices b and i refer to blood and saline respectively.

References

ANGELAKOS, E.T. (1964). Semiconductor pressure micro-transducers for measuring velocity and acceleration of intraventricular pressures. *Am. J. med. Electron.* **3**, 226

BAILEY, J.J., ITSCOITZ, S.B., HIRSHFELD, J.W., GRAUER, L.E. and HORTON, MARTHA R. (1974). A method for evaluating computer programs for electrocardiographic interpretation. 1. Application to the experimenal IBM program of 1971. *Circulation* **50**, 73

BLACKBURN, J.P. (1976). Computers in the intensive therapy unit. *Brit. J. Clin. Equip.* **1**, 122–131

BLEICH, H.L. (1969). Computer evaluation of acid-base disorders. *J. clin. Invest.* **48**, 1689

BONNER, R.E., CREVASSE, L., FERRER, M.I. and GREENFIELD, J.C. (1972). A new computer program for the analysis of scalar electrocardio-grams. *Comput. Biomed. Res.* **5**, 629

BORGSTEDT, M.M., GOODSON, J.M. and GILLIES, A.J. (1966). Computer program for gas volume reduction tables. *Anesthesiology* **27**, 185

BRAITHWAITE, M.A. and BRADLEY, R.D. (1968). Measurement of cardiac output by thermal dilution in man. *J. appl. Physiol.* **24**, 434

BRAZIER, M.A.B.(1961). *Computer Techniques in E.E.G. Analysis.* Amsterdam; Elsevier

CACERES, C.A., STEINBERG, C.A., GORMAN, P.A., CALATAYUD, J.B., DUBROW, R.T. and WEIHRER, A.L.(1964). Computer aids in electro-cardiography *Ann. N.Y. Acad. Sci.* **118**, 85

COLBECK. W.J., HILL, D.W., MABLE, S.E.R. and PAYNE, J.P. (1968). Electrocardiographic transmissions by public telephone. *Lancet* **2**, 1017

COLES, E.C. (1973). *A Guide to Medical Computing.* London; Butterworths

COWELL, T.K. and BRAY, D.G. (1970). Measuring the heart's output. *Electron. Power* **14**, 150

DUMMERMÜTH, G. and FLÜHLER, H.(1967). Some modern aspects in numerical spectrum analysis of multichannel electroencephalographic data. *Med. biol. Engng* **5**, 319

ERNST, E.A., LASDON, L.S., OSTRANDER, L.E. and DIVELL, S.S. (1973). Anesthesiologist scheduling using a set partitioning algorithm. *Comput. Biomed. Res.* **6**, 561–569

ERNST, E.A. and MATLAK, E.W. (1974). On-line computer scheduling of anesthesiologists. *Anesth. Analg. Curr. Res.* **53**, 854–858

GALLA, S.J., SCHWARZBACH, B.A. and BUCCIGROSSI, R. (1969). A computer program for analysis of anesthetic records. *Anesthesiology* **30**, 565

HILL, D.W. (1959). The rapid measurement of respiratory pressures and volumes. *Br. J. Anaesth.* **31**, 352

HILL, D.W. and BODMAN, R.I. (1968). The application of a computer sorting program to prostatectomy patients. *Br. J. Anaesth.* **40**, 785

HILL, D.W., HOOK, J.R. and BELL, E.G. (1961). A servo-operated respiratory waveform simulator. *J. scient. Instrum.* **38**, 100

HILL, D.W. and PAYNE, J.P. (1972). The use of analogue telephone data links for the transmission of physiological signals. *Br. J. Anaesth.* **44**, 562

HOFFER, E.P., KANAREK, D., KAZENNI, H. and BARNETT, G.O. (1973). Computer interpretation of ventilatory studies. *Comput. Biomed. Res.* **6**, 347–354

HOPE, C.E., LEWIS, C.D., PERRY, I.R. and GAMBLE, A. (1973). Computed trend analysis in automated patient monitoring systems. *Br. J. Anaesth.* **45**, 440

JENSEN, R.E., SHUBIN, M., MEAGHER, P.F. and WEIL, M.M. (1966). On-line computer monitoring of the seriously ill patient. *Med. biol. Engng* **4**, 265

KELMAN, G.R. (1966). Digital computer sub-routine for the conversion of oxygen tension into saturation. *J. appl. Physiol.* **21**, 1375

KELMAN, G.R.(1967). Digital computer procedure for the conversion of PCO_2 into blood CO_2 content. *Resp. Physiol.,* **3**, 111

KENNY, G.N.C. and DAVIS, P.D.(1979). The use of a microcomputer in anaesthetist teaching. *Anaesthesia* **34**, 583–588

KUBICEK, W.G., KARNEGIS, J.N., PATTERSON, R.P., WITSOE, D.A. and

MATTSON, R.H. (1966). Development and evaluation of an impedance cardiac output system. *Aerospace Med.* **37**, 1208

MENIN, S.J., BARNETT, G.O. and SCHMECHEL, D. (1973). A computer program to assist in the care of acute respiratory failure. *J. Am. med. Ass.* **223**, 308

MERGLER, H.W. and PRIMIANO, F.P. Jr.(1978). Microprocessor-based blood-gas analyser. *I.E.E.E. Trans. Ind. Electron. Control. Instrum.* **IECI-25**, 17−20

MOSTERT, J.W., MOORE, R.E. and MURPHY, G.P. (1969). Nomograms for estimation of peripheral resistance and work of the heart. *Anesthesiology* **30**, 569

MYERS, R.R., STOCKARD, J.J., FLEMING, N.I., FRANCE, C.J. and BICKFORD, R.G. (1973). The use of on-line telephone computer analysis of the EEG in anaesthesia. *Br. J. Anaesth.* **45**, 664

OSBORN, J.J., BEAUMONT, J.O., RAISON, J.C.A., RUSSEL, J. and GERBODE, F. (1969). Measurement and monitoring of acutely ill patients by digital computer. *Surgery* **64**, 1057

PAYNE, L.C. (1966). *An Introduction to Medical Automation.* London; Pitman

PORDY, L., JAFFE, H., CHESKY, K., FRIEDBERG, C.K., FALLOWES, L. and BONNER, R.E.(1968). Computer diagnosis of electrocardiograms. IV. A computer program for contour analysis with clinical results of rhythm and contour interpretation. *Comput. Biomed. Res.* **1**, 408

SANDMAN, A.M., HILL, D.W. and WILCOCK, H.A. (1973). An analogue pre-processor for the measurement by a digital computer of R-R intervals and R-wave widths. *Med. biol. Engng* **11**, 191

SHINOZAKI, T., ABAJIAN, J.C., HANSON, J.S. and TABAKIN, B.S.(1966). Linear calibration of pressure derivatives. *J. appl. Physiol.* **21**, 326

SOLBERG, H.E. (1973). A computer program for quality control of blood acid/base results. *Comput. Program. Biomed. (Amst.)* **3**, 79−86

TAYLOR, D.E.M. (1976). Human and computer assisted measurement and diagnosis in an intensive care unit. *Health Bull. (Edin.)* **34**, 180−182

VALBONA, C., PENNY, E. and McMATH, F. (1971). Computer analysis of blood gases and acid-base status. *Comput. Biomed. Res.* **4**, 623

WARNER, H.R. (1972). A computer-based information system for intensive care. In *Hospital Information Systems* (Ed. by G.A. Bekey and M.D. Schwartz). New York; Marcel Dekker

WESSEL, H.U., JAMES, F.W. and PAUL, M.H. (1966). Quantification of indicator dilution curves by special purpose analog computers. *Med. Res. Engng* **5**, 16

WESSELING, K.H., PURSCHE, R. and SMITH, N.T. (1976). A computer

module for the continuous monitoring of cardiac output in the
operating theatre. *Acta. Anesth. Belg.* **27**, *Suppl.* 327–341
WHELPTON, D.J. and WATSON, B.W. (1966). A respiration integrator.
Br. J. Anaesth. **38**, 233

3 Mechanics

Fundamental concepts

Mechanics may be defined as the subject in which is studied the conditions under which objects around us move or are at rest (Abbott, 1971). Much of mechanics is concerned with the study of the production and mode of action of forces. It impinges on the anaesthetist in connection with the action of pressure regulators and gauges, the action of automatic lung ventilators, respiratory mechanics and haemodynamics. It is important that anaesthetists have a clear understanding of the fundamental physical laws governing the interaction of various parameters.

Dimensional analysis

The fundamental dimensions of mechanics are mass (M), length (L) and time (T).

In addition to the study of force, for example, the contractility of the myocardium, the application of force is commonly encountered in terms of pressure, work and energy. These and all other mechanical quantities can be expressed dimensionally in terms of mass, length and time. For example, the dimensions of force are MLT^{-2}. If an equation relating mechanical quantities is to balance, the dimensions of the quantities on one side must be the same as those on the other side. A simple example occurs in Poiseuille's equation for the streamline flow of a liquid through a pipe, i.e.

$$\dot{Q} = \pi P r^4 / 8 \eta l$$

where $\dot{Q}$ is the flow rate of the liquid, r is the radius of the pipe, P the pressure drop along the pipe and η the viscosity of the fluid. The dimensions of viscosity may not be at once obvious. However, they can soon be derived by balancing the dimensions of the equation. The dimensions of $\dot{Q}$ are $L^3 T^{-1}$ (litres per second) and pressure is force per unit area, $(MLT^{-2})L^{-2}$, substituting in the equation,

$$[\eta] = MLT^{-2} L^{-2} L^4 / L^3 T^{-1} L$$

so that the dimensions of the viscosity are $MT^{-1} L^{-1}$. Apart from its use in deducing the dimensions of a particular quantity, the balancing of the dimensions in an equation provides a useful check on the accuracy of an equation, but will not take into account any errors appearing in numerical constants. For further reading, the references of Parkhurst (1964) and Porter (1958) should be consulted.

Units and definitions

Anaesthetists will encounter in hospital practice the English system of units which has been much used by engineers in the past and is still in common use by shopkeepers and the SI system of units which has now replaced the MKS system.

The English system of units

In the English system of units, the unit of mass is the pound, the unit of length is the foot and the unit of time is the second. The unit of force is the pound weight which is the force due to gravity acting on a mass of one pound. Although gas volume flows in anaesthetic practice are very seldom quoted in cubic feet per second as in industry, it has been general practice to have cylinder and pipeline pressure gauges calibrated in terms of pounds per square inch.

While new equipment is scaled in SI units, much older equipment abounds such as nitrous oxide cylinders with capacities quoted in gallons and pressure gauges scaled in pounds per square inch (p.s.i.). Indeed, in October 1979, the U.K. Consumer Affairs Minister announced a reprieve for gallons, pints, pounds, inches and other Imperial measures and said that no further compulsory metrication orders would be made in the United Kingdom. Thus while it would be much simpler to deal only with SI units in this book, it is still necessary to make mention of other systems of units.

The CGS system of units

The idea of a decimal system of units was proposed by Simon Stevin (1548–1620) who also developed the concept of decimal fractions. Following the French revolution, the statesman Talleyrand, advised by contemporary scientists, aimed at the establishment of an international decimal system of weights and measures à tous les temps, à tous les peuples'. It was based upon the metre as the unit of length (intended to be one millionth part of the distance from the North Pole to the equator at sea-level through Paris) and the gram. In 1837, the British Association for the Advancement of Science chose the centimetre and gram as the basic units of length and mass for scientific purposes. The adoption of the second as the unit of time led to the CGS system of units. An example of its use occurs with the measurement of left ventricular work quoted in gram-centimetres per second. In the SI system matters are simplified since all work is expressed in watts.

The MKS system of units

About 1900, practical measurements in metric units began to be based upon the metre, the kilogram and the second. In 1935, the International Electrotechnical Commission (IEC) accepted the recommendation of Professor Giorgi that the MKS system of mechanical units should be linked with the electromagnetic units by the adoption of one of the latter as a fourth base unit. The IEC adopted the ampere, the unit of electric current, as the fourth base unit in 1950 to give the MKSA system of units.

The SI system of units

Since 1875, all international matters concerning the metric system have been the responsibility of the Conférence Générale des Poids et Mesures (CGPM); this is also responsible for the Bureau International des Poids et Mesures (BIPM) at Sèvres in France. The kilogram is still defined in terms of the international prototype held at Sèvres, but the metre is now defined in terms of a number of wavelengths of a particular wavelength of light. The tenth meeting of the CGPM in 1954 adopted a rationalized and coherent system of units based upon the four MKSA units, the kelvin as the unit of temperature and the candela as the unit of luminous intensity. The eleventh conference in 1960 gave this system its full title of 'Système Internationale d'Unites' or SI units. It is the system which is coming into general adoption in the United Kingdom and many other countries, and is in official use by the United Kingdom's National Health Service. Following a lead from major learned societies, most scientific and medical journals now insist on the use of SI units. For these reasons questions on SI units are often asked in the Primary F.F.A.R.C.S. examination and anaesthetists taking this examination should be familiar with SI units.

The SI system of units is based on the metric system and is designed to:

(1) Provide a coherent system of units, i.e. one in which the product or quotient of any two unit quantities is the unit of the resultant quantity without the need to introduce any numerical factor.
(2) Ensure that the presentation of quantities and units is uniform in concept and style.
(3) Minimize the number of multiples and sub-multiples in common use.

It does not follow that SI units are neater or more convenient than those previously used, e.g. in the measurement of peripheral resistance. Here the CGS units are dyne-sec.cm^{-5} (dynes per cm^2)/(cm^3 per second). The corresponding SI units are $kN\ m^{-2}\ cm^{-3}$ s, or $kN\ m^{-5}$ s. In view of the international adoption of SI units the emphasis in this book will be placed firmly on SI units. However, mention will be made of the relevant equivalent units in other systems where these are appropriate in terms of practical situations.

SI base units

SI units for various quantities are derived from seven base units (*Table 3.1*).

TABLE 3.1

Quantity	SI unit	Symbol
Length	metre	m
Mass	kilogram	kg
Time	second	s
Electric current	ampere	A
Thermodynamic temperature	kelvin	K
Luminous intensity	candela	cd
Amount of substance	mole	mol

Derived SI units

These are obtained in the first instance by combinations of the base units and building up from these with base and derived units (*Table 3.2*). The coherent unit of volume is the cubic metre, but the litre is

TABLE 3.2

Quantity	Name	Symbol	Derivation
Frequency	hertz	Hz	$1 \text{ Hz} = \text{s}^{-1}$
Force	newton	N	$1 \text{ N} = 1 \text{ kg m s}^{-2}$
Work, energy, quantity of heat	joule	J	$1 \text{ J} = 1 \text{ N m}$
Pressure	pascal	Pa	$1 \text{ Pa} = 1 \text{ N m}^{-2}$

also recognized as an SI unit of volume. This is the unit of volume normally used in laboratory practice.

Prefixes for decimal multiples and sub-multiples of SI units

Decimal multiples and sub-multiples of SI units are formed by the use of prefixes (*Table 3.3*). The use of prefixes representing 10 raised

TABLE 3.3

Factor	Name	Symbol	Factor	Name	Symbol
			10^{-18}	atto-	a
			10^{-15}	femto-	f
10^{12}	tera-	T	10^{-12}	pico-	p
10^{9}	giga-	G	10^{-9}	nano-	n
10^{6}	mega-	M	10^{-6}	micro-	μ
10^{3}	kilo-	k	10^{-3}	milli-	m
10^{2}	hecto-	h	10^{-2}	centi-	c
10^{1}	deca-	da	10^{-1}	deci-	d

to a power which is a multiple of 3 is especially recommended. Widely used prefixes are mega, kilo, milli, micro and nano.

The combination of prefix and symbol is regarded as one new symbol, e.g. mm^3 means $(10^{-3} \text{ m})^3$ and not 10^{-3} m^3.

Only one prefix should be used to form decimal multiples or sub-multiples, e.g. 10^{-6} g is 1 μg not 1 mmg. In derived units, the prefix should be attached to one unit only, preferably in the numerator.

Care must be taken to avoid ambiguity, particularly when the symbol for a prefix is identical with that of a unit, e.g. N m for newton metre, not mN (10^{-3} N).

No space should be left between the symbol for a prefix and its unit, whereas a space should be left between symbols for derived units. An obvious example occurs with ms for milliseconds and m s for metres × seconds.

The symbol for a unit is unchanged in the plural and should not be followed by a full stop except at the end of a sentence, e.g. 8 mm and not 8 mm. or 8 mms. The solidus / or the word 'per' should only be used once in each unit. Where necessary, quantities can be raised to a negative power. For example, a pressure rise is wrongly expressed as $N/m^2/min$ which could be taken as $(N/m^2)/min$ or $N/(m^2/min)$. It should be written as $N\ m^{-2}\ min^{-1}$.

The decimal sign between digits is indicated by a full stop in typing. Commas are not used to divide large numbers up into groups of three, but a half space (whole space in typing) is left after every third digit, e.g. 502 499. If the numerical value of the number is less than unity, a zero should precede the decimal sign, e.g. 0.246 854 and not .246854.

When expressing a quantity by a numerical value and a unit, in most applications it is advisable to use a multiple or sub-multiple which yields a simple whole number lying between 1 and 999. For example, dimensions up to 0.99 metres can be expressed in millimetres. One microsecond is best expressed as 10^{-6} s and not 10^{-3} ms.

The SI symbol for 'day' (i.e. 24 hours) is 'd', but for clarity items such as urine output should be expressed preferably in terms of 'per 24 hours' (e.g. ml per 24 hours) since the expression 'per day' (e.g. ml d^{-1}) could be read as meaning 'between the hours of sunrise and sunset'.

For completeness, a reported measurement should include details of (a) the system; (b) the component; (c) the kind of quantity; (d) the numerical value; and (e) the unit, e.g.

arterial	blood halothane	mass concentration =	60		mg litre^{-1}
system	*component*	*kind of*		*numerical*	*unit*
		quantity		*value*	

Care must be taken to be sure that the name of any component is unambiguous. For acids and bases it is recommended that the designation of the maximally ionized form is used, e.g. for plasma measurements, the terms lactate and pyruvate are preferred to lactic acid and pyruvic acid.

SI units of concentration

The SI system includes two different types of unit of concentration

— mass concentration (grams per litre etc.) and amount of substance ('molar') concentration (mol per litre, millimol per litre, etc.). A choice has to be made between the two when reporting all measurements of concentration.

For substances having a defined chemical composition it is recommended that the concentration should be expressed in terms of the amount of substance. This arrangement may be applied to any defined particle such as an ion, atom, molecule or radical, but the nature of the particle must be self-evident in the report. In the past the equivalent concentration (e.g. mEq per litre) has been commonly used for reporting the results of monovalent electrolyte measurements (sodium, potassium, chloride and bicarbonate). Since this is not part of the SI system it should now be replaced by molar concentration. For sodium, potassium, chloride and bicarbonate the numerical values will be unaltered when expressed in the SI units of mmol per litre. Similarly, for other monovalent ions the numerical values for mEq per litre and mmol per litre will be identical. For non-monovalent ions the values will differ. A typical plasma sodium concentration of 140 mEq litre^{-1} becomes 140 mmol litre^{-1}.

Mass concentration is recommended for all protein measurements and for substances which do not have a sufficiently well-defined composition. The SI unit of mass concentration is expressed in terms of the litre, e.g. g litre^{-1}, mg litre^{-1}, whereas previously many measurements of mass concentration have been quoted in terms of 100 ml as the unit volume e.g. g/100 ml, mg/100 ml. For these measurements the numerical value will now increase by a factor of 10, e.g. a total serum protein concentration of 7 g/100 ml becomes 70 g litre^{-1}. In the case of proteins, the use of a molar concentration is impracticable since the molecular weight of the biologically active entity is uncertain. To avoid confusion in medical practice throughout the world the decilitre (100 ml) may be retained for expressing haemoglobin concentration in blood only, e.g. a normal blood haemoglobin concentration may be expressed as 14 g dl^{-1} or 140 g litre^{-1}. In the United Kingdom 14 g dl^{-1} is preferred.

Packed cell volume (PCV) will be expressed as a decimal fraction rather than as a percentage, e.g. 0.45 and not 45 per cent. For further details of the application of SI units in pathology readers should consult the *Journal of Clinical Pathology* **23**, 818 (1970) and Baron (1974).

The changeover to SI units will have marked effects in calculations concerned with pressure, energy, radiotherapy and nuclear medicine. The changes will be discussed individually in the appropriate sections of this book. It should be noted that temperature intervals on the SI system can be expressed in degrees Celsius ($^\circ$C).

Mass and weight

Mass is defined as 'the quantity of matter in a body' and is concerned with the amount of matter under consideration. Mass can be linked to the volume concerned via the concept of density. Density is defined simply as 'the mass of a unit volume of the material'. The density of substances relative to water, which is a convenient standard substance, is expressed in terms of their specific gravity – the mass of the substance divided by the mass of an equal volume of water. Both density and specific gravity are temperature dependent and should be quoted together with the temperature at which the measurement was taken. The dimensions of a volume are those of a length cubed, so that the dimensions of density are $M\,L^{-3}$ (i.e. $kg\,m^{-3}$).

If a light and a heavy object are held, one in each hand, the one with the greater mass is distinguished because it feels heavier. The sensation of weight arises from the action of the force of gravity. This is greater for the larger mass and needs to be offset by a correspondingly larger muscular effort. On earth, the universal availability of gravity makes it a convenient unit of force. Thus in the English system, the unit is the *pound weight.* Mistakenly, this is often contracted to one *pound.* The action of the earth's gravitational force is to cause a freely falling body to accelerate towards the earth's surface with a constant acceleration.

Length

The fundamental SI unit of length is the metre. It is SI practice to recommend the use of prefixes which raise 10 to a power which is a multiple of plus or minus three. Thus kilometres and millimetres are recommended, for example, whereas centimetres are not. This decision has an obvious impact on engineering drawings. The prefixes hecto, deca, deci and centi should be limited as far as possible to uses where the recommended prefixes are inconvenient.

Velocity and acceleration

The linear velocity of an object is expressed in terms of the distance it travels per unit time, e.g. metres second^{-1}, and has the dimensions of $L T^{-1}$. Electromagnetic blood flowmeters produce an output signal which is proportional to the blood stream velocity. Provided that the cross-section of the vessel in which the flow is measured is both constant and known, then the product of velocity and area gives the volume flow rate e.g. in litres per minute. When catheter-tip flow probes are used (Mills, 1963; Hartley and Cole, 1974), it may not always be easy to convert velocity to volume flow. This problem occurs in the ascending aorta due to turbulence.

Gas stream velocities can be measured directly by means of a pitot tube, but in anaesthesia a pneumotachograph is commonly employed. The cross-section of the pneumotachograph head is constant and the output is nearly always quoted in terms of a volume flow rate in litres per minute.

Acceleration is defined as the time rate of change of velocity. In studies on the contractility of the heart, an electromagnetic flow probe is often placed around the root of the ascending aorta. The output of the flowmeter gives the phasic blood volume flow in millilitres per minute. Using the signal from a left ventricular pressure transducer to gate an integrator, the flow signal can be integrated to give the stroke volume on a beat-by-beat basis. The acceleration of the blood stream can be found by feeding the flowmeter output into an electronic differentiating circuit. For accurate work it is desirable that the flowmeter should have a bandwidth of 100 Hz. The dimensions of acceleration are $L T^{-2}$. It can be written either as metres per second per second or as $m s^{-2}$. The acceleration due to gravity is approximately 9.81 m s^{-2} and is usually denoted by the symbol g. Transducers known as accelerometers are available for recording the acceleration of moving objects directly. These instruments can be composed of piezoelectric material such as barium titanate which produces an output voltage proportional to the acceleration applied across the crystal (Cobbold, 1974; Tims, Davidson and Timme, 1975). The high sensitivity piezoelectric accelerometer of Tims, Davidson and Timme (1975) has a sensitivity of 0.29 Vm^{-1} s^2 at frequencies up to 1 kHz.

Force

As in the English system of units, it is convenient to think in terms of a unit based on the force due to gravity. Thus the force due to gravity acting on a mass of one pound is called one pound-force, while that on a mass of one kilogram is called one kilogram-force or one kilopond. Since gravity varies by about 0.5 per cent over the earth's surface, units of force such as the pound weight which depend on the value of gravity can only be used for low accuracy work.

Newton's second law of motion states that when a given mass is accelerated, the acceleration produced is proportional to the magnitude of the applied force. This statement can be expressed in the form of the equation $F = kma$, where F is the force, k is a constant of proportionality, m is the mass and a is the acceleration.

Since k is a simple number, the dimensions of force are those of mass $\times$ acceleration, i.e. MLT^{-2}. By giving k a value of unity, it is possible to define a unit of force which is absolute and independent of gravity, i.e. a unit force will give unit mass unit acceleration. The SI unit of force is the newton which is that force which will give a mass of one kilogram an acceleration of one metre per second per second. A dyne is that force which gives a mass of one gram an acceleration of one centimetre per second per second. The dyne is the CGS unit of force and one newton $= 10^5$ dynes.

Pressure

Pressure is defined as 'force per unit area' e.g. newtons per square metre on the SI system. One newton per square metre is called one pascal. On the CGS system, the unit of force is the dyne per square centimetre while on the English system the pound weight per square inch is usually abbreviated to pounds per square inch (p.s.i.). It is better to use lbf in^{-2}, thus preserving the idea of a force. At present many existing hospital pressure gauges for anaesthetic gases are still scaled in terms of p.s.i., but the new gauges which are now being supplied in the United Kingdom are scaled only in terms of hundreds of kilopascals.

Thus the oxygen cylinder pressure gauge on a U.K. anaesthetic machine will now be scaled from 0–300 hundreds of kilopascals, i.e. 0–4350 p.s.i. gauge, with graduation marks at 20, 50, 100, 150, 200, 250 and 300 hundreds of kilopascals.

The nitrous oxide cylinder pressure gauge is calibrated from 0–100 in terms of hundreds of kilopascals i.e. 0–1450 p.s.i. gauge, with markings at 15, 54 and 100. The mark at 54 hundreds of kilopascals

(783 p.s.i.) is close to the pressure of 749 p.s.i. which is the pressure in a cylinder containing both liquid and gaseous nitrous oxide at 20 °C.

The carbon dioxide pressure gauge is calibrated from 0–100 in terms of hundreds of kilopascals with markings at 15, 57 and 100. The mark at 57 is equivalent to 827 p.s.i. which is close to the pressure of 825 p.s.i. found in a cylinder containing both gaseous and liquid carbon dioxide at 20 °C.

The cyclopropane pressure gauge is calibrated from 0–10 hundreds of kilopascals with markings at 5 and 10. The mark at 5 is equivalent to 72.5 p.s.i. which is close to the pressure of 78 p.s.i. found in a cylinder containing both liquid and gaseous cyclopropane at 20 °C.

Pressure gauges for hospital pipelines are now scaled from 0–10 hundreds of kilopascals (0–145 p.s.i.) with markings at 2, 3, 4, 6 and 10.

The mark at 4 hundreds of kilopascals is equivalent to 58 p.s.i. which is close to the normal pipeline pressure of 60 p.s.i.g.

Vacuum pipeline gauges are scaled in an anticlockwise direction either from 0–30 kilopascals (0–4.35 p.s.i.) or from 0–100 kilopascals (0–14.5 p.s.i.) depending on whether they are for low or high suction applications.

Whilst the anaesthetic equipment industry has adopted gauges scaled in hundreds of kilopascals i.e. Pa $\times$ 10^5, it is also feasible to work in terms of megapascals (10^6 Pa) as has been done in this book for simplicity. Thus an oxygen contents gauge could be scaled from 0–300 hundreds of kilopascals and could also be scaled 0–30 MPa.

The use of a column of liquid to measure pressure

In *Figure 3.1*, consider a column of liquid of density ρ and having a unit cross-sectional area. If the height of the column is h, then the volume of the column is ($h \times 1 \times 1$) and its mass is $h \times \rho$. The force

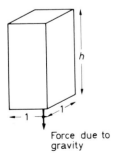

Force due to
gravity   Figure 3.1

due to gravity acting over the unit area is simply $F = g \times \rho \times h$, where g is the acceleration due to gravity. Taking the density of mercury as 13 600 kg per cubic metre at room temperature, the mass of a column 0.22 m (120 mm) high is $0.12 \times 10^{-4} \times 13\,600$ kg $= 0.1632$ kg if the cross-section is one square centimetre. The acceleration due to gravity is 9.81 metres per second per second so that the force on the 10^{-4} square metres area is $0.1632 \times 9.81 \times 10^4 = 16\,010$ pascals which is the same as 16.01 kPa. On this basis 1 mmHg = 133.5 pascals. Using an accurate figure for the density of mercury, the official relationship is that 1 mmHg = 133.32 pascals.

In respiratory measurements, pressures of the order of centimetres of water (inflation pressures) and millimetres of mercury (resistance to gas flow) are commonly encountered. Both centimetres of water and millimetres of mercury are used in the measurement of bladder pressure and central venous pressure. These units are still in use because of the ease with which water and mercury manometers are employed in clinical practice. It should be noted that the torr, which is numerically equally to one millimetre of mercury is not as SI unit.

The aneroid pressure gauges used to measure the inflation pressure generated by automatic lung ventilators are still being calibrated in centimetres of water.

In the United Kingdom, blood-gas tensions are now quoted in kilopascals rather than in millimetres of mercury. Since 1 kPa = 7.50 mmHg, a typical PCO_2 of 40 mmHg becomes 5.33 kPa and a typical PO_2 of 100 mmHg becomes 13.33 kPa. A blood-gas analyser would have a typical range for PCO_2 of 0.7–33.3 kPa and for PO_2 of 0–132.9 kPa.

Blood pressures are still measured in terms of the millimetre of mercury since this has been used for many years and clinicians across the world are familiar with the values. A typical arterial blood pressure of 120/80 mmHg would become 16/10.7 kPa.

Barometers

If a long glass tube, sealed at one end, is filled with mercury and inverted in a dish of mercury (*Figure 3.2*) the pressure of the atmosphere acting on the mercury surface in the dish will support a column of mercury whose height is such that the pressure it develops due to the effect of gravity is equal to the atmospheric pressure. Such an arrangement constitutes a Fortin barometer for measuring the atmospheric pressure. In practice the dish is replaced with a flexible

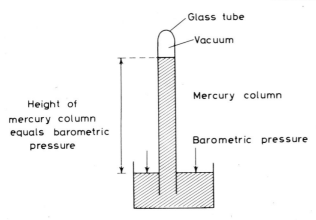

Figure 3.2. Principle of a Fortin barometer

container and this can be squeezed by means of a screw mechanism to set the level of the mercury surface at a fixed mark, the height of the column then being read with a vernier scale. With clean, dry, mercury in the tube, a vacuum exists in the tube above the top of the mercury column. This is known as a Torricellian vacuum. Suppose that some water was introduced into this space and the temperature of the barometer was 20 °C. The water vapour would exert a partial pressure of 18 mmHg at this temperature. This would cause the height of the mercury column to be reduced by 18 mm. For example, if without the water the column was 760 mm high, it would be reduced to 742 mmHg by the saturated water vapour.

Another form of barometer is the *aneroid* barometer. This is a diaphragm-type gauge using an evacuated capsule forming one side of the diaphragm as a reference pressure. Although not as accurate as the Fortin barometer, it is compact and does not contain mercury.

Gauge pressure and absolute pressure

On the majority of pressure gauges, such as those indicating the pressure in anaesthetic gas cylinders, the gauge is set to indicate zero when the pressure inside the cylinder is actually atmospheric (0.10133 $MN\ m^{-2}$ a, 14.7 $lbf\ in^{-2}$ a). Pressures referred to atmospheric pressure are known as gauge pressures and are written as $N\ m^{-2}$ g or $lbf\ in^{-2}$ g.* Pressures which are referred to a true zero pressure (vacuum) are

*Except where otherwise indicated, values are quoted in gauge pressures.

known as absolute pressures, e.g. N m^{-2} a or lbf in^{-2} a. A cylinder filled to a pressure of 12.41 MN m^{-2} g (1800 lbf in^{-2} g) would read 12.48 MN m^{-2} a (1815 lbf in^{-2} a) on an absolute pressure gauge. At this level of pressure the difference is likely to be relatively unimportant. However, in hyperbaric chambers operating at a few atmospheres pressure it is important to quote the units of pressure employed. For example, consider a hyperbaric chamber in which the pressure can be raised to 2 atmospheres above atmospheric. The chamber pressure can then be described as 2 atmospheres gauge or 3 atmospheres absolute, i.e. 3 ata. This unit is frequently encountered in the hyperbaric literature. A good description of the design of a hyperbaric operating room is that of Baker (1965).

Pressure gauges and regulators

The pressure gauges of the dial type encountered in anaesthetic practice are usually based upon either the Bourdon tube or a diaphragm. Bourdon tube gauges are used for an approximate measurement of the higher pressures, such as the filling pressures of gas cylinders. The action of the Bourdon tube is illustrated in *Figure 3.3*. The application

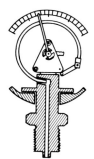

Figure 3.3. Bourdon tube gauge. (By courtesy of Drägerwerk, Lübeck)

to the inside of the metal tube of the pressure to be measured causes the tube to attempt to straighten out. The resulting motion is transmitted via a linkage to cause the pointer to move over the scale. The tube is usually made of a special alloy of copper.

In order to obtain the greater sensitivity required to measure pressures in the range of centimetres of mercury or water, use is made of diaphragm-type pressure gauges (*Figure 3.4*). The pressure to be measured is applied to one side of the metal diaphragm, the other side being at atmospheric pressure. The movement of the diaphragm is magnified through the linkage to actuate the pointer. This type of gauge is used to measure inflation pressures from an automatic lung ventilator. *Figure 3.5* illustrates an absolute pressure version of the

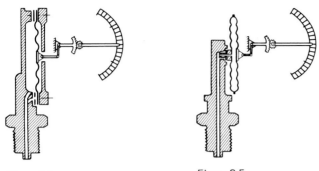

Figure 3.4   Figure 3.5

Diaphragm manometer. (By courtesy of Drägerwerk, Lübeck)

diaphragm manometer. Here the diaphragm forms one wall of an evacuated capsule. The diaphragm is vertical when the pressure on each side is equal and bows in towards the capsule when the pressure to be measured is greater than zero. The diaphragm motion is again sensed by a linkage and the reading is set to zero when the applied pressure is zero. This is the principle used in the aneroid barometer.

Pressure regulators

Pressure regulators or reducing valves are frequently encountered when it is necessary to step down a high pressure, such as that from a gas cylinder, to a lower pressure. As gas is withdrawn from the cylinder, so the inlet pressure applied to the regulator or valve will fall. The action of the pressure regulator is to hold the outlet pressure from the regulator sensibly constant over a wide range of inlet pressures. This compensatory action is not possible with a simple needle valve. It is also desirable to be able to withdraw gas from the regulator at a wide range of flow rates without markedly affecting the output pressure.

Figure 3.6 shows a simplified diagram of a single-stage pressure regulator. This is typical of the type fitted to oxygen cylinders. The version used on anaesthetic machines does not have a control knob for adjusting the outlet pressure but has a preset adjustment. By means of

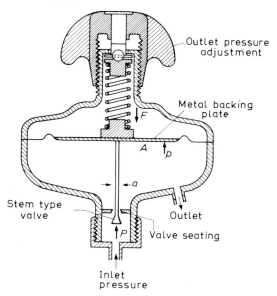

Figure 3.6. Single-stage regulator

the control knob and associated screw, a spring pressure can be applied to the metal backing plate on the rear side of the rubber diaphragm. This side is also connected to the atmosphere via vent holes cut in the regulator housing. The reduced outlet pressure of the regulator is applied to the other side of the diaphragm to give an opposing force. Acting on this assembly there is also a third force, which arises from the high inlet pressure to the regulator, acting against a small-area conical valve seating. Let the force exerted by the spring be F, the effective area of the diaphragm be A, the outlet pressure be p, the inlet pressure be P, and the effective area of the valve orifice be a.

Assume that initially the regulator is running in a state of equilibrium. As the inlet pressure is reduced perhaps due to the cylinder emptying, two effects occur: (1) The force acting on the conical valve decreases; (2) The pressure drop across the valve decreases. Hence in order to maintain the desired rate of gas flow, the valve must open further and the spring must relax. For many regulators, the second effect is small compared with the first. The regulator of *Figure 3.6* is of the *inverse acting type*, since both the high and the low pressures act in opposition to the spring. In each case, the force developed is equal to the product of the pressure multiplied by the effective area over which the force acts, thus $F=pA+Pa$. If the relaxation of the spring can be ignored, F can be assumed to remain constant. A change ΔP of the inlet pressure will be accompanied by a change of Δp in the outlet pressure. Under the new conditions $F=(p+\Delta p)A+(P+\Delta P)a$. By subtraction, $\Delta p=-\Delta P(a/A)$. The minus sign indicates that as the cylinder pressure falls, so the outlet pressure tends to rise. The magnitude of this effect depends on the ratio of the effective areas of the inlet valve to the diaphragm. In practice, the use of a large diaphragm gives rise to a

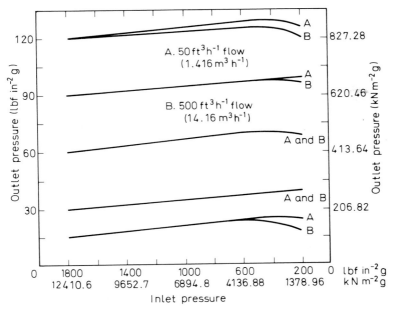

Figure 3.7. Pressure characteristic for a single-stage oxygen therapy regulator. (By courtesy of British Oxygen Co. Ltd)

bulky regulator, and the use of a small valve orifice limits the possible throughput of gas. Typical values for this ratio lie between 200 and 300 to 1. The effective area of a rubber diaphragm is about 0.7 to 0.9 of its actual area, while the effective area of a stem type of inlet valve is about 1.1 times the free area of the valve. *Figure 3.7* illustrates the variation of output pressure with inlet pressure for a typical single stage regulator. *Figure 3.8* shows the variation of outlet pressure with changing gas flow for the same regulator. When the resistance to gas flow of the apparatus being supplied is decreased, more gas flows from the regulator and the pressure balance across the regulator is upset. It can be shown that a change in output volume flow rate of ΔQ is related to the corresponding change in output pressure ΔP by an equation of the form $\Delta Q = Kr \, (\sqrt{P}) \, (A/S) \, \Delta P$ where r is the radius of the inlet valve,

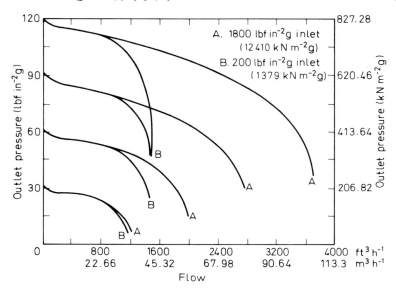

Figure 3.8. Flow characteristic for a single-stage oxygen therapy regulator. (By courtesy of British Oxygen Co. Ltd)

S is the spring stiffness (N m^{-1}), A is the effective area of the diaphragm, P is the inlet pressure and K is a constant. It is usual to incorporate a relief valve into the body of the regulator so that if any leakage occurs across the valve seat, a dangerous pressure cannot build up under the diaphragm.

In older types of British anaesthetic machines the outlet pressure of the cylinder regulators was set at 34.5 kN m^{-2} (5 lbf in^{-2}). In modern machines the outlet pressure is often set at 413.7 kN m^{-2} (60 lbf in^{-2}). This is the same as that of gas pipeline systems in British hospitals. It confers advantages in the standardization of equipment and allows the operation of gas-powered ventilators which are based upon the use of an entrainer. The anaesthetist should check for himself the outlet pressure provided by the regulators he is actually using; for example, the Airmed A-S II regulator is set to give 206.8 kN m^{-2} (30 lbf in^{-2}).

Flow restrictors are incorporated in anaesthetic machines fitted with 413.7 kN m^{-2} (60 lbf in^{-2}) pressure regulators. The restrictors are situated before the gas flowmeters in order to protect them from damage should the high pressure be suddenly applied to the flowmeter tubes. Gas cylinder valves should be opened slowly in order to lengthen the period during which compression of the gas between the cylinder valve and the pressure regulator occurs. This manoeuvre eliminates the formation of a shock wave. Modern practice is to incorporate the pressure regulator in the cylinder yoke block thus obviating the need for high-pressure tubing to connect the yoke and regulator.

Anaesthetic machines are also provided with one-way or backflow check valves whose function is to prevent the loss of gas occurring from an empty cylinder yoke or the transfer of gas from one cylinder to another when cylinders are connected in parallel. The check valves are usually mounted on the cylinder yokes but in some machines they are fitted on the low-pressure side of the reducing valves. The cylinder yokes are now of the pin—index non-interchangeable type to prevent

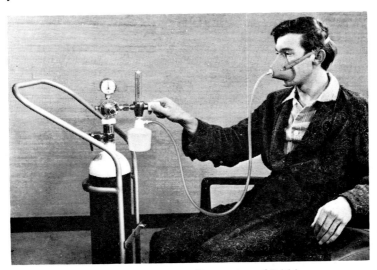

Figure 3.9. Oxygen therapy apparatus. (By courtesy of British Oxygen Co. Ltd)

the accidental connection of the wrong type of cylinder in a particular gas yoke. Sintered metal filters are provided at the inlet of the pressure regulators to protect them from the ingress of dirt or grit.

It is arranged that the output from the oxygen pressure regulators is fed not only to the oxygen flowmeter but also to a parallel path which provides the emergency flush supply. It is desirable that the flow available when the 'emergency oxygen' lever is activated should be not less than 35 litres per minute. This flow is fed directly into the anaesthetic circuit.

A number of oxygen failure devices have been devised to draw attention to a failure in the oxygen supply. It is desirable that the unit should be independent of a power source such as a battery and be unaffected by the back pressure produced by a ventilator in operation. Oxygen failure devices are discussed in Chapter 12.

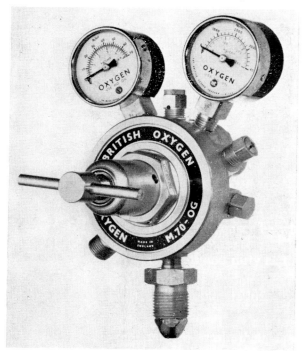

Figure 3.10. Two-stage pressure regulator. (By courtesy of British Oxygen Co. Ltd)

Single-stage regulators have a performance which is adequate for use with anaesthetic machines and oxygen therapy equipment (*Figures 3.7, 3.8, 3.9*). However, for the control of gas flows in laboratory experiments on respiratory apparatus and in instruments such as gas chromatographs, a better performance is necessary. In these cases a two-stage regulator is used (*Figure 3.10*). The output from the first stage regulator serves as the input for the second stage; the final variation, in output pressure, is greatly reduced by this means for an equivalent change in the inlet pressure. For a two-stage regulator the change in the output pressure is given by $\Delta p_2 = \Delta p_1 \, (a_1 a_2)/(A_1 A_2)$, where p_1 is the inlet pressure to the first stage, a_1 and a_2 are the effective areas of the inlet valves for each stage and A_1 and A_2 are the effective diaphragm areas.

Demand-type regulators

The type of regulator so far described is designed to deliver a substantially constant flow of gas against a wide range of inlet pressures. The supply of gas from the regulator is in the form of a steady stream.

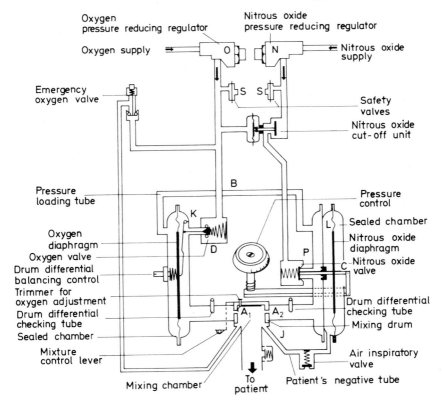

Figure 3.11. Schematic diagram of a Walton 5 dental anaesthetic machine. (By courtesy of British Oxygen Co. Ltd)

However, when it is required to supply gas to a spontaneously breathing patient, an economy of gas is obtained by the use of a demand system. Examples of demand systems occur in nitrous oxide—oxygen anaesthetic machines used in dental practice and the nitrous oxide—oxygen analgesic machines used in obstetrics.

A schematic diagram of a Walton 5 dental machine is given in *Figure 3.11*. The two-stage pressure regulators N and O reduce the pressure from the supply cylinders to 68.9 kN m^{-2} (10 lbf in^{-2}). Small variations occurring in the outlet pressures of the regulators are of no consequence since the pressures will be equalized later by the pressure-loading arrangement. The safety valves S act as a check on the pressure applied to the oxygen valve D and the nitrous oxide valve P in case of any creep in the outlet pressures of the reducing valves. These safety valves are set to blow off at a pressure of 89.6 kN m^{-2} (13 lbf in^{-2}). The nitrous oxide cut-off unit is arranged to interrupt the flow of nitrous oxide in the event of a failure in the oxygen supply. The negative pressure produced by the patient's inspiratory effort is transmitted via tube J to the sealed chamber L thus causing the nitrous oxide diaphragm to move over to the left. This motion is transmitted by means of a push-rod C to the nitrous oxide valve P which then opens to admit nitrous oxide from the supply to the mixing drum via the orifice A_2. The pressure acting at A_2 is fed via the pressure-loading tube B to cause the oxygen diaphragm and linkage K to move to the right, thus opening the oxygen valve D. Oxygen now flows from the supply to the mixing drum via orifice A_1. When the patient's inspiratory effort ceases the valve return springs shut the oxygen and nitrous oxide valves and stop the gas flow.

Any increase in the negative pressure developed by the patient will open up the valve ports further, resulting in an increase in the flow of gas through the mixer ports to the patient. The pressure drop across each orifice is arranged to be almost equal and is of the order of 2 cmH$_2$O at 10 litres per minute and 60 cmH$_2$O at 100 litres per minute for the 10 per cent N$_2$O setting. Any change in the nitrous oxide pressure at orifice A_2 produces a corresponding change in the oxygen pressure at A_1 because of the change in the loading on the oxygen diaphragm. This causes the pressure to be held almost equal at A_1 and A_2, of the order of 0.05 cmH$_2$O, over a wide range of gas flows and respiratory rates.

Rotation of the mixing drum (*Figure 3.12*) determines the relative apertures of A_1 and A_2. In this way the proportions of the gas mixture

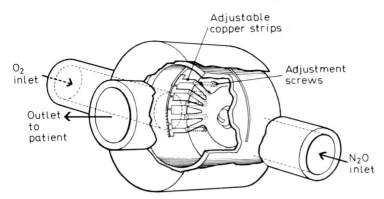

Figure 3.12. Mixing drum of the Walton 5 dental anaesthetic machine. (By courtesy of British Oxygen Co. Ltd)

delivered by the machine are under the control of the mixture control lever which rotates the drum. The dimensions of the drum are approximately 50 mm diameter by 25 mm wide with a wall thickness of 1.5 mm. The mixing valve consists of an outer chamber and a rotatable inner mixing drum or sleeve, both machined to fine tolerances. Two apertures are situated in the side wall of the mixer drum through which oxygen and nitrous oxide respectively can enter. The apertures work in conjunction with slots cut in the inner drum or sleeve valve. The slot which engages with the nitrous oxide inlet port is approximately 25 mm long by 1.5 mm wide. The slot for the oxygen port is of the same length but tapers in width from approximately 1.5 mm until at the other end it is so narrow that it is continued as a series of ten small holes. These cover the low end of the range, i.e. from 0–10 per cent oxygen in 1 per cent steps. Since grease or oil might tend to clog these holes, the need for these lubricants is eliminated by coating the inside of the mixing chamber with PTFE which has a low coefficient of friction. Gas-tightness is assured by the precision grinding of the drum. During the manufacturers' calibration the adjustment of the oxygen apertures to give accurately the desired gas mixtures is accomplished by means of five copper strips each adjustable by a screw (*Figure 3.12*). The first four strips cover 0–20 per cent in steps and the fifth, 20–50 per cent oxygen. The reason for the fifth strip covering a wider range is due to the scale on the Walton 5 machine being non-linear and becoming more compressed as the 50–100 per cent positions are approached. The delivery pressure ranges from 0–20 mmHg and can be varied by rotating the pressure control knob situated on top of the machine. This action causes a loading spring to operate on the outside of the nitrous oxide diaphragm. The increased pressure applied to the nitrous oxide side is transmitted to the oxygen side thus keeping the two gas pressures in balance. When the gas mixture from the machine enters the patient's lungs, the back pressure resulting from the combination of lung compliance and airway resistance is transmitted back to the nitrous oxide diaphragm. Movement of the diaphragm then overcomes the loading of the spring and shuts off the supply of the two gases. In the absence of back pressure when the machine is freely discharging to atmosphere, no load will be developed across either the diaphragm or loading spring — these components being largely inoperative. When the pressure control is not set to zero, and gas is being drawn from the machine by the patient's inspiratory efforts, the flow supplied depends upon the suction applied to the diaphragm. A minimum negative pressure of about 2 mmHg is required to initiate flow, and at −3.2 mmHg a flow of approximately 100 litres per minute is produced. The gas flow is increased if the pressure control knob is operated to increase the basic supply pressure to the mixer drum ports. Two 680-litre (24 ft^3) oxygen cylinders plus two 1820-litre (400 gallon) nitrous oxide cylinders are carried and the emergent mixture can be continuously varied between 100 per cent N_2O and 100 per cent O_2. Smith (1961a) has evaluated the performance of the Walton 5 machine in the laboratory.

Another interesting application lies in the administration of a 50/50 per cent v/v nitrous oxide–oxygen mixture for use by women in labour, particularly during domiciliary practice by midwives. The mixture, known as 'Entonox', is supplied in lightweight 500-litre cylinders to the demand valve, and from there to a facemask. The mixture is exhaled to atmosphere via an expiratory valve. The Entonox demand valve is shown in *Figure 3.13*. In this case the demand valve is supplied with a fixed pre-mixed gas mixture, whereas in the case of a dental anaesthetic machine, provision also has to be made to vary the composition of the mixture.

Referring to *Figure 3.13* the pressure of a 'full' cylinder of 50/50 nitrous oxide–oxygen is 13.44 MN m^{-2} (1980 lbf in^{-2}). This is reduced by a special kind of two-stage regulator in which the output from a conventional type of first stage is fed to a particularly sensitive second stage which serves as the actual demand valve. An inspiratory effort from the patient develops a negative pressure, and moves the sensing

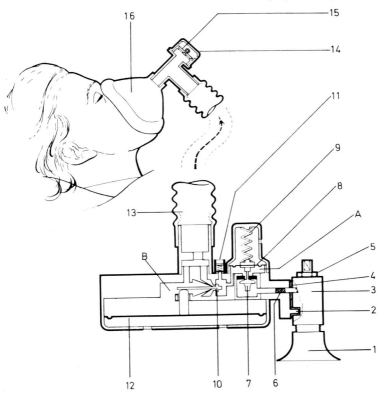

Figure 3.13. Schematic diagram of the Entonox analgesic apparatus. (By courtesy of British Oxygen Co. Ltd)

1. Cylinder (50% nitrous oxide/50% oxygen). 2. Yoke pin. 3. Non-interchangeable cylinder valve. 4. Bodok seal. 5. Gland nut. 6. Filter. 7. 1st stage valve. 8. Diaphragm. 9. Spring. 10. 2nd stage (tilting type) valve. 11. Safety valve. 12. Sensing diaphragm. 13. Corrugated tube. 14. Exhalation valve. 15. Diaphragm. 16. Face-mask. A. 1st stage reduction. B. 2nd stage reduction

diaphragm. This motion opens a tilting-type valve to release the gas during inspiration. Expiration closes the tilting-type valve and allows the expired gas to vent to atmosphere via a separate exhalation valve. For supplying the demand action, the tilting valve provides a second stage of pressure reduction. In comparison with most other regulators the main distinguishing function of this one is that it regulates the output pressure to a level slightly below atmospheric instead of substantially above it. The apparatus is capable of supplying a peak inspiratory flow greater than 275 litres per minute. During use the temperature of the Entonox demand valve may fall to below $-20\,^{\circ}C$, but this does not affect its functioning or the composition of the emergent gas mixture. Davies, Hogg and Rosen (1974a, b) discuss the resistance to breathing of Entonox demand valves and the acceptable upper limits of resistance to respiration of apparatus for inhalation analgesia during labour. Hogg *et al.* (1974) found that a laminar flow resistance of 0.26 cm of water per litre per minute gave a power dissipated in the apparatus of less than 1.68 W at 40 litres per minute for 99.9 per cent of the population studied. They recommended that the additional power required to inspire through the apparatus, with the ventilation occurring in mothers having analgesia, should not be greater than the additional power involved in breathing without apparatus at the greater ventilation found in mothers without analgesia.

Vacuum (suction) regulators

Pressure regulators are normally employed to provide a known, stable, positive presure. However, they can also be used to provide a known, stable, negative pressure. Such an application occurs in wall-mounted suction equipment for use in intensive care areas where a vacuum pipeline is available. *Figure 3.14* shows a cross-section of a wall-mounted suction controller and its associated collector jar. A high suction version of the controller provides a range of vacuum from 50–500 mmHg below atmospheric and will evacuate a 1.5-litre capacity jar to 400 mmHg below atmospheric in less than 4 seconds, whilst a low suction version will provide a vacuum in the range 0–150 mmHg below atmospheric and takes less than 2 seconds to evacuate a 1.5-litre jar to a vacuum of 130 mmHg below atmospheric. These performance figures are based on the availability of a wall suction pipeline outlet capable of passing 40 litres of free air at a line pressure of 500 mmHg below atmospheric pressure. Stands are available for the units to be either wall- or wall-rail-mounted.

Medical gas cylinders

The nominal pressure in a full cylinder of oxygen is 13.44 MN m^{-2} (1980 lbf in^{-2}), so that cylinders have to be carefully manufactured to withstand such high pressures and they must subsequently be regularly inspected and tested. Every five years each cylinder is subjected to a hydraulic test of 20.68 MN m^{-2} (3000 lbf in^{-2}) for oxygen, 23.17 MN m^{-2} (3360 lbf in^{-2}) for nitrous oxide or 22.75 MN m^{-2} (3300 lbf in^{-2}) for both oxygen and nitrous oxide if the cylinder is an 'S' type.

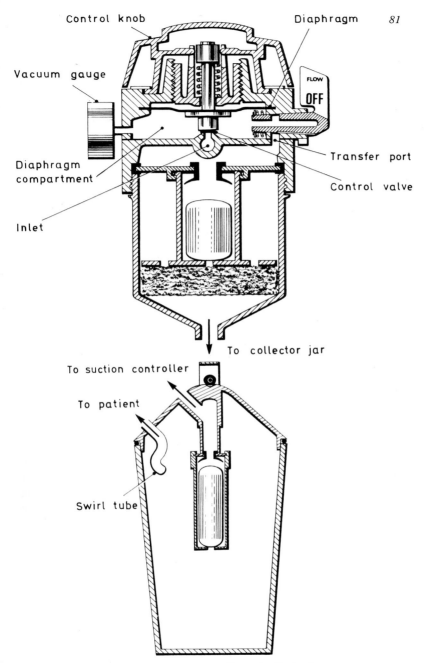

Figure 3.14. Cross-section of suction controller and collector jar.
(By courtesy of British Oxygen Co. Ltd)

Older cylinders, manufactured from 1946, are made from a steel containing 1.3–1.7 per cent of manganese. In the 1950s, a steel containing 0.4–0.9 per cent of molybdenum was introduced. The greater tensile strength of the molybdenum steel enabled the wall thickness, and hence the weight, of the cylinder to be reduced. The current practice is gradually to replace the older cylinders by flyweight models

TABLE 3.4. Nominal fully charged cylinder pressures at 15 °C

Gas	lbf in^{-2} g	kPa × 100	MPa
Air	1987	137	13.7
Carbon Dioxide	725	50.0	5.00
Cyclopropane	65	4.5	0.45
Entonox	1987	137	13.70
Helium	1987	137	13.70
Nitrous Oxide	638	44.0	4.40
Oxygen	1987	137	13.70

TABLE 3.5. Nominal free gas capacity at 15 °C and 760 mmHg in litres

British Oxygen Co. Cylinder Size	Oxygen	Nitrous oxide	Cyclo-propane	Carbon dioxide	Entonox
AA	–	–	36 (8 gall)	–	–
A	–	–	96 (20 gall)	–	–
B	–	–	180 (40 gall)	–	–
C	170 (36 gall)	450 (100 gall)	–	450 (2lb)	–
D	340 (72 gall)	900 (200 gall)	–	900	500
E	680 (24 cu. ft.)	1800 (400 gall)	–	1800 (7lb)	–
F	1360 (48 cu. ft.)	3600 (800 gall)	–	–	2000
G	3400 (120 cu. ft.)	9000 (2000 gall)	–	–	5000
J	6800 (240 cu. ft.)	–	–	–	–

manufactured from chrome-molybdenum steel according to the Home Office specification 'S' of 1961. This will prove to be of particular convenience to midwives, and ambulance crews using the Entonox premixed nitrous oxide–oxygen. The insides of steel medical gas cylinders are often coated with a film of red rust. This is capable of markedly absorbing vapours such as halothane. Hence, when selecting cylinders for the storage of accurately known vapour mixtures, it is desirable to choose cylinders made from a non-ferrous alloy rather than steel.

The measurement of physiological pressures

During surgery and intensive therapy, anaesthetists will often be concerned with the need to measure physiological pressures such as the systemic arterial blood pressure, pressures in the chambers of the heart and airway pressure. For pressures that vary relatively slowly, such as the central venous pressure, it is usual to employ a saline or mercury manometer, and for the monitoring of the airway pressure in conjunction with a ventilator an aneroid capsule manometer is adequate. However, a knowledge of the pressure waveform is often necessary, as in the recording of arterial pressures, and the obtaining of an electrical analogue of the waveform is essential for display on a cathode ray tube oscilloscope and for further processing such as the extraction of the systolic and diastolic pressures. Under these circumstances some form of pressure transducer is employed to transform the physiological pressure varying with time into a corresponding electrical signal. Substantial improvements in the design of pressure transducers in terms of reliability and safety have led to their being accepted as standard items in physiological measurement equipment. Usually pressure transducers operate with their pressure sensing portion in direct contact with the pressure to be measured. This approach is known as the direct measurement of pressure. In contrast, in indirect pressure measurement techniques, the measuring device is not in direct contact with the pressure concerned. An obvious example occurs with the various techniques for the indirect measurement of the arterial blood pressure.

Pressure transducers

From the viewpoint of the anaesthetist, contact is made between the pressure to be monitored and the transducer by means of a suitable tube in the form of a catheter or cannula. This is usually air-filled in the case of airway or oesophageal pressures and saline-filled in the case of blood pressures. The pressure is transmitted via this physical connection to operate on the sensitive diaphragm of the transducer. Thus the transducer is located outside the patient's body. Alternatively, the transducer can be mounted at the tip of a catheter so that its diaphragm is actually located at the site in the body where the pressure is to be measured. Having the transducer external to the body makes calibration and stability problems less severe, but the distortion of the pressure waveform arising from the inertia and friction introduced by the fluid column in the catheter may be a distinct limitation, e.g. when it is required to record an accurate left ventricular pressure waveform.

Various manufacturers have developed different types of pressure transducers for patient monitoring and physiological studies; for example the capacitance manometer, the linear variable differential transformer and bonded and unbonded strain gauge transducers. These have all produced creditable results, but current practice is concentrating on the unbonded strain gauge type. Unlike the capacitance and transformer types, this can easily be energized from either a stabilized d.c. or a.c. supply and can be adapted to provide a high degree of isolation of the patient's side of the diaphragm from the electrical circuitry of the transducer as required by hospital electrical safety regulations.

The principle of the unbonded strain gauge pressure transducer

Wire strain gauges were originally developed by engineers for the measurement of the small movements produced by tension and compression in beams and other structures. Strain is the increase in length per unit length resulting from the application of stress, i.e., force per unit area. The operation of a wire strain gauge follows from the fact that if a length of wire is stretched its electrical resistance increases due to the increase in length and the reduction in cross-sectional area. Conversely, if the wire is forced to contract, then its electrical resistance will decrease. The 'gauge factor' of a wire strain gauge is defined as $F=(r/R)/(\ell/L)$ where R is the original resistance of the gauge, r is the change in resistance of the gauge when stressed, L is the original length of the gauge and ℓ is the change in length due to the stress. Typical values of F are of the order of 2 to 3.

The cantilever beam illustrated in *Figure 3.15* provides a simple example of the operation of strain gauges. One strain gauge is firmly attached, or bonded, to the upper surface of the beam and a second gauge is bonded to the lower surface. The gauges are connected into opposite arms of a Wheatstone Bridge circuit as shown in *Figure 3.16*. Since the gauges are in opposite arms, changes in gauge resistance due to ambient temperature changes cancel. Applying a load to the far end

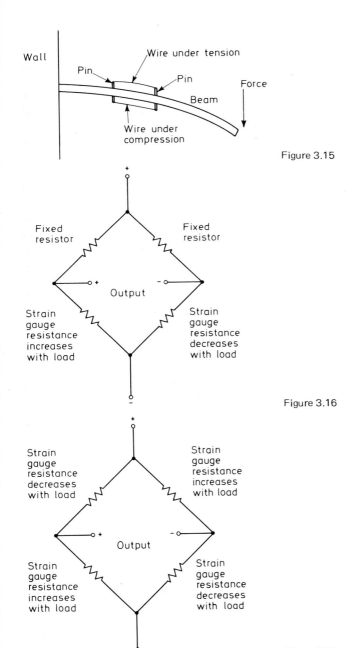

Wall

Wire under tension

Pin

Pin

Force

Beam

Wire under
compression

Figure 3.15

Fixed
resistor

Fixed
resistor

Output

Strain
gauge
resistance
increases
with load

Strain
gauge
resistance
decreases
with load

Figure 3.16

Strain
gauge
resistance
decreases
with load

Strain
gauge
resistance
increases
with load

Output

Strain
gauge
resistance
increases
with load

Strain
gauge
resistance
decreases
with load

Figure 3.17

of the cantilever increases the resistance of the upper gauge and decreases the resistance of the lower gauge, thus unbalancing the previously balanced bridge circuit. Because two of the four bridge arms consist of fixed resistors, this configuration is called a *strain gauge half bridge*. Twice the sensitivity can be obtained with the *strain gauge full bridge* of *Figure 3.17* in which all the four arms are active. Wire strain gauges are purely resistive and can be energized by either a well stabilized d.c. or a.c. source. For a.c. operation a carrier amplifier having an energizing oscillator and a demodulator is employed.

Higher gauge factors, which are of the order of 50 times those obtained with wire gauges can be obtained by the use of semiconductor strain gauges. However, care will be required to compensate for the greater temperature sensitivity and non-linearity of the semiconductor gauges. Single crystal silicon is used for the gauge material and is encapsulated with epoxy resin for protection from the environment. Doping of the silicon with phosphorus yields a negative resistance—strain characteristic while a positive characteristic is obtained by doping with boron. A suitable combination of gauge types is chosen to provide temperature compensation. Silicon gauges have been used in some forms of bonded strain gauge pressure transducer having a silicon diaphragm with the strain gauge deposited on its rear surface by integrated circuit manufacturing techniques. However, the unbonded strain gauge pressure transducer with semiconductor gauges gives a better electrical isolation.

Unbonded wire strain gauge pressure transducers

These have proved to be one of the most used transducers — for example, the Statham P23 range. The principle of their construction is shown in *Figure 3.18a*. Four strain-sensitive wires are connected to a pair of supporting frames, one of which can move inside the other. The inner frame moves and is attached to the pressure sensing diaphragm of the transducer while the outer frame is fixed. An initial tension is applied to the wires to maintain them under tension when the moving frame is at either end of its travel. Mechanical stops limit the travel and prevent over-stretching of the wires. A positive pressure applied to the diaphragm relative to atmospheric pressure will stretch wires B and C and relax wires A and D which comprise a strain gauge full bridge. The inner frame is spring-mounted to maintain it in a central position when there is atmospheric pressure on both sides of the diaphragm.

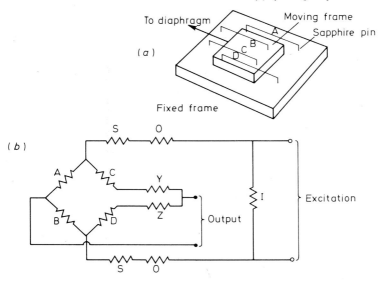

Figure 3.18

Additional resistors are located within the transducer's housing to allow for adjustment of the sensitivity and output voltage (*Figure 3.18b*).

The principle of the linear differential transformer pressure transducer
This type of pressure transducer is essentially an audio-frequency transformer having one primary and two secondary windings. The latter are connected in series opposition so that the beginning of one winding is connected to the finish of the other, *Figure 3.19*. The transformer has a moveable core of ferromagnetic material which is connected to the transducer's pressure sensing diaphragm. With atmospheric pressure on both sides of the diaphragm it is arranged that the core is centrally situated between the two secondary windings. The electromagnetic fields linking the primary to each of the secondaries which have equal numbers of turns are then identical so that the voltage induced in each secondary is equal. The fact that the secondaries are in series opposition ensures that their respective output voltages are opposite in phase and sum to zero.

The application of a pressure to the diaphragm moves the core to couple more of the electromagnetic field from the primary into one secondary than into the other. The amplitude of the resultant output signal will depend on the magnitude of the applied pressure, and its phase on which of the secondaries has the largest voltage induced in it, i.e. whether the pressure change was positive or negative with respect to atmospheric. The phase of the output signal from the combined secondaries will reverse as the diaphragm moves through the central

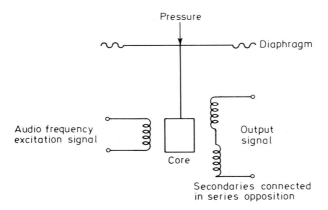

Figure 3.19

position. The output a.c. signal from the secondaries is fed into a phase-sensitive detector which produces a d.c. signal whose algebraic sign (positive or negative) depends on whether the pressure applied is above or below atmospheric and whose amplitude is proportional to the pressure change.

The transducer represents an electrical impedance since it is comprised of resistive and reactive (inductance and capacitance) elements. The device is powered by an amplitude stabilized a.c. supply of a few kilohertz, typically 2.4 kHz at 5 V. In practice, there will not be a complete absence of output signal at the null position of the diaphragm and core owing to the presence of harmonics of the excitation frequency. Their contribution to the output is nulled electrically by the user by means of the resistance and capacitance balance controls on the associated carrier amplifier used with the transducer. A differential transformer type of transducer can only be used on a.c. supply.

The pressure transducer cuvette

When the pressure transducer is of the type which is used external to the patient's body, the transducer's diaphragm interfaces with a small

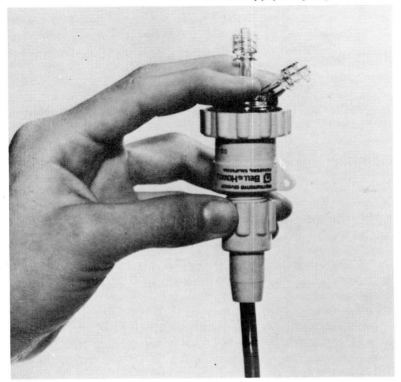

Figure 3.20. Blood pressure transducer fitted with a transparent
cuvette or 'dome'. (Courtesy of Bell & Howell Ltd)

volume chamber – the cuvette (also called a dome) – which is fitted
with two openings (*Figure 3.20*). These openings usually end in Luer–
Lok taper fittings to which can be connected three-way stopcocks. The
volume of the cuvette is designed to be as small as possible and the
shape is such as to facilitate flushing in order to remove any trapped
air bubbles. It is constructed from a transparent plastic so that the
presence of blood or bubbles in the cuvette can easily be observed.

There is an increasing tendency to provide the transducer with
disposable cuvettes in which the side making contact with the transducer's diaphragm is flexible. The packs of domes are pre-sterilized to
minimize the risks of infection and the plastic construction provides an
additional insulation between the metal diaphragm and the fluid
connecting with the patient. Fox *et al.* (1978) have confirmed that

both the type of dome and the method of its attachment to the transducer can affect the overall performance of the transducer. The opening facing the diaphragm is connected with the catheter or cannula leading to the patient. With the stopcock turned so that the connection with the transducer is occluded, the sidearm may be used to flush through the cannula or catheter with sterile heparinized saline to remove any bubbles or clots. It is important to shut off the connection with the transducer during this procedure as the use of small volume syringes may develop an over-pressure which could damage the transducer. The side connection of the cuvette is used for the application of atmospheric pressure for the setting of the baseline of the pressure recording and the application of known calibration pressures from a mercury sphygmomanometer. It can also be used for flushing the cuvette to remove bubbles, the sidearm of the other three-way stopcock then being open to the atmosphere. Before connection of the system to a patient, the dome—transducer assembly and the stopcocks should be checked for leaks at a pressure which is not less than the highest systolic pressure likely to be encountered. Leaks can allow the patient's blood to leak back into the cuvette which is undesirable from the viewpoint of sterility.

The presence of markedly compressible air bubbles will spoil the frequency response of the system. The best results are obtained with taps which are in good condition and of the screw fitting type and the cuvette and tubing filled with saline made with freshly boiled water.

When cleaning the transducer, the diaphragm should be gently swabbed with a cotton ball containing hydrogen peroxide or sterile water. Transducers should not be steam autoclaved but sterilized with a room temperature chemical solution such as Cidex or Zephiran or by a gas sterilization process. When ethylene oxide gas is used, the transducer should be completely dry both inside and out in order to inhibit the formation of toxic ethylene glycol. When a transducer is in clinical use, strict precautions must be observed at all times to prevent contamination of the taps and cuvette with an organism such as pseudomonas. The Millar catheter tip pressure transducer can also be sterilized with ethylene oxide gas or Cidex or Zephiran. It must be not autoclaved or exposed to gamma radiation or formaldehyde vapour solutions.

Calibration of pressure transducers

When the transducer is mounted external to the patient's body, calibration and checking of the baseline level is an easy matter. Calibration is normally performed by means of a sphygmomanometer bulb and a mercury or saline filled manometer depending on the pressure range to be covered. It may be necessary to calibrate both an associated panel meter and a chart recorder. Many transducer bridge amplifiers have a calibration control scaled in terms of 100 mmHg pressure. This functions by unbalancing the bridge circuit by a known amount. It is simple and convenient to operate, but it must never be allowed to replace a manometer since errors may creep in.

Conventionally, blood pressure is referred to atmospheric pressure at the level of the heart. A correction of -7.8 mmHg should be applied for each 100 mm the site of measurement is below the level of the heart. Transducer housings often carry a mark to indicate the position of the diaphragm so that this can be placed relative to the heart. The reference level may change if the patient's position alters and this becomes of importance when measuring low pressures such as the central venous pressure (Debrunner and Bühler, 1969).

Catheter tip transducers can only be calibrated outside the body with respect to a mercury sphygmomanometer by placing the transducer inside a plastic 'dome' fitted with a silicone rubber fluid seal and a female Luer fitting.

The performance of modern physiological pressure transducers

In order to provide quantitative data for a discussion on pressure transducers it is instructive to look at the stated performance specification for a modern device, such as the Type 746 pressure transducer by Siemens Ltd. This is a bonded semiconductor strain gauge transducer designed for the measurement of liquid pressures in the range -10 to $+300$ mmHg (-1.33 to $+40$ kPa) so that the possible applications include the measurement of intraventricular, intra-arterial and intra-venous blood pressures as well as intracranial, intra-abdominal and intra-uterine pressures. The pressure transducer's cuvette (*Figure 3.21*) is designed to have a conical shape to provide a strong swirling action during flushing to ensure the complete removal of any physiological fluids and air that may have remained in the cuvette.

The quoted sensitivity of the type 746 transducer is 50 μV per volt per cmHg and the volume displacement or compliance is 0.06 mm^3 per 100 mmHg. The non-linearity is ± 1 per cent of full scale and the temperature drift is 0.05 mmHg $^\circ$C^{-1} for the baseline and 0.04 per cent $^\circ$C^{-1} for the response to subsequent applied pressure. The maximum operating temperature is 55 $^\circ$C, the weight is 175 g and the insulation is tested to 10 000 V d.c.

The 746 transducer is fitted with a pre-sterilized disposable cuvette (dome). The materials used in the cuvette and its associated diaphragms can be autoclaved. Since pre-sterilized cuvettes are employed, the actual body of the transducer does not need cleaning or sterilizing, eliminating the possibility of damage to the transducer from mishandling. However, to maximize the safety factor of the device the transducer and part of

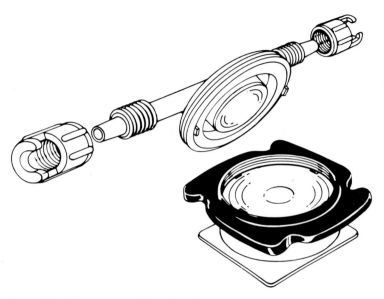

Figure 3.21. Siemens Type 746 physiological pressure transducer showing disposable cuvette. (Courtesy of Siemens Ltd)

the connecting cable can be submerged in a sterilizing solution. The inlet and outlet ports of the cuvette are fitted with Linden nuts and the Siemens stopcock set includes a number of adaptors having different connection fittings. The main elements of the 746 transducer are the receptor with pressure sensing diaphragm and locking ring, the disposable cuvette with its insulating diaphragm and the overlap-nuts (*Figure 3.21*).

The transducer assembly is easily mounted horizontally in the transducer holder, after which the sterilized stopcocks can be mounted and the liquid system can be filled. The rugged construction of the device is designed to effectively eliminate shift of the baseline arising from knocks or blows.

The rubber diaphragm of the cuvette isolates the fluid system from the transducer's pressure sensitive diaphragm both in regard to electrical and bacteriological safety. Additionally, the internal electrical components are completely insulated from the transducer's housing. The 746 will withstand the effects of d.c. defibrillation on the patient. It is claimed that there is no need to recalibrate when the transducer is changed for another of the same type.

The Siemens Pressure Amplifier Type 863 has been designed mainly for use with the Type 746 transducer, and has pressure ranges of 10, 20, 40, 100, 200 and 400 mmHg. The direct coupled d.c. amplifier has an input impedance of more than 10 megohms and a temperature drift in combination with the 746 of less than 0.2 mmHg $^{\circ}C^{-1}$. The excitation voltage for the transducer is 6 V d.c. adjustable by ±5%, and the frequency range is 0–1 kHz. The output signal level is 0–1.4 V, with an output impedence of less than 1 Ω. By depressing a push-button the electrical mean pressure can be obtained and low-pass filters are available for upper cut-off frequencies of 5, 10, 20 and 60 Hz (3 dB point) with slopes of −12 dB per octave. Auxillary units can be supplied to provide outputs corresponding with the systolic and diastolic pressures and dP/dt or $(dP/dt)/P$ for cardiac contractility measurements.

The Model 1280C physiological pressure transducer by Hewlett Packard is a differential transformer transducer covering the range −100 to +400 mmHg (−13 to +53 kPa), *Figure 3.22*. Typical

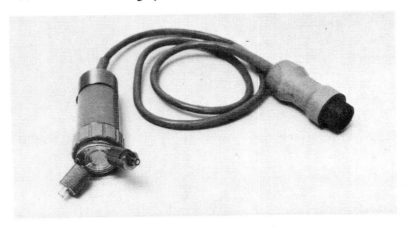

Figure 3.22. Hewlett Packard Type 1280C physiological pressure transducer. (Courtesy of Hewlett Packard Ltd)

applications include the measurement of blood pressure, intracranial pressures, intra-uterine pressures and internal gas pressures. The quoted thermal drift is 0.15 mmHg $°C^{-1}$, overload pressures +3000 mmHg and −100 mmHg (+400 kPa to −13.3 kPa), and the sensitivity is 40 μV V^{-1} mmHg^{-1} ± 1 per cent. The hysteresis is quoted as less than 0.1 per cent and the non-linearity is less than 1 per cent of full scale. The input impedance is typically 175 Ω and the output impedance 300 Ω. The operating temperature is 5–54.5 °C. The Model 1280C has an internal volume of 0.5 ml when used with a disposable dome and a volume displacement of 0.04 mm^3 per 100 mmHg. Its weight is approximately 320 g. The leakage current flowing from the transducer via the fluid-filled catheter to earth is quoted as less than 2.5 μA r.m.s. at 115 V 60 Hz. The materials used in the construction of the 1280C are not corroded by saline solution or by most chemical and gas sterilization procedures. Ringer's solution may be corrosive under some conditions. An adequate time must be allowed for ethylene oxide gas, if used for sterilization, to be released from the plastic materials.

Martin *et al.* (1973) give details of an automatic system for the calibration of blood pressure transducer amplifiers. The zero balance and gain are set in a single sequence and calibration is completed within a period of one minute.

Sandman and Hill (1974) and Francis (1974) describe analogue circuits for the separation of the systolic and diastolic pressures from the arterial pressure waveform produced by a blood pressure transducer.

Littler *et al.* (1972) developed a portable direct arterial pressure monitoring system based on a miniature tape recorder which can be worn by the patient for continuous monitoring. The performance of the arrangement has been assessed by Goldberg, Raftery and Green (1976) who found it to be satisfactory for the recording of pressure but not waveforms. Measurements were made in 104 studies on 100 patients with no major complications and a high degree of patient acceptability.

The use of pressure transducers with catheters

For the measurement of blood pressure at peripheral sites such as the radial artery, the pressure transducer is connected to the patient's artery via a short flexible plastic cannula and a three-way stopcock. For the measurement of pressures at more distant sites, such as in the chambers of the heart, two possibilities exist: the use of a conventional

pressure transducer external to the patient's body and in communication with the site of measurement via a fluid-filled catheter; or the use
of a miniature transducer mounted at the tip of a catheter (Millar and
Baker, 1972). The two situations are quite different in terms of
frequency response and calibration requirements.

In the case of the external transducer, a regular checking of the
baseline setting and of the calibration presents no problems since a
sphygmomanometer and atmospheric pressure can easily be applied to
the transducer. However, the frequency response of the transducer
alone is seriously degraded by the effects of the inertia and friction of
the fluid column filling the catheter. Geddes (1970) gives the following
formula for the undamped natural frequency response of the transducer—
catheter combination:

$$f_0 = 1.4 \times 10^3 \; d/(V_d L p)^{\frac{1}{2}}$$

where f_0 is in hertz, d is the catheter diameter in centimetres, L is the
catheter length in centimetres, V_d is the volume displacement of the
transducer alone in mm^3 per 100 mmHg and p is the density in $g \; cm^{-3}$
of the fluid filling the catheter. It is eveident that the highest natural
frequency is obtained by the use of the shortest possible catheter
having the largest possible internal diameter. In practice, anatomical
considerations will normally determine the choice of the catheter
dimensions. Since f_0 varies as $(V_d)^{-\frac{1}{2}}$, the use of a transducer with
a stiffer diaphragm and thus a smaller volume displacement will
produce a higher natural frequency at the expense of a less sensitive
transducer.

When a step increment of pressure is applied to the transducer—
catheter combination, the deflection of the associated pen recorder will
normally execute a damped oscillation about its final settling position
(*Figure 3.23*). The damping factor of the system is defined as the ratio
of successive pressure oscillations in the same direction when a pressure
step has been applied to the system. In order to obtain the optimum
frequency response for a given transducer and catheter, the damping
factor should be adjusted to a value of 0.7. It can be varied by placing
an adjustable restriction in the fluid-filled line (Ardill, Fentem and
Wellard, 1967).

When the catheter has a miniature pressure transducer mounted at
its tip, the frequency response is uninhibited by the presence of a fluid
filled catheter and extends out to approximately 1000 Hz making it

possible for the transducer to pick up heart sounds as well as the arterial pressure waveform.

The baseline for the recorder and the calibration of the catheter-tip pressure transducer are performed before the device is inserted into

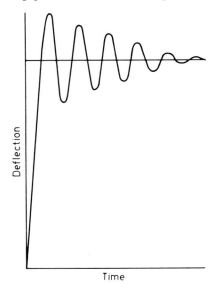

Time   Figure 3.23

the patient's cardiovascular system. When this has occurred, the transducer cannot be exposed to known pressures without removing it from the patient. Hence, the design of the transducer and the components used in its construction are most important in order that its calibration can be relied upon while in use.

Unusual pressure waveforms

Unusual or markedly distorted blood pressure waveforms may arise from a number of physiological conditions, but they may also prove to be artefacts. For example, a damped arterial pressure waveform may arise from the presence of thrombus in the catheter, air bubbles, a loose connection, kinking of the catheter, impinging of the catheter tip against the blood vessel or arteriospasm. Notches may appear on the waveform due to resonances arising from air bubbles close to the transducer or the use of long tubing which is too compliant. It is important to be alert for artefacts and to be able to distinguish them from true physiological conditions.

Indirect methods for the measurement of arterial blood pressure

An obvious need exists for techniques capable of measuring the systolic and diastolic pressures indirectly without recourse to an arterial puncture. The apparatus can be rapidly placed in position on a patient who suffers minimum inconvenience. The drawbacks are that the time interval required to establish successive readings may be too long to allow the following of rapid changes in blood pressure, and there may be a significant discrepancy between direct and indirect readings at systolic pressures of less than about 70 mmHg. This follows since the pressure which is measured will depend on variables such as the arterial wall compliance, the location and size of the cuff and the magnitude of the pulse pressure. These effects will be subject dependent (Van Bergen *et al.*, 1954).

Depending upon the technique adopted, a single or double cuff is placed around a limb and inflated to a pressure in excess of the subject's systolic pressure and gradually deflated, preferably linearly with time. The Riva–Rocci–Korotkoff technique is the oldest and relies on the fact that pulsations are detectable with the use of a stethoscope placed over an artery distal to the cuff when the intra-arterial pressure just exceeds the cuff pressure. The cuff pressure when these Korotkoff sounds are first evident corresponds to the systolic pressure. The detection of the diastolic point is not so clear-cut and relies on the disappearance or muffling of the sounds; this is the auscultatory method.

The inflation and deflation of the cuff can be automated using a timer and a reservoir of compressed air. The detection of the sounds can be accomplished by placing a microphone in a pocket of the cuff. Another approach relies on the use of beams of ultrasound to detect the pulsating motion of the artery walls when the systolic pressure exceeds the cuff pressure (Hochberg and Saltzman, 1971). Systems for the automated indirect measurement of blood pressure are available which give an light-emitting diode digital display of the systolic and diastolic pressures and the pulse rate. If an ectopic beat is detected an arrhythmia warning light is activated.

The oscillotonometer technique of Von Recklinghausen (1906) is widely used by anaesthetists for the indirect measurement of blood pressure. A double cuff arrangement is used to obtain a greater sensitivity. The basic principle is to sense the sudden increase in the volume oscillations of the cuff which occurs at the systolic pressure and the sudden decrease in their amplitude which happens at the diastolic point.

In practice two cuffs, an upper and a lower (*Figure 3.24*) are used with the oscillotonometer. The instrument's case contains two pressure sensitive capsules 1 and 2. The diaphragm of capsule 1 is relatively stiff and its interior is at atmospheric pressure. Capsule 2 is more sensitive than capsule 1 and so is compressed more readily for a given applied pressure. Each capsule is connected to one end of a pivoted bar which in turn actuates the pointer.

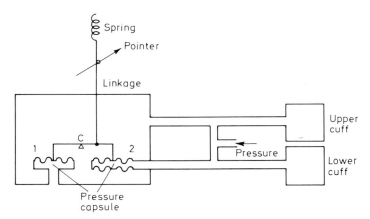

Figure 3.24

To determine the blood pressure, both the cuffs and the interior of the case are inflated to a pressure which is in excess of the patient's systolic pressure. The inflation pressure is shown on the pointer via capsule 1; capsule 2 is unaffected since the same pressure is applied to both its interior and exterior. The cuff pressure is then released in small steps and after each decrement a lever on the oscillotonometer is operated manually to detect the presence of the systolic point. Moving the control lever switches out the upper cuff as seen in *Figure 3.25,* while the case remains at the upper cuff pressure. Blood passing beneath the upper cuff produces pressure pulsations in the lower cuff which are transmitted via capsule 2 to the pointer. The systolic point is detected by the sudden increase evident in the pulsations.

When the systolic pressure has been noted, the control lever is moved back to its original position and the pressure of the upper cuff dropped to something in excess of the likely diastolic pressure. The diastolic point is taken as the pressure at which the pulsations suddenly decrease in amplitude.

In more modern forms of oscillotonometer, the pressure can be dropped continuously starting above the systolic presure and the oscillations can be observed without the need to change over the position of the control lever. In this version, the two cuffs are connected via a fine bore capillary tube which offers sufficient resistance to the pulsatile airflow but which allows the steady pressure to be changed slowly in both cuffs. As before, when the systolic and diastolic points have been detected, the lever is returned to its original position to cause the pressure to be read from the pointer.

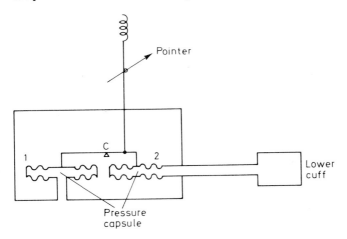

Figure 3.25

Geddes *et al.* (1977) have shown that the lowest cuff pressure which gives maximum amplitude of the oscillations correlates closely with the mean arterial pressure. Ramsey (1979) described an automatic system based on this principle for monitoring the mean arterial pressure in man. The instrument automatically inflates a standard blood pressure cuff and determines the mean arterial pressure by measuring the cuff pressure oscillations as the cuff pressure is reduced by discrete amounts. The discrete cuff deflation allows the oscillation data obtained at each cuff pressure to be tested for artefacts and averaged, thus greatly enhancing the rejection of artefacts. This arrangement was tested on the bicep and ankle in 28 studies involving 17 subjects having intra-arterial catheters in position. Averaging the mean errors from each of the 28 studies, there was an overall mean error of -0.28 mmHg with a standard deviation of 4.21 mmHg. The correlation coefficient was 0.98

and the instrument gave good results in a wide variety of clinical subjects and physiological states.

Meldrum (1978) has also reported on a commercial system based on a microprocessor for finding the mean arterial pressure in terms of the pressure at which the maximum amplitude of the pulsations occurs. He points out that an important factor to be borne in mind when considering the significance of this technique is that mean arterial pressure is found from the tracing obtained with an arterial pressure transducer by dividing the area under the pressure waveform by the baseline time over which the area was measured. The mean arterial pressure, however, is not the simple arithmetic average of the systolic and diastolic pressures. In practice, an approximation is often taken to be diastolic + 1/3 (systolic—diastolic). For a subject with a systolic pressure pulse of relatively short duration, the mean arterial pressure may lie quite close to the diastolic pressure. Meldrum found that in a comparison of the standard auscultatory method with the maximum oscillation method in a hypertensive and a hypotensive subject, the mean pressure was approximately one third of the pulse pressure above diastolic for the hypertensive but approximately half way between systolic and diastolic for the hypotensive. This result would be expected since a hypotensive individual is likely to have a less sharply peaked pressure waveform. The microprocessor determines the mean pressure for each beat and hence tends to overcome beat-to-beat variations.

Winn, Hildebrandt and Hildebrandt (1977) have described a semi-automatic blood pressure monitor utilizing an electronic sphygmo-manometer. The microphone is placed under an occluding arm cuff to detect the Korotkoff sounds and a pressure transducer measures the cuff pressure, which is reduced at a steady rate of 2—6 mmHg per heartbeat. A gate circuit is incorporated to reject spurious pulses.

Alexander, Cohen and Steinfeld (1977) have examined the criteria for the choice of an occluding cuff for the indirect measurement of blood pressure. They point out that to attain accuracy, the cuff must operate so that the intra-bladder pressure is always the same as the pressure applied by the tissues of the arm to the artery wall. The results of an analysis showed that the pressure applied to the artery wall is markedly influenced by longitudinal motion of the arm tissue which must be constrained in order for there to be accurate pressure trans-mission. A wide cuff effectively accomplishes this under its central region. Criteria were established for the design of occluding cuffs and versions for clinical use have been produced from a plastic film in a variety of lengths and widths.

Kassam, Johnston and Cobbold (1977) describe a fully automatic system for the control of the blood pressure cuff which incorporates a pneumatic control system, an integrated silicon pressure transducer and a digital read-out.

Work and power

Work is done when a force moves its point of application. Clearly work must be done in lifting a cylinder of gas from a rack to an anaesthetic machine against the force of gravity. The dimensions of work are those of force×distance, i.e. ML^2T^{-2}, in the SI system the metre-newton or joule. In the CGS system the unit of work is the erg=1 dyne-cm and 1 joule=10^7 ergs. The unit of work in the English system is the foot-pound (a force of one pound weight acting through a distance of one foot).

From the physiological aspect, an obvious application of mechanics occurs in the process of respiration. There is also a substantial interest in haemodynamics and the action of inotropics drugs upon the heart. With the advent of electromagnetic blood flowmeters and catheter-tip pressure transducers, anaesthetists are now often involved in quantitative studies of the effects of drugs upon the circulatory system.

Work cost of breathing

It is interesting to consider the work required to move a volume v of gas against a pressure p. For convenience, let the volume v be shaped as

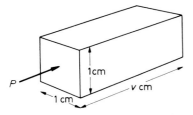

Figure 3.26

in *Figure 3.26*, i.e. having a unit cross-sectional area and a length v. The pressure p is applied to the unit area giving rise to a force P which acts through a distance v to move the gas, so that the work done is Pv. In the SI system the respiratory work can be expressed in joules.

Cooper (1961) found it convenient to use the cm-kilopond as the unit of respiratory work, since if a pressure of 1 cm of water is caused to move 1 litre of gas, the work done is 1 cm-kilopond. Others have taken the metre-kilopond as their unit of respiratory work. One metre-kilopond = 9.81 joules. Thus the work done in moving a tidal volume of 0.5 litres against a mean pressure of 10 cmH$_2$O is 0.05 metre-kilo-ponds = 0.49 joules. If the respiratory rate is 15 per minute, i.e. once every 4 seconds, the respiratory power is ¼ × 0.49 J = 0.125 watts. Similar considerations occur in the calculation of cardiac work.

Cardiac work

Consider the calculation of left ventricular work. The work done per minute is considered to be due to the mean aortic pressure acting over a distance equal to that which would contain the cardiac output in a volume having unit cross-sectional area. At present, in many papers, cardiac work is quoted in the units of gram-metres per minute. This results from expressing the mean blood pressure in grams weight per square centimetre and assuming that this acts over a distance in metres obtained by multiplying the cardiac output in litres per minute by 10 (litres/10=metres). Strictly speaking, the units of gram-metres per minute are those of cardiac power (power is defined as the rate of doing work) rather than cardiac work. The corresponding unit in the SI system is the watt. For a patient in shock with a mean arterial pressure of 50 mmHg and a cardiac output of 1.5 litres per minute, the cardiac work is 1.068 gram-metres per minute or 0.175 watts. For a mean arterial pressure of 85 mmHg and a cardiac output of 6.64 litres per minute, the cardiac work is 7.675 gram-metres per minute or 1.26 watts.

It is instructive to look at this last calculation in more detail. The mean arterial pressure is 85 mmHg = 8.5 cmHg. The force per square centimetre due to this pressure is given by

(mass of Hg in kg) × (acceleration due to gravity)

$$= \frac{8.5 \times 13.6}{1000} \times 9.81$$

$$= 1.134 \, N$$

The minute volume of 6.64 litres can be contained in a volume 1 cm^2 × 66.4 m long.

Work = force × distance

= 1.134 × 66.4 J

Power = work ÷ time

= 1.134 × 66.4/60

= 1.254 W

Thus the cardiac work in watts

$$= \frac{(\text{Mean arterial pressure in mmHg}) \times (\text{Cardiac output in l/min})}{449.7}$$

approximately (i.e. neglecting the filling pressure).

Respiratory resistance

The work cost of breathing is concerned with the effort required to ventilate the lungs. To do this, work must be done against three main forces. These are (a) the elastic resistance of the lungs, defined as the force tending to return the lungs to their original size after an inspiration; (b) the force required to move non-elastic tissues, i.e. the rib cage, diaphragm and contents of the abdomen; (c) the force required to overcome resistance to gas flow through the tracheobronchial tree, and through any external breathing apparatus.

The transpulmonary pressure is the pressure difference existing between the airway (mouth) and the pleural space. It is designated P_{tp}. If any external apparatus is present, there will exist across this an additional pressure drop P. Thus the total pressure difference required to overcome resistance is $P_T = P + P_{tp}$. For simplicity, the patient's respiratory system can be considered in terms of a frictional airway R_L in series with an elastic lung of compliance C_L. As an approximation, during inspiration $P_{tp} = V/C_L + R_L \dot{V}$ and $P = R\dot{V}$ where R is the external resistance and $\dot{V}$ is the volume flow rate at the time considered. If V is the volume of gas in the lungs above the functional residual capacity (the volume of the quiescent lungs when no pressure difference exists between the alevoli and the atmosphere) at that time, then the pressure in the lungs required to overcome the compliance is $P_c = V/C_L$. The total non-elastic pulmonary resistance R_L includes both the airway resistance and the resistance of non-elastic tissues. The resistance of the non-elastic tissues is usually fairly constant and changes in R_L usually arise from changes in the calibre of the airways. For spontaneous respiration it can be seen that $P_T=P+P_{tp}=R\dot{V}+V/C_L +R_L\dot{V}$. Thus the pressure required to inflate a lung to a given volume depends both on the elasticity of the lung and the rate of gas flow. At low respiratory frequencies, with a low average gas velocity, the pressure drop required to overcome resistance to gas flow is small and most of the pressure is available to inflate the lung. At the points of zero gas flow during the respiratory cycle the flow-resistive pressure drop becomes zero. Inertial components of the pressure drop are then negligible and P_{tp} is a function of lung compliance alone.

The frictional resistance to deformation of non-elastic lung tissues offers a resistance to gas flow of about 30–40 per cent of the total airway resistance (McIlroy *et al.*, 1955). The total airway resistance of about 1.6 $cmH_2O\ l^{-1}$ s in normal adults has about 50 per cent of its value contributed by the nasal passages, 20 per cent by the remaining upper airways and the balance from the low airways (bronchi and bronchioles). Hildebrandt and Young (1965) provide a concise account of the anatomy and physics of respiration. The time constant of a lung is given by the product $R_L C_L$ in seconds where the values apply to that lung. In cases of marked pathology of a lung the values need not be the same for each lung. The time constant is the time interval in which inflation would be complete if the initial flow rate remained constant. This definition is of interest when ventilation is performed by means of a constant-flow ventilator. With a constant-pressure ventilator and during spontaneous respiration, the rate of inflation decreases with a rise in alveolar pressure and inspiration will be 95 per cent complete at the end of three time constants. The presence of different time constants in different parts of the lungs gives rise to a maldistribution of the inspired gases.

The time constant approach lends itself to a simple estimation of R_L – the total non-elastic pulmonary resistance. The patient either expires into a conventional spirometer (Comroe, Nisell and Nims, 1954) or the lungs of the relaxed patient are inflated by means of a suitably weighted spirometer (Newman, Campbell and Dinnick, 1959; Bodman, 1963). In both cases the patient must have been given a muscle relaxant drug. For both techniques the curve of expired or inspired volume respectively against time approximates to a simple exponential curve. The static compliance is given by the ratio tidal volume/inflation pressure. When gas is forced out of the lungs the time constant   is equal to the time taken for 63 per cent to be discharged.

Similarly, when gas if forced in, the time constant equals the time required to introduce 63 per cent of the tidal volume. The resistance is given by time constant × inflation pressure/ tidal volume. If the time constant is measured in seconds, the tidal volume in litres and the inflation-pressure in centimetres of water, then the units of resistance are centimetres water per litre per second. Since 1 $cmH_2O = 98.1$ N m^{-2}, these values can easily be converted into units of newtons per square metre per litre per minute.

Bodman (1963) measured expiratory flow resistances in paralysed patients during urological surgery. In three patients less than 36 years of age he found normal values ($1.2-3.2$ cmH_2O 1^{-1} s). This contrasts with values as high as 16 cmH_2O 1^{-1} s found in older patients some of whom had an impaired respiratory function. The figures exclude the resistance of the endotracheal tube and connections ($4.8-9.2$ cmH_2O 1^{-1} s). In five patients Newman, Campbell and Dinnick (1959) found an expiratory resistance that was almost double the inspiratory resistance.

The pressure required to inflate a lung is given by $P_t = \dot{V}(R + R_L) = V/C_L$. As the lung is inflated and a plot made of volume against mouth pressure, the pressure will consist of two components; one part overcoming the compliance, the other overcoming the resistance to gas flow. Don and Robson (1965) made use of a constant-flow ventilator, so that here a plot of mouth pressure against time is equivalent to a plot of mouth pressure against inspired volume. After a definite time the flow is abruptly stopped (*Figure 3.27*). The mouth or tracheal

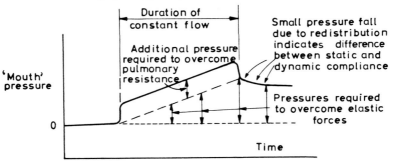

Figure 3.27 Plot of mouth pressure against time for a constant flow ventilator. (After Don and Robson, 1965)

pressure is continuously recorded. The static pressure obtaining when the flow ceases is the elastic pressure component for that tidal volume. This can be subtracted from the dynamic pressure recorded just prior to the cessation of flow to give the pressure drop used to overcome the flow resistance. From a knowledge of this pressure drop and the volume flow rate of the ventilator, the flow resistance can be deduced. The static compliance is found from the tidal volume and the static pressure when the flow is stopped. The methods so far described measure the total pulmonary resistance (airway plus pulmonary tissue resistance).

The measurement of airway resistance alone can be accomplished by means of a body plethysmograph (Dubois, Bothelo and Comroe, 1956). Basically, the patient is seated inside a sealed container and inhales from the external atmosphere via a pipe. Because of his airway resistance, the pressure of his alveolar gas falls below atmospheric, his thorax expands and causes a rise in the box pressure. Using a pneumo-tachograph and a pressure transducer, a plot of pressure gradient versus respiratory flow rate is produced on a cathode-ray tube screen and the airway resistance is deduced from the slope of the figure.

The additional resistance to breathing imposed upon a patient by external apparatus should be of particular concern to the anaesthetist. In general, it is desirable to make it as small as possible. The obvious points to look for are the choice of an adequate lumen endotracheal tube, the clenching of teeth on the tube or the obstruction of the tube by a foreign body, the absence of kinks in the tubing and the avoidance where possible of sharp bends. Hinforomi (1965) has measured the resistance to airflow of a number of anaesthetic equipment components, and Smith (1961b, c) discusses the effects of added resistance to respiration.

It should be recalled that care needs to be taken in the measurement of the resistance to gas flow of breathing apparatus, for example, it can happen that the resistance of a complete apparatus is less than the sum of the resistances of its individual components! A simple T-piece is often used to provide a pressure-tapping for a manometer. At the higher gas flow rates, a significant venturi effect may be produced, resulting in a reduction in the pressure recorded. Pressure tappings are better made by means of a series of small holes spaced around the circum-ference of the tube in question, the holes communicating to a small annular chamber which is connected to the manometer. Sharp bends or changes of bore arising when a complete apparatus is assembled may also give rise to a significant difference between the resistance of the complete apparatus and its separate parts. When measuring the resistance of a pipe or connector it is desirable that the emergent flow on leaving the object in question should not vent directly to atmos-phere (unless it will do so in use), but should continue through the distal pressure tapping via another length of pipe to atmosphere. This will eliminate possible effects due to sudden expansion of the gas on leaving the pressure tapping.

Consider the simple case of the work cost of moving a certain tidal volume against a fixed external resistance to breathing. By plotting the pressure at the mouth against the gas volume moved at that time over a complete respiratory cycle, a pressure–volume loop is obtained (*Figure 3.28*). The total work done per cycle is equal to the sum of the

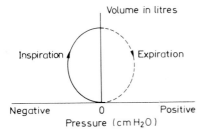

Figure 3.28. Pressure–volume loop for a respiratory cycle against an external frictional resistance

instantaneous products of pv, i.e. to the area contained within the loop. This can be calculated by dividing the area into strips of equal width dv and multiplying in each case by the appropriate value of the pressure p, and then adding up all the products of pdv. In terms of the calculus technique of integration discussed in the first chapter, it is now possible to write

$$\text{Work} = \int \left(p \; \frac{dv}{dt} \right) \; dt.$$

In the simplest case, the output voltage from the manometer of a pneumotachograph (proportional to the volume flow rate dv/dt) is integrated and displayed on the Y-axis of a long-persistence cathode-ray tube oscilloscope, and the output voltage from a pressure transducer connected to a mouthpiece is displayed simultaneously on the X-axis. The pressure transducer is connected across the external resistance and the area of the loop represents the work cost of moving gas against this resistance. If the work cost of breathing against the external airway resistance plus the anatomical airway resistance is to be measured, then the pressure transducer is connected between the distal end of the external resistance and an oesophageal balloon. The pressure in the oesophagus approximates to the intrapleural pressure (Mead *et al.*, 1955). The resulting $P–V$ loop on the oscilloscope screen is then photographed and its area measured with a planimeter (Lewis and Welch,

1965). A planimeter is a mechanical device consisting of two jointed arms. The end of one arm acts as a pivot and this arm also carries a wheel whose revolutions can be counted with a vernier dial. The free end of the second arm carries a point which is moved around the periphery of the loop causing the wheel on the other arm to rotate. The difference between the dial readings at the start and finish of the loop is proportional to the area of the loop. The planimeter dial can be calibrated by running the point round the perimeter of a known rectangular area.

A more elegant method is to multiply together automatically the instantaneous values of the pressure and volume flow rate, and then feed the voltage representing the product into an integrating circuit. The output of the integrator then indicates the work. A servo-multiplier

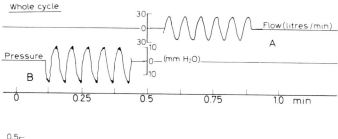

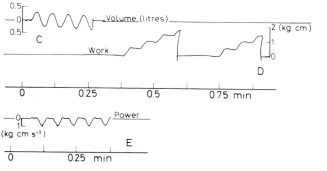

Figure 3.29

was used by Merrifield, Hill and Smith (1967) to compare the work cost of breathing through two types of emergency anaesthetic apparatus. The work required to perfuse a Gardner Universal vaporizer with the tidal volume from a sine-wave pump is shown in *Figure 3.29* taken from their paper. Engström and Norlander (1962, 1966) employed a Hall-effect multiplier in their studies on respiratory power and work. This type of investigation is conveniently performed with a small general-purpose analogue computer using a solid state multiplier. A good account of this technique is that of Fletcher and Belville (1966).

Cooper (1961) found that with a 20-litre minute volume, the total rate of frictional work performed by his subjects wearing a closed-circuit breathing apparatus was some 5 J per minute. In the case of the lungs, in addition to the frictional work which must be performed to move the respired gases, there is an expenditure of energy in doing work on non-elastic tissues. Cooper shows how to distinguish between the frictional and elastic components of work in the pressure-volume diagram of a respiratory cycle.

Power

Power is defined as the rate of doing work and has dimensions of $ML^2 T^{-3}$. An instantaneous value for the power being developed during respiration can be obtained by continuously multiplying together the appropriate values of volume flow rate and pressure. For spontaneous respiration, Engström and Norlander (1962) found a respiratory power requirement of approximately 0.2 watts. In electrical practice the unit of power is the watt (W) and this is the SI unit of power. One metre-kilopond per second equals 9.81 W. One horsepower equals 746 W or 550 foot-pounds per second. The work output of bicycle ergometers used in exercise tolerance studies is usually expressed in watts. Typically, two output ranges would be provided from the electrical generator which comprises the load against which the patient works — 0–200 and 0–400 watts. The output power of a surgical diathermy set is also quoted in terms of watts into a specified load impedance. Typical quoted powers lie in the range 200–500 W. The lowest tracing in *Figure 3.29* shows the power required to perfuse a Gardner Universal vaporizer with a tidal volume from a sine-wave pump.

Energy

Energy is defined as the capacity for doing work, and in effect it represents a certain amount of stored work, and its dimensions will be those of work (ML^2T^{-2}). All forms of energy are interchangeable. The

SI unit of energy is the joule (J). A small electric spark which could set off an explosion can be produced by only microjoules of energy, whereas the energy stored in the charged high-voltage capacitor of a d.c. defibrillator would be of the order of 100 joules (100 watt-seconds). Larger amounts of electrical power used to be expressed in terms of kilowatt-hours, since the product (watts $\times$ time) is a measure of the total amount of energy used. In the SI system the kilowatt-hour is now replaced by the megajoule (MJ) which equals 10^6 joules. The unit of heat energy was the calorie, but in the SI system this is now replaced by the joule where one calorie=4.186 joules. Nutritionists have also agreed to abandon the calorie.

A body may possess mechanical energy in two ways: (1) By virtue of its stored (stationary) energy with respect to other bodies in its vicinity (*potential energy*); or (2) As a result of its motion (*kinetic energy*). For example, an automatic ventilator can impart kinetic energy to the gas inflating the patient's lungs by virtue of the potential energy stored under pressure in the driving gas cylinder.

The electrical energy stored in a d.c. defibrillator is given by the equation E joules = $\frac{1}{2}CV^2$ where C is the capacity of the high voltage capacitor in farads and V is the d.c. voltage to which it has been charged. For an energy of 100 J, a 16 microfarad capacitor would have to be charged to 3536 volts and for 400 J a 16 microfarad capacitor would have to be charged to 7071 volts. In a practical d.c. defibrillator the values of the capacitance, resistance and inductance of the output circuit are chosen to provide what is hoped to be the most effective waveform. Losses in the circuit mean that the energy delivered to the patient is less than the energy stored in the capacitor. Flynn, Fox and Bourland (1972) found that an average of 60 per cent of the stored energy was delivered to the patient in 23 defibrillators. Patton and Pantridge (1979) found no evidence of a need for defibrillators for use with man having a stored energy of more than 400 J. Out of 24 patients resuscitated, the mean value of the peak current required for defibrillation was 0.35 ± 0.03 (SE) amperes per kilogram body weight. There was no apparent correlation between the current required and body weight.

Energy aspects of respiration

Respiration represents an example of a control system which operates in its normal mode to utilize a minimal amount of energy. Normal breathing can be regarded as a relaxation oscillation, the inspiratory

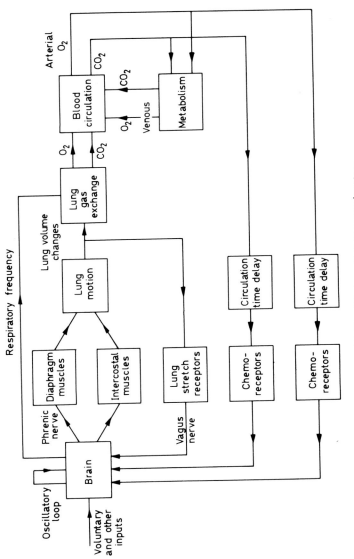

Figure 3.30. Simplified respiratory control system

muscles expanding the lungs and this expansion in turn giving rise to an increased inhibitory feedback from proprioceptors. A reciprocal inhibition within certain cell groups in the respiratory centre tends to maintain the motorneuronal discharge for a short period. After this period the discharge ceases, the muscles contact passively like a stretched spring, and the proprioceptive discharge decreases (Milsum, 1966). The respiratory cycle then recommences. This is obviously a simplified system, since expiration has been assumed to be passive. The inspiratory effort is largely produced by the combined action of the diaphragm innervated by the phrenic nerve and of the intercostal muscles innervated by the intercostal nerves (*Figure 3.30*). The main feedback pathway is believed to be from the stretch receptors of the lung tissue via the vagus nerve, the respiratory centre being largely in the medulla. The respiratory centre contains inspiratory and expiratory sets of motor neurones which reciprocally inhibit each other to produce a bistable control element. Hence, respiration will continue when the vagus is cut, although it is slower and deeper.

When the lungs expand as a result of muscular action, they store potential energy since the elastic tissues act in part as a spring. They

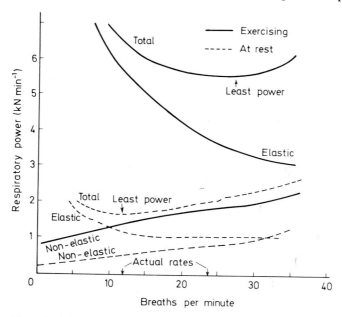

Figure 3.31. Work cost of breathing as a function of respiratory rate

also act as viscous-type energy dissipators since the movement of the lung tissues dissipates energy as does the flow of inspired gas. The total inspiratory work is the sum of these components. During passive expiration, the potential energy of the spring effect is returned and dissipated in the motion of the tissues and the motion of the expired air against the expiratory resistance. *Figure 3.31* taken from Christie (1953) shows the variation of both elastic and non-elastic work (represented as power) with respiratory frequency for a subject at rest and exercising. It can be seen that in each case, the subject adjusted his breathing rate so that his power consumption was minimal. The alveolar ventilation was 4 litres per minute at rest and 12 litres per minute while exercising.

Myocardial contractility

For a given cardiac output and heart rate, the pumping action of the heart expels a mass of blood with each stroke into the pulmonary circulation and the aorta. By Newton's second law of motion, the acceleration of the blood is proportional to the cardiac force acting. The acceleration of the blood leaving the left ventricle can be measured directly by means of a cuffed electromagnetic flow probe placed around the root of the ascending aorta. The frequency response of the flowmeter should preferably extend out to 100 Hz. The output signal from the flowmeter is proportional to the instantaneous blood velocity. This signal is fed into an electronic differentiating circuit to produce an output signal which is proportional to the acceleration of the blood. Assuming that the hydraulic resistance of the ascending aorta is reasonably constant throughout systole, then the pressure in the left ventricle should be proportional to the blood velocity, and the differential of the presure (dp/dt) is related to the myocardial contractility. Schaper, Lewi and Jageneau (1965) found that dp/dt as measured with a catheter-tip pressure gauge placed in the left ventricle shows a positive maximum during the isovolumetric contraction phase prior to the onset of flow (*Figure 3.32*). During the ejection of the stroke volume, the left ventricular pressure does not change markedly, so that dp/dt falls almost to zero. Owing to the fall in the left ventricular pressure occurring during the isovolumetric relaxation phase, dp/dt exhibits a negative maximum at this time. Schaper and colleagues showed that during contraction, dp/dt is not determined by the magnitude of the aortic blood pressure, and that during relaxation dp/dt depends upon the strength of the preceding contraction, the end-diastolic dimensions of the heart and the origin of the depolarizing potential. Mason (1969) discusses the usefulness and limitations of the rate of rise of instantaneous pressure (dp/dt) in the left ventricle in the evaluation of myocardial contractility in man, while Gersh *et al.* (1970) attempted to

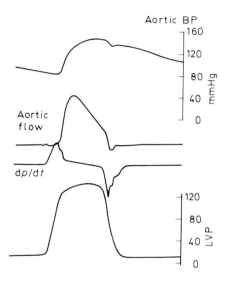

Figure 3.32. Variation over a single heart beat of the aortic pressure, aortic flow, rate of change of left ventricular pressure and left ventricular pressure. (After Schaper *et al.*, 1965)

correct for pre-load and after-load by using (dP/dt)/P where P is the instantaneous value of the left ventricular pressure. Noble (1966) showed that the maximum acceleration of blood from the left ventricle is a contractility index which reflects the pump function of the heart. In dogs, Welham *et al.* (1978) found good correlations between the maximum rate of change of the thoracic electrical impedance, the peak aortic velocity, the peak aortic acceleration and the peak rate of change of aortic pressure (dp/dt) of 0.954, 0.950 and 0.937 respectively as the combined correlation coefficients obtained from five dogs.

Van der Bos *et al.* (1973) discuss problems with the use of indices of myocardial contractility, while a good account of the myocardial contractile state and its role in the response to anaesthesia and surgery is that of Siegal (1969). Siegal makes the point that alteration in the velocity-dependent aspects of the force—velocity relationship and in the duration of the active state are the fundamental differences between the inotropic mechanism involving a true change in myo-cardial contractility, and the Frank–Starling mechanism which does not involve a change in contractility.

Changes of an inotropic nature result in an alteration of the acceleration of the isometric myocardial force as given by the magnitude of the *isometric time tension index* (ITT). ITT=$(dp/dt)_{max}/$IIT where $(dp/dt)_{max}$ is the maximum rate of change of increasing left ventricular pressure and IIT is the *integrated systolic isometric tension*. In *Figure 3.33*, IIT is the shaded area under the left ventricular pressure

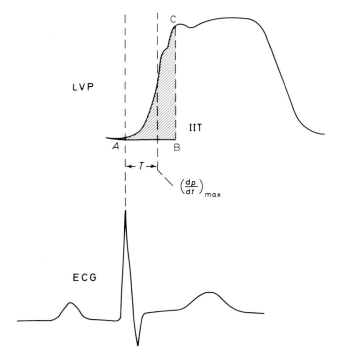

Figure 3.33. Calculation of the isometric time tension index

curve defined as follows: if T is the time in seconds from the peak of the preceding R-wave to the time corresponding to the maximum slope of the increasing left ventricular pressure waveform, 50 per cent is added to the value of T to give the interval AB, and the area is calculated lying under the pressure curve from the start of its upslope to point B. This area in (mmHg×seconds)=IIT. Since the dimensions of $(dp/dt)_{max}$

are mmHg s^{-1} the dimensions of ITT are s^{-2}. Typically, if $(dp/dt)_{max}$ =2000 mmHg s^{-1} and AB=50 ms, and the ordinate BC=75 mmHg, then ITT=2000/[½×(50/1000)×75]=1067. Increases in myocardial length due to the Frank–Starling mechanism do not alter the value of the ITT. The effect in the dog of a linearly increasing blood arterial halothane concentration on the heart rate, stroke volume, cardiac output, left ventricular work, aortic and systemic arterial pressure, total systemic resistance and isometric time tension index is described by Gil-Rodriguez, Hill and Lundberg (1971). The only variable in which a statistically significant change was not obtained was the total systemic resistance.

References

ABBOTT, P. (1971). *Teach Yourself Mechanics*, p. 13. London; English Universities Press

ADLER, L. and BURN, N. (1967). A warning device for failure of the oxygen supply. *Anaesthesia* 22, 156

ALEXANDER, H., COHEN, M.I. and STEINFELD, L. (1977). Criteria in the choice of an occluding cuff for the indirect measurement of blood pressure. *Med. Biol. Engng & Comput.* 15, 2–10

ARDILL, B.L., FENTEM, P.H. and WELLARD, M.J. (1967). An electromagnetic pressure generator for testing the frequency response of transducers and catheter systems. *J. Physiol. Lond.* 192, 19P

BAKER, W.W. (1965). Hyperbaric operating theatre. *Wld med. Electron. Intrum. Lond.* 3, 81

BARON, D.N. (1974). SI units in pathology: the next stage. *Med. Lab. Technol.* 31, 1

BASKETT, P.J.F., HYLAND, J., DEAVE, M. and WRAY, G. (1969). Analgesia for burns dressing in children. *Br. J. Anaesth.* 41, 684

BODMAN, R.I.(1963). Clinical applications of pulmonary function tests. *Anaesthesia* 18, 355

CHRISTIE, R.V. (1953). Dyspnoea in relation to the visco-elastic properties of the lung. *Proc. R. Soc. Med.* 46, 381

COBBOLD, R.S.C.(1974). *Transducers for Biomedical Measurements: Principles and Applications.* New York; Wiley

COMROE, J.H., NISELL, O.I. and NIMS, R.G. (1954). A simple method of concurrent measurement of compliance and resistance to breathing in anaesthetized animals and man. *J. appl. Physiol.* 7, 225

COOPER, E.A. (1961). Behaviour of respiratory apparatus. *Med. Res. Memo. natn. Coal Bd med. Serv.* 2, 11

DAVIES, J.M., HOGG, M.I.J. and ROSEN, M. (1974a). Upper limit of resistance of apparatus for inhalation anaesthesia during labour. *Br. J. Anaesth.* **46**, 136

DAVIES, J.M., HOGG, M.I.J. and ROSEN, M. (1974b). Resistance of Entonox valves. *Br. J. Anaesth.* **46**, 145

DEAL, C., OSBORN, J.J., ELLIS, E. and GERBODE, F.(1968). Chest wall compliance. *Ann. Surg.* **167**, 73

DEBRUNNER, F. and BÜHLER, F. (1969). Normal central venous pressure—significance of reference point and normal range. *Br. med. J.* **3**, 148–150

DON, H.F. and ROBSON, J.G. (1965). The mechanics of the respiratory system during anaesthesia. *Anaesthesiology* **24**, 168

DUBOIS, A.B., BOTHELO, S.Y. and COMROE, J.H.(1956). A new method of measuring airway resistance in man using a body plethysmograph. *J. clin. Invest.* **35**, 327

ENGSTROM, C.G. and NORLANDER, O.P.(1962). A new method for analysis of respiratory work by measurement of the actual power as a function of gas flow, pressure and time. *Acta anaesth. scand.* **6**, 49

ENGSTROM, C.G. and NORLANDER, O.P. (1966). Respiration analyser for assessment of respiratory power and work. *Proc. 2nd European Congress of Anaesthesiology, Copenhagen*, **1**, 175

FLETCHER, G. and BELVILLE, J.W. (1966). On-line computation of pulmonary compliance and work of breathing. *J. appl. Physiol.* **21**, 1321

FLYNN, C.J., FOX, F.W. and BOURLAND, J.D. (1972). Indicated and delivered energy by d.c. defibrillators *J. Assoc. Advancement Med. Instrum.* **6**, 323–324

FOX, F., MORROW, D.H., KACKER, E.J. and GILLIELAND, T.H. (1978). Laboratory evaluation of pressure domes containing a diaphragm *Anesth. Analg.* **57**, 67–76

FRANCIS, G.R. (1974). An improved systolic—diastolic pulse separator. *Med. Biol. Engng* **12**, 105–108

GEDDES, L.A. (1970). *The direct and indirect measurement of blood pressure.* Year Book Publishers, Chicago

GEDDES, L.A., CHAFFEE, V., WHISTLER, S.J., BOURLAND, J.D. and TACKER, W.A. (1977). Indirect mean blood pressure on the anesthetised pony. *Am. J. Vet. Res.* **38**, 2055–2057

GERSH, B.J., PRYS-ROBERTS, C., REUBEN, S.R. and BAKER, A.B. (1970). The relationship between depressed myocardial contractility and the stroke output of the canine heart during halothane anaesthesia. *Br. J. Anaesth.* **42**, 566

GIL-RODRIGUEZ, J.A., HILL, D.W. and LUNDBERG, S. (1971). The correlation between haemodynamic changes and arterial blood halothane concentrations during halothane-nitrous oxide anaesthesia in the dog. *Br. J. Anaesth.* **43**, 1043

GOLDBERG, A.D., RAFTERY, E.B. and GREEN, H.L. (1976). The Oxford continuous blood pressure recorder: technical and clinical evaluation. *Postgrad. Med. J.* **52**, Suppl. 7, 104–109

HARTLEY, C.J. and COLE, J.S. (1974). A single-crystal ultrasonic catheter-tip velocity probe. *Med. Instrum.* **8**, 241

HILDEBRANDT, J. and YOUNG, A.C. (1965). Anatomy of physics of respiration. In *Physiology and Biophysics.* Ed. by T.C. Ruch and H.D. Patton. Philadelphia; Saunders

HINFOROMI, B.K. (1965). The resistance to airflow of tracheostomy tubes, connections and heat and moisture exchangers. *Br. J. Anaesth.* **37**, 454

HOCHBERG, H.M. and SALTZMAN, M.B. (1971). Accuracy of an ultrasound blood pressure instrument in neonates, infants and children. *Curr. Ther. Res.* **13**, 482–488

HOGG, M.I.J., DAVIES, J.M., MAPLESON, W.W. and ROSEN, M. (1974). Proposed upper limit of respiratory resistance for inhalational apparatus used in labour. *Br. J. Anaesth.* **46**, 149

KASSAM, M., JOHNSTON, K.W. and COBBOLD, R.S.C. (1977). An automatic multi-function pressure cuff control. *Can-Med Prog. Technol.* **5**, 157–160

LEWIS, F.J. and WELCH, J.A. (1965). Respiratory mechanics in postoperative patients. *Surg. Gynec. Obstet.* **120**, 305

LITTLER, W.A., HONOUR, A.J., SLEIGHT, P. and SCOTT, F.D. (1972). Continuous recording of direct arterial pressure and electrocardiogram in unrestricted man. *Br. med. J.* **iii**, 76–78

MARTIN, R.W., WEIL, M.H., SHUBIN, H., PALLEY, N., CARRINGTON, J.H., BISERA, J. and BOYCKS, E.C. (1973). Automated calibration of blood pressure signal conditioners. *I.E.E.E. Trans. Biomed. Engng* **BME-20**, 60–62

MASON, D.T. (1969). Usefulness and limitations of the rate of rise of instantaneous pressure (dP/dt) in the evaluation of myocardial contractility in man. *Am. J. Cardiol.* **23**, 516–527

MEAD, J., McILROY, M.B., SELVERSTONE, N.J. and KRIETE, B.C. (1955). Measurement of intra-oesophageal pressure. *J. appl. Physiol.* **7**, 491

MELDRUM, S.J.(1978). A new instrument for the automatic determination of mean arterial blood pressure. *J. Med. Engng & Technology* **2**, 243–244

MERRIFIELD, A.J., HILL, D.W. and SMITH, K. (1967). Performance of the Portablease and the Fluoxair portable anaesthetic equipment: with reference to use under adverse conditions. *Br. J. Anaesth.* **39**, 50

MILLAR, H.D. and BAKER, L.E. (1972). A stable ultra-miniature catheter-tip pressure transducer. *Med. Biol. Engng* **11**, 86

MILLS, C.J. (1963). An intraluminal electromagnetic flowmeter. *J. Physiol. Lond.* **167**, 2

MILSUM, J.M. (1966). *Biological Control Systems Analysis,* p. 409. New York; McGraw-Hill

NEWMAN, H.C., CAMPBELL, E.J.M. and DINNICK, O.P. (1959). A simple method of measuring the compliance and the non-elastic resistance of the chest during anaesthesia. *Br. J. Anaesth.* **31**, 282

NOBLE, M.I.M., TRENCHARD, D. and GUZ, A. (1966). Measurement of the significance of the maximum acceleration of blood from the left ventricle. *Circ. Res.* **19**, 139–147

OSBORN, J.J., BEAUMONT, J.O., RAISON, J.C.A. and ABBOTT, R.P. (1966). Computation for quantitative on-line measurements in an intensive care ward. In *Computers in Biomedical Research* 3, 207. (Ed. by R.W. Stacy and B.D. Waxman). New York; Academic Press

PADMORE, G.R.A. and NUNN, J.F. (1974). SI units in relation to anaesthesia. *Br. J. Anaesth.* **46**, 236

PARKHURST, R.C. (1964). *Dimensional Analysis and Scale Factors.* London; Chapman and Hall

PATTON, J.N. and PANTRIDGE, J.F. (1979). Current required for ventricular fibrillation. *Br. med. J.* **1**, 513–514

PORTER, A.W. (1958). *The Method of Dimensions.* London; Methuen

RAMSEY III, M. (1979). Noninvasive automatic determination of mean arterial pressure. *Med. Biol. Engng & Comput.* **17**

SANDMAN, A.M., and HILL, D.W. (1974). An analogue pre-processor for the analysis of arterial blood pressure waveforms. *Med. Biol. Engng* **12**, 360–363

SCHAPER, W.K.A., LEWI, P. and JAGENEAU, A.H.M. (1965). The determinants of the rate of change of the left ventricular pressure (d*p*/d*t*). *Arch. Kreislaufforsch.* **46**, 27

SIEGAL, J.H. (1969). The myocardial contractile state and its role in the response to anaesthesia and surgery. *Anaesthesiology* **30**, 519

SMITH, W.D.A. (1961a). The performance of a Walton 5 anaesthetic machine. *Br. J. Anaesth.* **33**, 440

SMITH, W.D.A. (1961b). The effects of external resistance to respiration. Part 1. General Review. *Br. J. Anaesth.* **33**, 549

SMITH, W.D.A. (1961c). The effects of external resistance to respiration. Part II. Resistance to respiration due to anaesthetic apparatus. *Br. J. Anaesth.* **33**, 610

SNOOK, R. (1969). Resuscitation at road accidents. *Br. med. J.* **4**, 348

TIMS, A.C., DAVIDSON, R.I. and TIMME, R.W. (1975). High sensitivity piezoelectric accelerometer. *Rev. Sci. Instrum.* **46**, 554–558

VAN BERGEN, F.H., WEATHERHEAD, D.S., TRELVAR, A.E., DOBKIN, A.B. and BUCKLEY, J.J. (1954). Comparison of indirect and direct methods of measuring arterial blood pressure. *Circulation* **10**, 481–490

VAN der BOS, G.C., ELZINGA, G., WESTERHOF, N. and NOBLE, M.I.M. (1973). Problems in the use of indices of contractility. *Cardiovasc. Res.* **7**, 834–848

VON RECKLINGHAUSEN, H. (1906). Unblutige Blutdruchmessung. *Arch. Exper. Path. and Pharmakol.* **5**, 325–504

WELHAM, K.C., MOHAPATRA, S.N., HILL, D.W. and STEVENSON, L. (1978). The first derivative of the transthoracic electrical impedance as an index of changes in myocardial contractility in the intact anaesthetised dog. *Intensive Care Med.* **4**, 43–50

WINN, R., HILDEBRANDT, J.R. and HILDEBRANDT, J. (1977). Semi-automatic blood pressure monitor utilizing an electronic sphygmomanometer. *J. Appl. Physiol. Respir. Environ. Exercise Physiol.* **43**, 379–381

4 Automatic lung ventilators and respirators

The need to supply the ventilatory requirements of patients suffering from respiratory insufficiency is widespread, and has resulted in a profusion of mechanical devices designed to produce or supplement ventilation. Because the inspiratory phase of respiration can be induced either by the application of a positive pressure to the lungs, or by the application of a negative pressure to the outside of the thorax, it is possible to divide the machines into two main categories. The negative pressure system has been commonly employed with patients suffering from a chronic respiratory insufficiency such as may arise from poliomyelitis or as a result of a chest injury and the apparatus used is known as a body respirator. On the other hand, acute cases of respiratory insufficiency, such as may occur during surgery or with patients in a coma, are treated with automatic lung ventilators which apply a positive pressure rhythmically to the lungs through a face-mask, endotracheal tube or tracheostomy. It is with the positive pressure machines that anaesthetists are more likely to be concerned, but anaesthetists in specialist units are managing patients with a long-term respiratory insufficiency by means of a body respirator. However, anaesthetists will be much more concerned with the routine use of positive pressure machines in conjunction with muscle relaxants. Positive pressure ventilators are also used in intensive care units over extended periods.

Body respirators

There are three main types of body respirator. With the cabinet or tank respirator (Drinker and McKhann, 1929) the patient is enclosed in a

121

rigid airtight box up to his neck. The rhythmic production of a negative pressure in the box at the desired respiratory frequency will suck air into the lungs. *Figure 4.1* shows a modified cabinet respirator (Kelleher, 1961) which has provision for rotating the patient from the supine to the prone position and producing a 15-degree head-down tilt which permits efficient physiotherapy and drainage of secretions. Bower *et al.* (1950) advocate the combination of a cabinet respirator and a positive pressure lung ventilator.

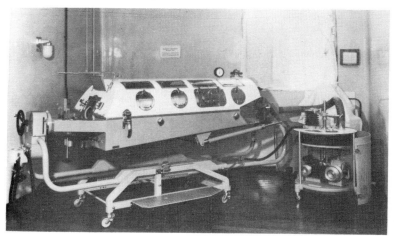

Figure 4.1. Cabinet respirator having provision for rotating the patient from the supine to the prone position and providing a 15 degree head-down tilt. (By courtesy of Cape Engineering Company)

For patients who are not so severely paralysed, a cuirass ventilator may be used to assist respiration, perhaps only at night. A rigid shell or cuirass is placed around the front of the patient's chest, and a rhythmic negative pressure applied to its interior. Provision may also be made, by means of an inflatable waistcoat, to provide positive pressure to the patient's back in order to assist expiration. The ventilatory efficiency of the cuirass ventilator in the case of totally paralysed chronic poliomyelitis patients has been discussed by Collier and Affeldt (1954).

Patients whose respiratory requirements are less stringent can obtain a greater degree of freedom of movement than is possible in a cuirass by means of an intermittent positive pressure abdominal respirator or belt. One form of this, described by Adamson *et al.* (1959), consists of an elastic inflatable flat bladder built into an abdominal corset. As the bladder is inflated, the abdominal wall is compressed and the diaphragm rises causing expiration. When the bladder deflates the abdominal contents and diaphragm fall as a result of gravitational pull and inspiration occurs passively. As a patient's respiratory efficiency increases, he might progress from a cabinet respirator to a cuirass and then to a belt.

Automatic lung ventilators

Although there are many makes of positive-pressure automatic lung ventilators available, it is possible to classify the majority of them into one or other of two main classes: *constant flow* or *constant pressure generators*. In the simpler models of ventilator, the changeover from the inspiratory to the expiratory phase will be initiated either when the ventilator has delivered a pre-set volume of gas, or when the inflation pressure has risen to a pre-set value. Once the flow pattern of gas into the lungs has been established it will take place under the influence of a pressure differential. This differential, depending upon the type of machine and its settings, can occur between a positive pressure and atmospheric pressure, a positive pressure and a negative pressure (negative phase) or between a positive pressure and a lower positive pressure. In the more complicated ventilators, the cycling of the ventilator may be controlled by an electronic or electromechanical timing unit — a pre-set volume being delivered subject to a pre-set maximum inflation pressure or by a combination of pressure and time cycling. Broadly speaking, two forms of construction exist. Small size ventilators, often gas powered, are intended for use in the recovery room or intensive care unit, or during surgery in conjunction with a separate anaesthetic machine. Larger size, electrically powered ventilators often include an anaesthetic machine and humidifier, and are designed to operate for long periods with the minimum of attention. They are intended for use with patients suffering from chronic respiratory insufficiency in major surgery. Alarm signals may be incorporated to indicate the advent of a mains power supply failure, the disconnection of a breathing tube or the onset of respiratory obstruction (Lamont and Fairley, 1965).

Compliance

The expansion of the lungs under the influence of the positive pressure applied by the ventilator can be expressed in terms of the patient's respiratory compliance. For a patient having an intact chest, the total value of the compliance is determined by the elastic properties of the lungs and of the chest wall. The slope of the line which results from plotting the external force (pressure) against the resulting increase in volume gives a measure of the stiffness or distensibility of the lungs and thorax (Comroe *et al.*, 1962). This is the 'static' compliance measured when the transpulmonary pressure is constant. A 'dynamic' compliance is obtained when the subject is breathing. Compliance is defined as 'the volume increase produced by each unit pressure increase in the alveoli' (Mushin *et al.*, 1969). It is normally expressed in terms of litres per centimetre of water pressure (litre/cmH$_2$O). Mushin *et al.* take a typical value for the total compliance of chest wall plus lungs to be 0.05 litre/cmH$_2$O (the compliance of the chest wall, and of the lungs each

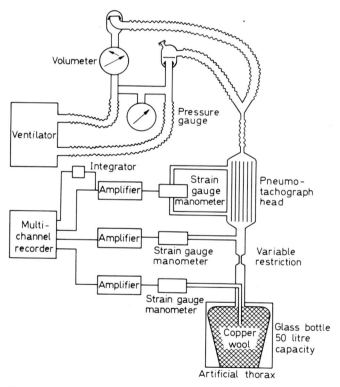

Figure 4.2. Schematic diagram of the apparatus used for evaluating the performance of an automatic ventilator in the laboratory. (Reproduced from Hill (1966) by courtesy of Springer-Verlag, Berlin-Heidelberg-New York)

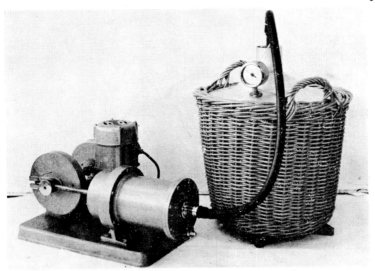

Figure 4.3. Artificial thorax suitable for simulating the compliance of an adult patient, connected to a sine-wave respiration pump

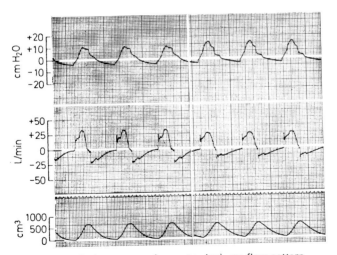

Figure 4.4. Inflation pressure (upper tracing), gas flow pattern (middle tracing) and tidal volume (lower tracing) waveforms obtained from a Dräger Spiromat 66 ventilator. On the left are the patterns before an increase is made in the airway resistance. Originally, at a flow of 25 litres per minute, the pressure drop across the orifice was 10 cmH$_2$O, and then it was increased to 14 cmH$_2$O. (Reproduced from Hill (1966) by courtesy of Springer-Verlag, Berlin-Heidelberg-New York)

approximate 0.1 litre/cmH$_2$O). The value of the total compliance is used in calculations associated with intermittent positive pressure respiration. With this value of total compliance, an increase in alveolar pressure of 10 cmH$_2$O will produce a volume increase within the alveoli of 500 ml. It is important to notice that for a given value of compliance, once the inflation pressure is fixed, then the tidal volume is determined also. A test object of known compliance is needed for the experimental investigation of the performance of ventilators. A suitable device, a glass carboy filled with copper wool, is described by Hill and Moore (1965). The volume of the carboy is 51.7 litres, and assuming a barometric pressure of 760 mmHg, its compliance is 0.05 litre cmH$_2$O^{-1}. As will be mentioned later, the carboy is filled with copper wool in order to eliminate any adiabatic effects. The experimental arrangement of such an artificial thorax to test a ventilator is illustrated in *Figure 4.2* and the artificial thorax connected to a sine-wave pump is shown in *Figure 4.3*. The waveforms obtained from a Dräger Spiromat 66 ventilator are given in *Figure 4.4* (Hill, 1966).

Pressure and flow generators

Positive pressure generated by the ventilator during the inflationary phase is applied to the lungs via the patient's upper airway and tracheobronchial tree. A resistance to gas flow results, and until equilibrium is attained, the pressure in the lungs will be lower than the inflationary pressure applied to the airway by the ventilator. Peslin (1969) discusses the physical properties of ventilators during the inspiratory phase.

By making the assumption that the airway resistance and compliance are constant, it is then possible to think in terms of a simple electrical analogy for the process of ventilation. The lungs can be regarded as a capacitor connected to a generator via a resistor. In pneumatic terms this is equivalent to a compliance in series with an airway resistance. Mushin *et al.* (1969) assume standard conditions of a compliance of 0.05 litres per cmH$_2$O in series with an airway resistance of 6 cmH$_2$O per litre per second. In the case of a ventilator which is a flow generator, the electrical generator should be a constant current generator. Here, changes of external circuit resistance will not appreciably alter the circuit current which is determined by the characteristics of the generator. A ventilator of the constant flow type will give rise to a gas flow pattern which is relatively independent of changes occurring in the resistance to flow. The pressure available at the outlet of the ventilator is arranged to be substantially above the backpressure built up in the lungs, perhaps 300 cmH$_2$O or more. A built-in resistance to flow may be needed to limit the maximum flow rate to a safe value. The value of the resistance encountered will determine the rate of rise of pressure at the airway and lungs. Provided that a pre-determined inflation pressure is not exceeded, such a ventilator will deliver a set

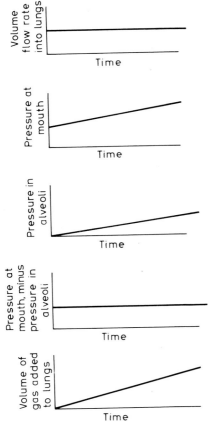

Figure 4.5. Ideal pressure, volume and flow relationships for a constant-flow type of ventilator

tidal volume in spite of changes in compliance and resistance. It is said to be 'compliance compensated'. It cannot, however, compensate for the action of any leaks which may be present in the breathing circuit. Howells (1963) points out that in more than 1000 cases he never encountered an established leak. However, changes in compliance are

common, as for example when the surgeon leans on the chest and
because of this the compensating action of a flow generator is a
desirable property. Assuming a constant compliance, the pressure in the
lungs will rise linearly with the constant increase in lung volume
produced by a constant flow generator. For a constant airway
resistance and a constant flow rate, there will exist a constant
difference between the pressure at the mouth and in the lungs. These
facts are illustrated in *Figure 4.5*.

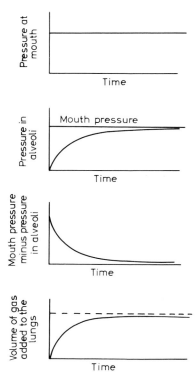

Figure 4.6. Pressure, volume and flow
relationships for a constant-pressure
type of ventilator

When a pressure generator type of ventilator is employed, the
pressure and volume in the lungs rise exponentially to limiting values as
shown in *Figure 4.6*. It is assumed that the output pressure of such a
ventilator is not substantially above the pressure required to inflate the
lungs. A possible value might be 35 cmH$_2$O. The difference in pressure
between the mouth and the lungs falls to zero exponentially, since if
sufficient time is allowed the pressure in the lungs will become equal

to that developed by the ventilator. If a leak develops around the endotracheal tube, a constant pressure type of generator which is pressure cycled will go on supplying gas until the pre-set pressure level is reached or until it is not able to supply any more gas. An increase in compliance will reduce the tidal volume which has to be delivered in order to reach the pre-set pressure.

The actions of pressure and flow generation can be distinguished by considering the effects on the action of the ventilator of a severe obstruction to the gas flow, perhaps the kinking of a tube. In a pressure generator, the pressure will continue to follow the pre-set pattern of the machine, the volume delivered now being greatly diminished. In a flow generator, the pressure will rise to a high value, the maximum of which the machine is capable, in order to try to maintain the flow as nearly as possible at the original value.

The use of an inspiratory pause

An inspiratory pause can be produced by arranging that the required tidal volume is delivered in a time appreciably shorter than the pre-set period of inspiration. A wait occurs with the patient's lungs inflated before the ventilator commences its expiratory phase. Referring to *Figure 4.7*, the tidal volume is delivered over the time interval OA.

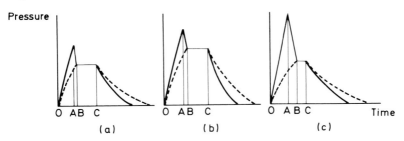

Figure 4.7. The variation with time throughout a ventilatory cycle of the upper airway pressure and alveolar pressure during intermittent positive pressure ventilation of a patient with (a) a normal airway resistance and compliance; (b) a normal airway resistance and a low compliance; (c) an increased airway resistance and a normal compliance (solid line, upper airway pressure; dashed line, alveolar pressure)

During the next period AB, the pressure in the airway and the alveolar pressure come into equilibrium. The period BC when the pressures are equal is the inspiratory pause time. At point C, expiration occurs. The provision of an inspiratory pause is a useful feature as it allows an estimate to be made of the alveolar pressure. In the IMV Pneumotron ventilator, the inspiratory pause can be adjusted from 0 to 3 seconds.

For a given tidal volume, the equilibrium pressure attained during the inspiratory pause will be a measure of the total compliance (lungs plus rib cage) of the patient. Thus for a patient with a low compliance, the equilibrium pressure will be higher (*Figure 4.7(b)*) than would be the case for a patient with a normal value of compliance (*Figure 4.7(a)*). For a patient with an increased value of the airway resistance (*Figure 4.7(c)*), there will need to be an increased pressure difference between the upper airway pressure and the alveolar pressure to supply the same tidal volume, but since the compliance has not changed the equilibrium pressure will be the same.

An inspiratory pause is also known as an inspiratory hold. The steady pressure developed during the pause has time to ventilate partially blocked alveoli and can markedly improve the distribution of inspired gas in the lungs. The increased mean intrathoracic pressure which is produced by this waveform may give rise to circulatory problems in some patients.

Ventilatory parameters

The five main parameters involved in intermittent positive pressure ventilation are *minute volume, tidal volume, ventilatory rate, inflation pressure* and *compliance.* These are linked by the relationships:

minute volume = ventilation rate × tidal volume

tidal volume = inflation pressure × compliance

The inflation pressure is usually taken as the airway pressure obtaining over the final portion of the inspiration period.

In practice, only four of these parameters will be under the control of the anaesthetist since the compliance must usually be taken as it occurs. Because of this, the inflation pressure will determine the tidal volume. Since minute volume and ventilation rate are related, in the finish there are only two independent variables. In ventilating patients with abnormal lungs and airways the choice of inspiratory flow rate is important. A high flow rate from a pressure-cycled ventilator may not drive sufficient volume into the lungs if the inflation time constant is too long. Slower flow rates are less likely to produce turbulence and will give a larger tidal volume, while requiring less pressure drop to over-come airway resistance. Some ventilators, such as the Cape 2000, provide a valve to adjust the inspiratory flow rate.

Minute volume dividers

In addition to the broad classification into pressure and flow gene-rators, it is possible to describe some types of ventilator as minute volume dividers. In these types, the total minute volume of gas fed into the ventilator is pre-set, often from the flowmeters of an anaesthetic machine, and the patient cannot obtain more, even by triggering the ventilator. Once the minute volume has been set, this determines the tidal volume and inflation pressure, leaving only the rate to be set. A number of ventilators provide metering arrangements for measuring the minute volume. Once this has been adjusted at a known rate, the tidal volume and inflation pressure follow automatically.

The application of negative pressure during the expiratory phase

In a number of ventilators, provision is made to apply suction to the patient's airway during each expiration. This has the effect of reducing the mean intrapulmonary pressure and can increase the rate of fall of pressure in the lungs during expiration. This facility may be valuable when narrow bore endotracheal tubes are used with children. It can also prove to be beneficial in increasing the venous return to the heart. Mushin *et al.* (1969) discuss the advisability of employing a negative phase and point out that it should be used with great caution with emphysematous patients. Watson, Smith and Spalding (1962) state that a negative phase during expiration can be expected to help the cir-culation only in patients whose circulatory reflexes are impaired.

Whilst a number of ventilators designed for use during anaesthesia offer the facility of a negative end-expiratory pressure (NEEP), this facility is not provided on the current comprehensive ventilators designed especially for intensive care unit use. The use of NEEP has become regarded as obsolete because it promotes atelectasis with but marginal reductions in the expiratory time required. A more favoured technique is to control the inspiratory flow rate as a function of pressure in order to increase the rate of expiration in a patient with airway collapse since an excessive pressure gradient will promote airway collapse.

The application of a positive end-expiratory pressure (PEEP)

Under some circumstances, such as the ventilation of infants suffering from the respiratory distress syndrome or patients who have inhaled vomit, there are advantages in arranging to have the end-expiratory pressure positive with respect to atmospheric. This pressure pattern yields the highest mean airway pressure and assists in preventing lung collapse. The application of PEEP can be obtained by adding a suitable water column to the outlet of the ventilator's expiratory line (Trinkle, 1971) or by terminating the line with a valve having an adjustable and calibrated closing pressure. For example, in the Pneumotron Series 80 ventilator a PEEP variable between 0 and 18 cm of water can be applied. Johnston, Donovan and Macdonnel (1974) discuss the use of PEEP during assisted respiration.

The use of a continuous positive airway pressure (CPAP) with spontaneous respiration

During automatic ventilation of the lungs, the use of a PEEP attachment with the ventilator ensures that the airway pressure will at all times be positive with respect to atmospheric pressure throughout the ventilatory cycle. The distension of the lungs by this technique has proved beneficial in the treatment of babies suffering from the respiratory distress syndrome. When the baby is able to breathe spontaneously, a similar effect may be obtained by the application of a continuous positive airway pressure (CPAP). Gregory *et al.* (1971) have shown that this situation can be most easily achieved by placing the head in a small chamber which is then pressurized to between 2 and 20 cm of water above atmospheric. In one commercial version, a cylindrical Perspex chamber is employed fitted with a disposable, transparent, plastic neck seal. A pressure of 10 cm of water is obtainable with a flow of gas into the head box of approximately 7 litres per minute. Pressure limitation is accomplished by the use of dead weight relief valves ranging from 5 to 20 cm of water in 5 cm increments. An alarm can be fitted to sound if the pressure falls below a pre-set level.

The action of CPAP is to improve the infant's arterial oxygen tension and consequently the oxygen content of the inspired air can be reduced. CPAP has also been administered via a face mask, endotracheal tube or a nasal cannula making use of the fact that newborn infants only breath through the nose (Theilade, 1978).

Patient triggering

An automatic lung ventilator normally cycles continuously at a pre-set ventilatory rate. After the administration of a muscle relaxant drug when spontaneous respiration commences to return, it is desirable to have the facility for allowing the patient's attempts at respiration to trip the ventilator over into the inspiratory phase so that it delivers a full tidal volume to the patient. By backing up the patient's voluntary efforts, this triggering action encourages the 'weaning' of the patient from the ventilator. The ventilator is first adjusted to cycle at the minimum respiratory frequency with an appropriate choice of tidal volume. If, between the cycles of the ventilator, the patient should attempt an inspiration, then the small negative pressure which he produces, of the order of 1 cmH_2O, is caused to deflect a sensitive diaphragm. The movement of the diaphragm or 'trigger' operates a switch or valve and makes the ventilator change directly to the start of a new inflation. Because of the basic rate set on the machine, if the patient should fail to continue his attempts at respiration, he is not left in an apnoeic state. The sensitivity of the trigger must not be so great that it can be operated by small movements of the corrugated tubing connecting the patient to the ventilator.

Intermittent mandatory ventilation (IMV)

Intermittent mandatory ventilation is another technique to assist in the weaning of patients from fully controlled ventilation to spontaneous respiration (Lawler and Nunn, 1977). In the IMV mode the ventilator provides a mandatory breath at pre-set time intervals and between the breaths the patient is able to breath spontaneously. In electronic flow metering ventilators such as the IMV Pneumotron and the Servo Ventilator a flow cycling inhibitor arrangement is used to synchronize the mandatory breaths with the spontaneous inspiratory phase. The frequency of the IMV breaths can be gradually reduced by the operator to enable the patient to co-ordinate a gradual transference from mandatory to spontaneous breathing; in the case of the Servo Ventilator the range is from one in two to one in ten breaths being mandatory.

The Puritan–Bennett MA-2 ventilator offers a sophisticated IMV arrangement in which the ventilator delivers demand breaths whose tidal volume is proportional to the patient's inspiratory effort and mandatory breaths whose volume is determined by the IMV volume control setting. Both demand and mandatory breaths are triggered by the patient's inspiratory efforts. However, during any mandatory breath interval in which the patient fails to trigger a breath, the ventilator automatically delivers a mandatory breath thus maintaining the IMV rate which has been pre-set.

The Cape 2000 ventilator has pre-set mandatory breath intervals of 15, 30, 60 or 90 seconds with a nominal inspiratory time of 2.5 seconds. The low airway pressure alarm is put out of action during the use of the IMV mode, but the high pressure and mains failure alarms continue in operation.

Sighs

In intensive care ventilators the facility for producing an extra large tidal volume (a sigh) at predetermined intervals is provided in order to periodically distend the lungs. The sigh is arranged to be synchronous with the patient's inspiration. A typical arrangement allows the time between successive sighs to be adjustable between 1 and 30 minutes continuously, the sigh duration to be between 0.5 and 5 seconds and the sigh volume between 200 and 2000 ml. A push button control can be provided for the manual initiation of a sigh and it is arranged that changes in the tidal volume or the airway pressure due to a sigh will not set off the alarms. The role of sighs in relation to the surface tension of the lungs is discussed on page 200. In some ventilators multiple sighs (1, 2 or 3) can be provided.

Controlled ventilation

In the majority of cases, ventilators are set to operate in the 'controller' mode. A controller is a lung ventilator which operates continuously and independently of the patient's inspiratory effort. The ventilator establishes a pre-set respiratory pattern, the ratio of inspiration to expiration time being usually in the range 1 : 1.5 to 1:2. In pressure-cycled ventilators such as the Bird and Cyclator, a pressure-sensitive valve is tripped when the inflation pressure reaches a pre-set value, this causing the ventilator to start the next expiratory phase. In volume-cycled ventilators such as the Howells and Beaver, when the bellows reach a pre-set excursion, the ventilator is tripped into the next expiratory phase. In time-cycled ventilators such as the Cape and Dräger Narcose Spriomat, a timing unit automatically changes over the inspiratory and expiratory phases at a predetermined rate. A full account of many makes of ventilator is given by Mushin *et al.* (1969).

Jain (1974) has performed an analysis of assisted respiration based on the use of a linear, first-order lung model and applying to it rectangular, sine-wave and ramp input pressure waveforms. The criteria of a simultaneous minimization of the average alveolar pressure and the ventilatory work per minute was used. Jain found that a rectangular

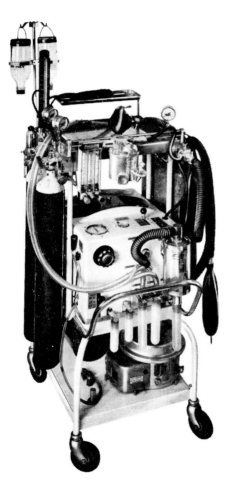

Figure 4.8. The East-Radcliffe anaesthetic machine fitted with an East-Radcliffe ventilator and humidifier. (By courtesy of H. G. East & Co. Ltd)

input pressure waveform resulted in the least work done by the patient when triggering the ventilator for a given magnitude of spontaneous effort and respiratory rate. Wald *et al.* (1968) have carried out a theoretical study of controlled ventilation.

In order to bring out the difference in operation of a *constant pressure* and a *constant flow* ventilator, attention will first be concentrated on two ventilators, the Radcliffe and the Manley Pulmovent. A description will then be given of the Cape 2000 ventilator which is a flow generator with time cycling subject to an overriding pressure or tidal volume limit.

The Radcliffe ventilator (*Figure 4.8*) (Russell *et al.*, 1956) is a time-cycled constant pressure generator, having an optional negative phase available during expiration. Referring to *Figure 4.9*, during inspiration

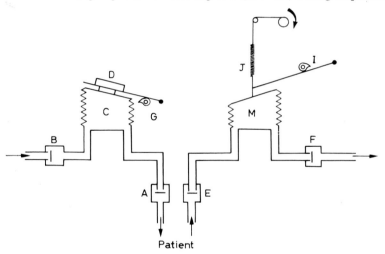

Figure 4.9. Schematic diagram of the Radcliffe ventilator with negative phase

valve A is open and the non-return valve B is closed. The bellows C are compressed by the weight D to give a constant pressure commensurate with the inflation pressure and discharge their contents into the patient. The maximum capacity of the bellows is 1400 ml. When the time-cycling mechanism changes over to expiration, valve E opens and valve A closes. These are poppet valves operated by the cycling mechanism. The patient expires to atmosphere via valve E and non-return valve F. Meanwhile, the bellows C are refilled by the action of cam G which lifts the arm and weight D, entraining gas through valve B. During inspiration, bellows M are emptied by the action of cam I. If required a subatmospheric pressure can be produced in bellows M by the action of spring J to give a negative pressure phase. Since the Radcliffe applies a constant inflationary pressure, the resulting tidal volume will depend on the value of the patient's compliance. Hence the Radcliffe does not compensate for compliance changes, but will compensate for leaks up to the limiting volume of bellows C. The inspiratory/expiratory ratio is fixed at 1:2, an electric motor and gears providing a choice of seven respiratory rates. The inflation pressure can be adjusted by altering the number and position of weights attached to the hinged arm of bellows C. An aneroid manometer indicates the inflation pressure, and the resulting tidal volume can be measured with a built-in Wright respirometer.

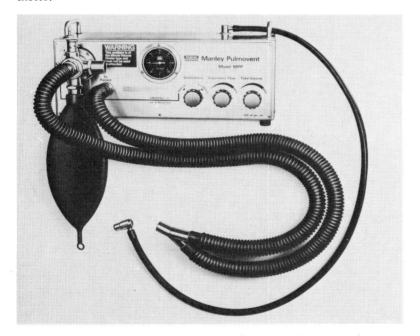

Figure 4.10. The Manley Pulmovent ventilator. (Courtesy of the Medishield Corporation)

The Manley Pulmovent (*Figure 4.10*) is a constant flow generator which can provide an inflation pressure of up to 70 cm of water. It is not fitted with a patient trigger and functions as a minute volume divider, and is entirely gas powered. The Pulmovent can be used either during anaesthesia or in an intensive care unit. The minute volume of ventilation is determined by the gas volume flow rate entering the ventilator either from the outlet of an anaesthesia apparatus or from a pipeline or air pump via a flowmeter. This minute volume must not exceed 20 litres per minute otherwise the ventilator may cease to cycle. The tidal volume control allows a bellows to expand to the required volume, the ventilatory frequency is then automatically set as the result of the minute volume divided by the tidal volume. The inspiratory flow control determines the inspiratory time. This necessarily also determines the ratio of inspiration to expiration time since the total time from the commencement of inspiration to the end of expiration has been established by the setting of the tidal volume and the ventilatory frequency.

The Pulmovent Model MPT provides the option of a negative pressure phase during expiration. Expiration is divided into a passive and an active phase of equal duration. During the passive phase expiration is to the atmosphere, the patient exhaling spontaneously. During the second phase expiration can be increased by the application of a subatmospheric pressure which can be varied from 0 to −10 cm of water. Alternatively the whole of the expiratory phase may be retarded by the application of a positive pressure up to + 10 cm of water (PEEP). The ventilator is volume cycled during inspiration and time cycled during expiration.

The main specifications of the Pulmovent are: minute volume 2 to 20 litres; tidal volume 150 to 1200 ml; frequency 10 to 60 per minute; inspiratory pressure 0 to 70 cm of water; expiratory pressure +10 to −10 cm of water; inspiratory flow 10 to 180 litres per minute.

Inspiratory phase

Referring to *Figure 4.11,* in the inactive condition bellows B1 and B2 are both collapsed, valves V1, V2, V4 and V5 are closed and valve V3 is open. With the automatic/manual mode selectors both set to the automatic position and a gas supply connected, gas enters the ventilator at the gas inlet and flows directly into bellows B1 and to the bellows safety valve.

The gas pressure expands bellows B1 against the action of their springs and as the bellows expand they operate an adjustable mechanical linkage which is connected to inspiratory valves V1 and V2. In

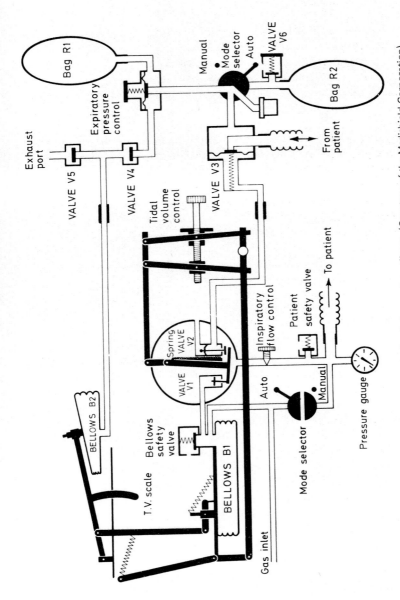

Figure 4.11. Schematic diagram of the Manley Pulmovent ventilator. (Courtesy of the Medishield Corporation)

addition, bellows B2 are also linked to bellows B1 and expand at the same time.

The adjustable linkage is moved by the tidal volume control so that immediately the bellows expand sufficiently to accomodate the selected tidal volume, the linkage opens valves V1 and V2 and allows the contents of bellows B1 to flow into the inspiratory flow control. The chosen inspiratory flow passes via the patient outlet to the patient. This flow is monitored by the pressure gauge and the patient safety valve.

Additionally, when valves V1 and V2 open, gas flows from the inspiratory valve via valve V2 into the expiratory valve where it closes valve V3 against the action of its spring, hence closing the expiratory circuit from the patient.

As the bellows empty they gradually return to the collapsed condition due to the action of their springs. The linkage closes valves V1 and V2 and also opens the vent to allow the pressure in the expiratory valve to vent to atmosphere. Valve V1 shuts off the inspiratory circuit and valve V3 opens due to the action of its spring to open the expiratory circuit.

Expiratory phase

With valves V1 and V2 closed and valve V3 open, the patient expires via valve V3 to the expiratory pressure control valve and bag R1. This is the passive expiratory phase and it can be either positive or negative depending on the setting of the expiratory pressure control valve.

During the expiratory phase bellows B1 are filling with fresh gas. As they expand bellows B2 are also expanded to create a subatmospheric pressure which opens non-return valve V4. Bag R1 now discharges into bellows B2 via valve V4 during the first half of the expiratory phase period. As bellows B2 expand at twice the rate of bellows B1 this interaction ensures that the active and passive expiratory phases are of an approximately equal duration.

When bag R1 is emptied by bellows B2, the pressure determined by the expiratory pressure control valve is applied to the patient and this pressure can be positive, atmospheric or subatmospheric depending upon the setting of the valve. Subatmospheric pressure is only applied during the second half of the expiratory phase while positive pressure is applied throughout expiration.

As bellows B2 expand due to the gas entering from bag R1, they operate a tidal volume scale. Bellows B1 are filling with fresh gas during the expiratory phase and when they collapse to initiate a subsequent inspiratory phase bellows B2 also collapse and open exhaust valve V5. Expired gas now flows to atmosphere via valve V5 during the current inspiratory phase or it may be ducted away by the action of bellows B2. Exhaled gases can be pumped away for a distance of up to 10 metres through a 25 mm diameter tube.

The inspiratory–expiratory sequence continues automatically until the gas supply is turned off or the Manual mode is selected.

Manual ventilation

In this mode fresh gas flows via the mode selectors and the patient outlet directly to the patient. As the gas takes the path of least resistance, bellows B1, the inspiratory valve and the inspiratory flow control are all bypassed and the expiratory pressure control valve, bag R1, valves V4 and V5 are all shut off by the expiratory circuit mode selector. Thus bellows B1 and B2 remain in the collapsed condition, valves V1 and V2 remain closed and valve V3 remains open. The patient expires via valve V3 and the expiratory circuit mode selector into bag R2. The patient's ventilation can be manually controlled by bag R2 and valve V6.

The entire expiratory circuit of the Pulmovent is externally mounted to allow it to be easily detached for autoclaving.

It is interesting to note that Sykes and Lumley (1969) found in anaesthetized patients undergoing open-heart surgery with automatic ventilation of the lungs that the ratio of dead space volume to tidal volume (V_D/V_T) was significantly less when the inspiration time was 1.5 seconds than when it was 0.5 or 1 second. In each case the sum of inspiration + expiration times equalled 3 seconds. They point out that when the duration of inspiration is reduced, pressure equilibrium is not achieved between the mouth and alveoli for alveolar units with long time constants and alveolar units with short time constants are consequently over-ventilated. This results in an uneven distribution of ventilation and the accentuation of inequalities in ventilation/perfusion ratios. The effect is manifest as an increase in the alveolar dead space and venous admixture effect. There is also likely to be an increase in the patient's anatomical dead space which contributes in part to the change observed in the physiological dead space. The volume of the anatomical dead space depends on the transpulmonary pressure at the end of inspiration (Shepard *et al.*, 1957) and this is related to the lung compliance and tidal volume. Watson (1962) reported a reduction in dynamic lung compliance in patients inflated with a short inspiration period. In one patient it was reduced from about 50 ml cmH_2O^{-1} to 35 ml cmH_2O^{-1} when the duration of inspiration was reduced from 1.0 to 0.5 seconds. For a constant tidal volume the transpulmonary pressure and anatomical dead space will increase if the lung compliance falls. Sykes and Lumley (1969) felt that the reduction in dynamic compliance arose from a maldistribution of the inspired gas resulting

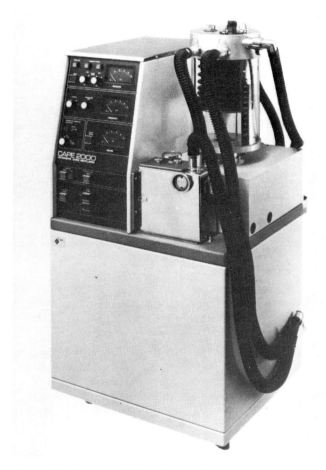

Figure 4.12. The Cape 2000 ventilator. (Courtesy of Cape Hospital Equipment)

from a scatter of time constants in the alveolar units. The use of a relatively slow inflation may be beneficial in the case of subjects suffering from gas distribution problems. However, for patients having a low cardiac output, i.e. having perfusion problems, a short inspiratory period with a higher flow rate results in a lower mean intrathoracic pressure and thus less interference with the venous return.

Bushman and Robinson (1968) point out that the lumen of the inspiratory hose from a ventilator can be smaller than that of the expiratory hose and this led them to the design of a double-lumen concentric ventilator hose. This is supplied with the Harlow ventilator, and also with the Pneumotron Series 80 and IMV Pneumotron ventilators. The use of a coaxial breathing circuit fitted with a scavenging valve to remove the effluent gases is described by Henville and Adams (1976).

The Cape 2000 ventilator by Cape Engineering Ltd (*Figure 4.12*) is a time-cycled flow generator which has been specially designed for intensive care and respiratory therapy applications. It is intended for open circuit use and has continuous and independent controls for tidal volume, inspiratory flow rate, airway pressure relief, inspiratory/ expiratory ratio, and the percentage of oxygen in the inspired gas mixture. For accurate mixture control the Quantiflex mixer unit described on p. 191 is employed. The expired volume is measured with a turbine-type transducer which feeds a panel meter. A second meter indicates the ventilatory frequency and a third meter displays the airway pressure. The volume meter can be switched to read either tidal volume (0–2 litres) or minute volume (0–25 litres). Upper and lower airway pressure alarms and a mains failure alarm are fitted. The high pressure alarm is instantaneous, but the low pressure alarm is given a 14 second delay.

With reference to *Figure 4.13,* a two-stage compressor (21) provides air at a nominal pressure of 13.8 kPa to the ventilating head via an electronically controlled shuttle valve (22). The compressed air passes into the pressure chamber (9) of the ventilating head, compresses the patient bellows (8) thus forcing the air or air and oxygen mixture in the bellows to the patient via the uni-directional valve (11) and the electrically heated humidifier (15). The inspiratory section of the ventilating head incorporates an inspiratory flow control (12) and a manual positive pressure relief valve (14) which can be adjusted between 20 and 70 cm of water. During the inspiratory phase the pressure-operated expiratory valve (17) is closed. During the expiratory

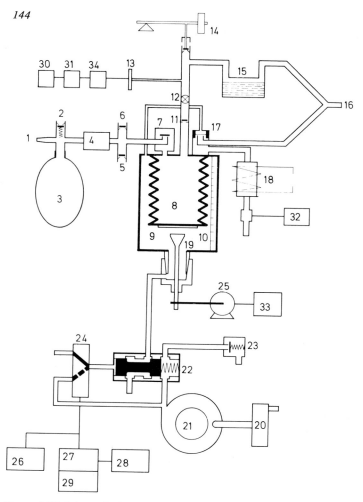

Figure 4.13. Schematic diagram of the Cape 2000 ventilator. (Courtesy of Cape Hospital Equipment)

1. Oxygen inlet. 2. Air inlet. 3. Storage bag. 4. Inspiratory filter. 5. Safety valve (air). 6. Relief valve (excess pressure). 7. Uni-directional valve. 8. Bellows. 9. Pressure chamber. 10. Volume scale. 11. Uni-directional valve (inspiratory). 12. Flow control valve. 13. Line filter (pressure monitor). 14. Manual positive pressure valve. 15. Humidifier. 16. Patient tubing & Y-piece. 17. Pressure operated expiratory valve. 18. Heated expiratory filter. 19. Bellows stop. 20. Compressor pre-filter. 21. Compressor. 22. Shuttle valve. 23. Spill valve. 24. Solenoid valve. 25. Volume control servo motor. 26. I.M.V. control. 27. Frequency control. 28. Frequency meter. 29. I.E. ratio control. 30. Ventilation failure alarm. 31. Pressure meter. 32. Tidal/minute volume meter. 33. Volume control. 34. Pressure monitor sensor

phase the pressure-operated expiratory valve (17) opens and the patient expires via this valve and a heated bacterial filter (18). At the same time the patient bellows are refilled with air or an air plus oxygen mixture via the inspiratory bacterial filter (4). The electronic control system provides a simple adjustment of ventilatory rate and the inspiration / expiration ratio. The tidal volume is adjusted by limiting the travel of the bellows against a scale on the bellows chamber.

A PEEP valve is located on top of the ventilating head and is adjustable between 0 and 20 cm of water. The ratio of inspiration time to expiration time is pre-set at 1:1, 1:2, 1:3 or 1:4 and selected by means of the appropriate control. The majority of the controls are located on the main control panel, but additional controls for inspiratory flow, maximum inflation pressure and PEEP are located on top of the ventilating head.

The patient system, including the complete ventilating head, the humidifier tank, breathing tubes and connectors are all fully auto-clavable in high temperature steam up to 140 °C. The only exception is the diaphragm of the pressure operated expiratory valve which is disposable and is easily removed before autoclaving.

Another powerful ventilator, which has been designed specifically for the ventilation of patients suffering from a chronic respiratory insufficiency is the Bennett Model MA-1. It is also a time-cycled flow generator, but uses a built-in bellows spirometer to measure the delivered tidal volume. The tidal volume range is 0–2000 ml with a frequency of 6 to 60 breaths per minute. The inflation period is set by the flow rate setting (10 to 100 litres per minute) and by the resistance and compliance of the patient and the connecting hoses. The timer sets the total duration of the ventilatory cycle, the balance being the expiratory time. A warning light shows when expiration time exceeds inspiration time.

Flow transducer controlled ventilators
The availability of compact respiratory gas flow rate sensors of the pneumotachograph or rotating vane type has led to their incorporation into electronically controlled volume-cycled ventilators. These sensors are small in size compared with the conventional bellows used for dispensing the tidal volume and thus permit the construction of compact ventilators for mounting at a bedside. The fact that a relatively compliant bellows is no longer interposed between the respiratory flow generator and the patient also means that the flow pattern actually

generated will reach the patient. A sophisticated form of this type of ventilator is the Medishield IMV Pneumotron. This is a true volume-cycled automatic lung ventilator designed primarily for use in intensive care. Three inspiratory flow waveforms can be selected: increasing flow, constant flow or decreasing flow. The delivered tidal volume remains almost constant regardless of any changes in the inspiratory phase time, the airway pressure, inspiratory waveform or flow rate.

The IMV Pneumotron has now largely replaced the Pneumotron Series 80 described in the third edition of this book. It is primarily intended for use in intensive care and three distinct modes of operation are available permitting planned stages of the patient's respiratory support from fully controlled ventilation, through gradually diminishing intermittent mandatory ventilation with patient triggering available until adequate spontaneous respiration is restored but with the ventilator's alarm circuits fully operational. The IMV Pneumotron may also be adapted for use during anaesthesia and may be powered from a 12 volt supply for use in an ambulance.

One turbine-type flow transducer is used to measure the pre-set tidal volume delivered to the patient, while a second transducer monitors the expired tidal volume and this is continuously compared with the delivered value. Any significant difference between the two values indicates a leak somewhere in the patient's circuit. The difference value is displayed on the inspired (delivered) tidal volume meter. The expired minute volume is displayed continuously on a separate meter which is provided with upper and lower limit alarm settings. The presence of a leak will result in a lower than normal value of the expired minute volume which can thus be arranged to generate an alarm. Alarms are available for a high or low minute volume, a high differential between the inspired and expired minute volumes, failure of either gas supply (air, oxygen or nitrous oxide) or the electrical mains.

The flow transducers are miniature turbines in which the rotational speed of the rotor is proportional to the velocity of the gas passing through the turbine. By means of a segmented disc coupled to the rotor and having alternate clear and opaque segments, the rotation of the rotor periodically interrupts a beam of light falling on to a photo-transistor. The rate of production of electrical pulses from the photo-transistor is proportional to the gas flowrate, while the number of pulses counted in a given time is proportional to the volume of gas passing in that interval.

Referring to *Figure 4.14*, oxygen and air (or nitrous oxide) at supply pressures of 300 to 400 kPa pass through a balancer (1) the output

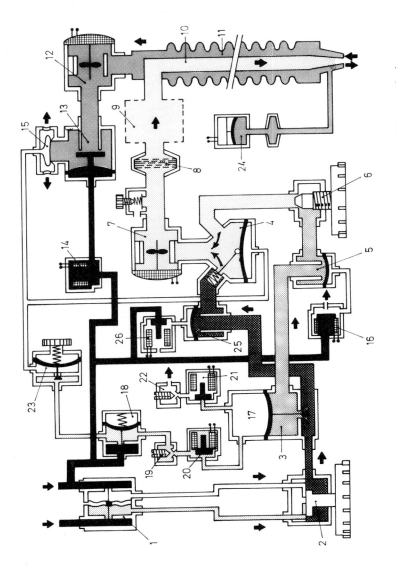

Figure 4.14. Schematic diagram of IMV Pneumotron. (Courtesy of the Medishield Corporation)

pressures of which are equal to whichever is the lower of the supply pressures. The two gases are then fed to a blender (2) adjustable from 21 to 100 per cent of oxygen and then to a fluid loaded gas regulator (3) – which provides the inspiratory flow control – and also to a demand valve (4) through which the patient can inspire spontaneously.

The gas output from the waveform regulator (3) passes to the gate valve (5) and thence through the inspiratroy control valve (6) after which it enters the demand valve chamber and the patient's circuit. On leaving the demand valve, the mixed gas passes through a flow transducer (7), a filter (8), a humidifier (9) and via the inner tube of the coaxial patient hose to the patient.

Expired gas passes along the outer corrugated tube of the coaxial hose (11) through a second flow transducer (12), through the expiratory valve (13) (activated by the solenoid-operated pilot valve (14)) and finally to atmosphere via the PEEP valve (15) if this is in use.

Electrical pulses generated by flow transducer (7) feed the circuits which activate the gate valve (5) via the solenoid-operated patient valve (16) to start and stop the flow of gas to the patient during the inspiratory phase.

If the pressure upstream of the flow control valve (6) i.e. the output pressure of regulator (3) is held constant, the flow at any particular setting of the flow control valve will be constant throughout the inspiratory phase. If a non-constant inspiratory flow is required, this is arranged by varying the fluid loading pressure in chamber (17) of regulator (3) so as to alter the output pressure. Thus, a decreasing flow waveform is obtained by arranging that the pressure in chamber (17) will be at maximum during the expiratory phase, being fed from a small regulator (18) via a pre-set needle valve (19) and a solenoid pilot valve (20) which is open, solenoid valve (21) being shut. At the start of inspiration, the main gate valve (5) is opened to allow gas to flow to the patient. The solenoid valve (21) simultaneously opens and the pressure in the chamber slowly decreases until the flows through needle valves (19) and (22) are in equilibrium. At this point, the pressure in chamber (17) is approximately halved, hence the output pressure of regulator (3) is also reduced, resulting in a drop in flow through valve (6). At the end of inspiration solenoid valve (21) closes and chamber (17) refills ready for the next inspiration.

When the ventilator is set up to generate an increasing flow waveform, solenoid valve (20) is shut during the expiratory phase and valve (21) is open, thus the pressure in chamber (17) is zero as also is the output pressure from regulator (3). At the start of inspiration solenoid valve (21) closes and valve (20) opens allowing the gas pressure in chamber (17) to increase at a rate determined by the setting of needle valve (19). Thus the pressure of regulator (3) will gradually rise and the flow through valve (6) will increase from zero to the maximum allowed by the setting of the control valve (6).

The output pressure of regulator (18) is approximately 150 kPa and in addition to providing the loading pressure in chamber (17) it also supplies the PEEP–CPAP regulator (23). This is a low pressure regulator, the output of which is adjustable between 0 and 20 cm of water. It is used to load simultaneously the PEEP valve (15) via a silicone rubber balloon and the fluid loading chamber of the demand valve (4), thus providing the CPAP function.

Although the demand valve (4) normally requires an inspiratory effort of between 0.5 and 1 cm of water to initiate the flow, increasing the output pressure of PEEP regulator (23) biases the diaphragm of the demand valve (4) and converts it into a continuous flow device. In these circumstances an equivalent expiratory pressure has to be exerted to shut-off the demand valve and this is made possible because the PEEP valve (15) is simultaneously and automatically loaded to the same pressure. Any gas drawn off by the patient is balanced by a compensating flow from the demand valve thus maintaining the CPAP level.

In addition to monitoring the airway pressure, transducer (24) is employed to operate a patient electronic trigger whose sensitivity is adjustable between 0 and 4 cm of water. At the low sensitivity end of this range, gas would normally tend to pass preferentially through the more sensitive demand valve so that when the patient trigger is selected, the demand valve is isolated by means of valve (25) and the solenoid pilot valve (26).

In order to cycle the ventilator, output pulses from the inspiratory flow sensor are fed to a pulse counter which produces a stepwise rise in voltage on a storage capacitor. The capacitor voltage is continuously compared with a fixed reference voltage which has been set by the manually adjustable tidal volume control. When the voltage on the capacitor equals the reference voltage, a comparator generates a signal which closes the inspiratory valve and starts the expiratory phase of the ventilatory cycle. Only when the required number of pulses have been generated will the ventilator change over to expiration. The changeover is unaffected by the duration of inspiration, the gas flow rate or variations in the flow rate occurring during inspiration.

The IMV Pneumotron has controls for tidal volume (0.2 to 1.4 litres), inspiratory pause time (0 to 3 seconds), ratio of inspiration time to expiration time (1:1 to 1:3), the percentage air—oxygen mixture (21 to 100 per cent), peak inspiratory flow rate (10 to 80 litres per minute), patient trigger (0 to 4 cm of water), positive end-expiratory pressure (PEEP) and continuous positive airway pressure (CPAP) (both 0 to 20 cm of water) and safety pressure override.

The safety pressure override control may be used to convert the ventilator from volume cycling to pressure cycling, but its main purpose is to handle sudden increases which may arise in the patient's airway resistance, perhaps due to bronchial spasm. The control is set to a pressure value which is slightly higher than the mouth pressure developed when the ventilator is volume cycling normally. The control then remains inoperative until a sudden increase in the airway resistance causes the airway or mouth pressure to rise when the override temporarily converts the ventilator to a pressure cycling mode. When the airway pressure reduces, the ventilator reverts to a volume cycling mode. During the pressure cycling mode, the tidal volume will have become reduced and this will cause the inspiration time to be reduced. The inspiratory—expiratory time ratio circuit will then correspondingly reduce the expiratory time resulting in an increase in the ventilatory frequency and the maintenance of the pre-set tidal volume. In the absence of the override, the airway pressure might rise to an excessive value.

The IMV Pneumotron's audible alarms can be muted for 15 seconds to allow for patient nursing procedures. A key switch allows a permanent muting. In order to be able to generate rapidly changing flow waveforms, the static compliance of the ventilator alone is less than 0.5 ml per 1 cm of water. All the external components of the ventilator are made from materials which are either disposable or which can be autoclaved. A coaxial pair of breathing tubes is used, together with a Fisher Paykel hot water humidifier. Electrical outputs are available for the tidal volume, minute volume, inspiratory flow, expiratory flow and airway pressure.

Another example of an electronic ventilator with a small compressible volume and controlled by pressure and flow transducers is the Siemens Servo Ventilator which is proving of considerable value both for therapy and teaching purposes in intensive care units. The feedback system continuously compares the pre-set values of the ventilatory pattern with those recorded by the flow and pressure sensors and operates to make them equal. IMV settings are available corresponding with one half, one fifth and one tenth of the pre-set minute volume.

The IMV ventilation is always synchronized with the patient's spontaneous respiration. A sigh can be switched in to give a doubled tidal volume once every 100 breaths. The working pressure (the highest pressure available for ventilation) can be set between 10 and 100 cmH_2O. Triggering is adjustable from -20 to $+45$ cm of water. The inspiratory time can be set between 15 and 50 per cent of the ventilatory cycle and the pause time between inspiration and expiration between 0 and 30 per cent of the cycle. The range of inspiratory to expiratory times is from 1:6 to 4:1. The expiratory circuit of the Servo Ventilator can easily be disconnected for autoclaving.

Ventilators such as the Pneumotron and the Servo Ventilator which have a small compressible volume and can generate rapidly changing respiratory waveforms need to be used with a humidifier which also has a small compressible volume if the waveform is to be transmitted to the patient. An internal compliance for the humidifier of less than 1 ml per cmH_2O pressure is possible with a good design.

The monitoring of respiratory mechanics

Ventilators fitted with pressure and flow transducers lend themselves to the on-line calculation of the respiratory mechanics variables. If the delivered pressure, the patient's airway pressure and the instantaneous gas flow rate are known then the resistance of the airways plus connecting tubing can be calculated as the pressure drop divided by the flow rate and expressed in terms of cm of water per litre per second for inspiration or expiration. The compliance of the lungs and chest wall can be calculated from a knowledge of the volume increment passed into the airway for a given increase in airway pressure. These calculations can be performed with a hard-wired unit connected to the Servo Ventilator and displayed on a breath-by-breath basis or fed to a pen recorder. It is also possible to display the end expiratory and peak inflation pressures and the inspiratory pause pressure. These derived variables can be of great value in the management of patients with severe respiratory problems.

Digital computers have been used as part of extensive patient monitoring systems in intensive care units and in some cases the monitoring of respiratory mechanics has been a feature. Osborn *et al.*'s (1969) system continuously monitored the respiratory mechanics of patients on automatic ventilators and changes in the compliance provided evidence of the patient tending to fight the ventilator. Lewis *et al.* (1972) also calculated respiratory mechanics, blood gases, cardiac output, ECG arrhythmias, arterial pressures, body temperature and respiratory and heart rates.

Humidifiers

It is useful for ventilators intended for the treatment of patients suffering from a chronic respiratory insufficiency to incorporate a humidifier. This is often of the 'bubble' type as shown in *Figure 4.8*. The principles of various types of humidifier are dealt with in Chapter 5. British Standard 4494:1970 deals with the specification for humidifiers for use with breathing machines. It states that the humidifier used shall be capable of delivering gas with a moisture content of not less than 33 mg per litre (equivalent to a relative humidity of not less than 75 per cent at 37 °C) at the patient's end of the delivery tube when the input gas temperature is 10 °C to 25 °C, the input relative humidity is zero, the minute volume delivered is in the range 5 to 20 litres and the inspiratory—expiratory phase time ratio is 1:2. The relative humidity of the humidified gas shall be measured after the gas has passed through a 1-metre length of 22 mm bore corrugated rubber tubing. The gas temperature measured at the point of entry to the patient must not fluctuate by more than plus or minus 2°C from the set temperature when the minute volume is varied between 5 and 20 litres and must not exceed 39 °C at any time. The resistance to gas flow of the humidifier should not be more than 30 mmH$_2$O (290 N m^{-2}) at a steady flow rate of 30 litres per minute.

The Cape 2000 intensive care ventilator employs a hot water bath type of humidifier which has an autoclavable stainless steel tank with a capacity of 2240 ml and a water surface area of 15 500 square millimetres. It should be filled with distilled or sterile water to a level half way up the sight glass. The heater power is 150 watts and the tank temperature is set at 60 ± 2 °C. With standard tubing the temperature at the patient's Y-piece is then 37 ± 1 °C. The tank is provided with a high temperature cut-out set at 70 °C and a lamp indicator. The humidifier takes 30—40 minutes to heat up to its operating temperature.

Geevalghese *et al.* (1976) have investigated the inspired air temperature produced by a number of immersion heater humidifiers and found that humidifiers with a fixed temperature thermostatic control performed consistently though most gave rise to inhaled air temperatures greater than 37 °C.

Ventilators are often fitted with an ultrasonic humidifier. In this type, radio frequency power is supplied to a piezoelectric transducer which then vibrates at a frequency of the order of 1.4 MHz. The resulting ultrasonic vibrations are focused on to a container holding sterile water or medication. The intense agitation of the fluid by the focused beam produces a mist of liquid particles which is claimed have a narrow distribution of particle diameters, resulting in a uniform penetration of the lungs. Powerful ultrasonic humidifiers can produce large amounts of water vapour and care must be taken in their use. One solution is to use a bubbler humidifier and an ultrasonic humidifier for alternate hours.

Robinson (1978) points out that ultrasonic humidifiers have not achieved the clinical acclaim that their producers expected. This is because little of the inspired water is in the vapour phase and the necessary cooling of the respiratory tract to produce vapour has deleterious effects on cilial action. Robinson (1978) goes on to say that there is also an increase in the airways resistance and a danger of water intoxication, particularly in infants. Difficulties have been experienced in obtaining a precise control of the output of ultrasonic devices.

Chase, Kilmore and Trotta (1961) discuss the respiratory water loss occurring in anaesthetic systems. Chase, Trotta and Kilmore (1962) describe some simple methods of humidifying non-rebreathing anaesthetic gas systems. Han and Lowe (1961) found the mean expired humidity in a series of nine anaesthetized patients to be 23.4 mg l^{-1}, that is, approximately 12 ml of water per hour. The loss was proportional to the minute volume. When a humidifier or heat exchanger was used to raise the water content of the inspired air to 14 mg l^{-1}, the patients were in a state of respiratory water balance. The mass of water vapour was estimated condensing in a cold trap as described by Burch (1965).

Nebulizers

Nebulizers are sometimes used with ventilators and assisters in respiratory therapy to generate aerosols of various medications. In general, nebulizers are designed to deliver a maximum number of particles per minute in a specified size range whilst humidifers are designed to deliver a maximum amount of water vapour with a minimum content of water particles. Simple scent-spray-type nebulizers are in common use, but ultrasonic types are also encountered. Broncho-dilator, mucolytic, proteolytic and antibiotic aerosols are required for particular conditions. A detailed account of nebulizers and the role of aerosol therapy is given by Egan (1973). A typical maximum output from an ultrasonic nebulizer would be 6 cm^3 of mist per minute at minute volumes of up to 25 litres per minute.

Assisters

Assisters are ventilators which have only a patient triggering facility and do not cycle continuously as a controller. They assist the respiration of spontaneously breathing patients by operating in response to the patient's inspiratory effort. They are useful in cases of respiratory insufficiency where the patient is unlikely to become apnoeic and particularly for patients on aerosol drug therapy. *Figure 4.15* shows an

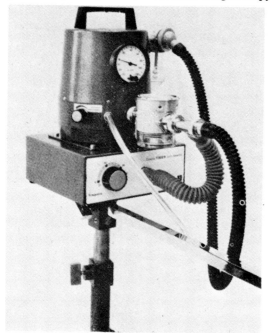

Figure 4.15. Dräger 'Assistor' fitted with a nebulizer, respirator and electronic cycling unit. (By courtesy of Drägerwerk, Lübeck)

assister by the Dräger Company which is fitted with a nebulizer for drug therapy. Wright (1958) describes a low-output nebulizer designed to inject nebulized water and drugs into the main gas stream via a side limb. It can produce just over 50 per cent saturation of the gas at 24 °C (Robinson *et al.*, 1969). The assister is powered from an oxygen cylinder or pipeline and entrains additional air, the minimum oxygen concentration administered to the patient never being lower than 50 per cent. The assister is shown mounted on top of an auxiliary electronic time-cycling unit which can be fitted to the assister in order to convert it into a controller. The timer unit is provided with a separate patient trigger diaphragm which is designed to be more sensitive than that already fitted into the assister. This arrangement ensures that the patient's respiratory efforts will fit into the cycling of the timer unit.

Fluid-logic controlled ventilators

A new development in ventilator design stems from the use of pneumatically powered logic circuits. These can be based either upon conventional poppet valves to control the gas flows (Burchell, 1957) or upon the use of 'fluid logic' elements. It is possible to produce gas powered analogues of many electronic circuits such as R—C oscillators, amplifiers, bistables, univibrators and logic gates. Thus the basic timing circuit generating the respiratory frequency might be the analogue of an R—C oscillator or a stable multivibrator. This feeds a univibrator to set the inspiration—expiration ratio. A sensitive pneumatic amplifier could sense the reverse flow arising from the patient attempting an inspiration, and this could initiate the next inflationary phase in the triggered mode. Such a system is inherently robust since the various elements consists only of poppet valves or fluid-logic elements made from channels moulded into small plastic blocks. While the poppet valve system uses moving parts, its gas consumption can be relatively low since when a valve is closed no gas passes. The fluid-logic system uses no moving parts, the various actions consisting only of the switching of gas streams. However, the gas consumption of a complete system tends to be high, and if a high degree of sensitivity is obtained in an amplifier by pulsing its jets at an audio frequency, this tends to produce a noisy combination. The pneumatic analogue of capacitance is volume and at respiratory frequencies, the volumes required are of the order of litres. Vince and Brown (1965) have outlined a scheme for a fluid-logic ventilator based upon a 12 Hz oscillator in a time-cycled arrangement. A series of binary counting stages totals the number of pulses generated by the oscillator. This number is continuously compared with a time interval which has been manually pre-set. When a correspondence of the values occurs, air is diverted into or out from the patient's lungs.

A simple fluid-logic bistable pressure-cycled ventilator

A simple, pressure-cycled ventilator using fluid logic has been described by Straus and Meyer (1965) and by Woodward *et al.* (1964). It is based upon a wall attachment fluid bistable element. Normally, a jet of gas issuing from a rectangular or circular nozzle into a stationary gas spreads outwards as it moves forwards in a downstream direction

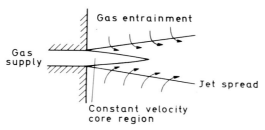

Figure 4.16. Normal undeflected jet of gas

(*Figure 4.16*). This is due to entrainment of the stationary gas into the moving jet in a momentum exchange process. If a wall in the device restricts the entrainment of gas on one side of the jet, then the local pressure on that side of the jet becomes reduced, causing the jet to be deflected towards the boundary (Parker, 1967; Klain and Smith, 1976; Duffin, 1977). The Coanda wall-attachment effect and jet-interaction principles are dealt with in more detail by Conway (1971). With a suitable positioning of the wall, the gas jet will re-attach itself to the wall further down, enclosing a region of low pressure (*Figure 4.17*). It is possible to deflect the jet into another stable region by applying a small control gas flow to the region of low pressure. This is now a bistable element with two stable positions.

In *Figure 4.18* is illustrated the basic method of operation of a pressure-limited ventilator powered by a bistable fluid device. There are no moving parts and the arrangement can operate with patient triggering. When the input control valve is opened, the gas to be inspired is

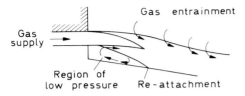

Figure 4.17. Re-attachment of the gas jet in the
deflected position

passed through the power nozzle and flows into the left output receiver
channel. It is deflected over into the left output channel because of the
action upon it of gas entrained through the right control nozzle, the set-
screw fitted to the left control nozzle ensuring that gas is first entrained
preferentially from the right-hand nozzle. From the left output, the gas
flows to the patient via a face-mask or endotracheal tube. As the inflationary pressure builds up, a portion of the gas is fed back to the left

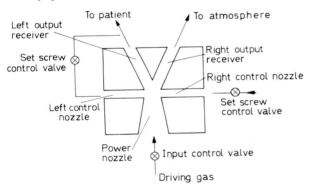

Figure 4.18. Schematic diagram of a pressure-limited ventilator
powered by a bistable fluid amplifier. (By courtesy of Harry
Diamond Laboratories)

control nozzle via the feedback line. When a sufficient pressure
differential has been created between the left and right control nozzles,
the gas flow direction changes over from the left to the right output
receiver. This results in the entrainment of gas through the left output
receiver, and the consequent production of a negative phase during
expiration. The falling inflationary pressure reduces the feedback flow,
and the gas stream again becomes deflected over to the left output
receiver causing the respiratory cycle to recommence. During the
expiratory phase of the ventilator, an attempted inspiration by the

patient will reduce the feedback flow and trigger the ventilator over into the next inspiratory phase, by switching the flow over into the left receiver. In this design, the fluid amplifier is moulded entirely from plastic and is smaller than a packet of cigarettes.

A fluid-logic volume-cycled ventilator

The design of a volume-cycled ventilator is of necessity more complicated than for the pressure-cycled type, since it must involve a volume-sensitive element. In *Figure 4.19*, opening of the input control valve allows the gas supply to be connected to the power nozzle and flow into the left output receiver, and from this into the cylinder. The piston moves forward, compressing the bellows and forcing the respired gases into the lungs. When the pre-set tidal volume has been reached, a trip situated on the bottom plate of the bellows activates the upper excursion-limiting trigger. This trigger opens a normally closed valve and allows gas from the driving supply to flow into the left control nozzle. When sufficient pressure difference has been created between the left and right control nozzles, the direction of flow changes over from the left to the right output receiver. The flow now entrains gas from the cyclinder, pulling back the piston, and expanding the bellows. The normally open inspiratory valve shuts, the gas mixture to be inhaled flows into the bellows via the one-way flap valve. The patient exhales through the expiratory valve. When the bellows has completed its filling, the bottom plate of the bellows activates the bottom stroke-limiting trigger, causing the power stream to be deflected back into the left output receiver and cycling recommences.

A patient triggering facility is available with this ventilator. A negative pressure produced by an attempted inspiration operates the patient trigger unit to entrain gas from the atmosphere or other suitable source to direct the power stream over to the left output receiver. With a driving gas pressure of 30 lbf in^{-2} (207 kN m^{-2}) gauge the tidal volume can be varied between 300 and 1000 ml at rates between 5 and 50 breathes per minute. The ventilator is volume limited with a maximum pressure set by the pressure of the driving gas.

In spite of their attractions of a small size and rugged construction, fluid-logic ventilators have not achieved a widespread popularity in civilian applications. This appears to be because they are somewhat wasteful of gas as gas must always keep flowing through them in contrast to valve types. There is also the fact that the gas passages are

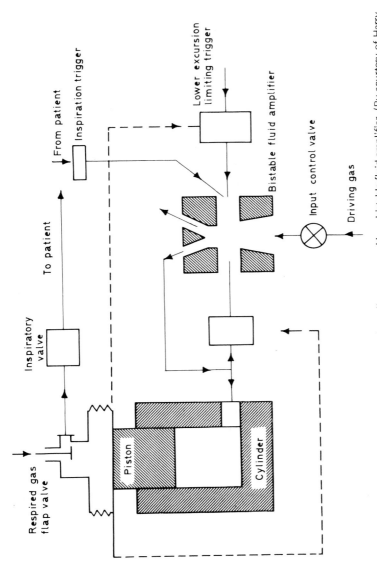

Figure 4.19. Schematic diagram of a volume-limited ventilator powered by a bistable fluid amplifier. (By courtesy of Harry Diamond Laboratories)

narrow and the device characteristics can be changed by the presence of grit or other foreign material.

However, Manson, Ross and Dundas (1979) describe a paediatric ventilator with a fluidic control system which is based on the use of fluidic industrial control modules made by the Corning Glass Corporation. These are made from an inert ceramic material by a photographic process, the logic circuit being constructed from standard modules attached to a Corning manifold. The gas consumption of the entire logic circuit is approximately 30 litres per minute and the consumption of the alarm systems is approximately 10 to 12 litres per minute. The system is basically a T-piece occluder. Inspiratory and expiratory time, inflation pressure limit, PEEP, CPAP and the inspiratory flow rate are independently variable and IMV is available. Warning systems are provided for failure of the driving gas, low airway pressure and the inspiratory pressure limit. The breathing circuit is isolated from the control and warning systems for ease of sterilization.

Hillyer and Johnston (1978) found that an unexpectedly high oxygen concentration reading from an oxygen analyser in the circuit revealed an unsuspected leak of oxygen through a perforation of the bellows of a fluidic ventilator powered by oxygen.

The use of pneumatic valves

Because of the problems which arise in the use of fluid-logic ventilators for routine clinical work development has proceeded with the use of ventilators based on pneumatic valves in the switching circuits. An example occurs in the Penlon Oxford Ventilator. In this device the driving gas and the patient's gas are kept completely separate. Referring to the schematic diagram of *Figure 4.20* it can be seen that the driving gas operates a linear actuator which expands or compresses a rubber bellows over a pre-set stroke length and with a pre-set velocity in both directions. The driving gas supply should be at a pressure of 60 lbf in^{-2}g (413.7 kN m^{-2}) and a volume flow rate of 4–12 litres per minute is required. The bellows has two one-way valves attached to it so that gas is drawn in during the expansion of the bellows and delivered to the patient during the compression stroke. The ventilator is thus volume-cycled with a stroke volume range of 200–1200 ml in the adult version and 50–300 ml by changing to a smaller bellows for use with infants. The inflation flow rate can be pre-set between 200 and 100 ml per second in the case of the adult bellows, the values being

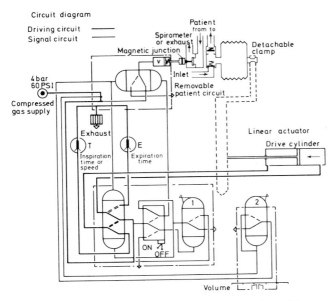

Figure 4.20. Schematic diagram of the Oxford Ventilator. (By courtesy of Penlon Ltd)

approximately halved for the infant bellows. By varying these values the ratio of inspiratory to expiratory time can be adjusted. The range of ventilatory frequencies varies with the tidal volume. With a 1000 ml tidal volume and an inspiratory/expiratory ratio of 1:2, the range of frequencies is 20—75 breaths per minute. The tidal volume calibration is based upon a compliance of 50 ml per cmH_2O pressure and an air-way resistance of 5 cmH_2O per litre per second. The pneumatic circuit connected to the driving gas also operates an inflating valve which is automatically closed at the start of the inflation stroke and opened at the end of inflation. There is also an on/off switch which is arranged so that the bellows will always complete an inflation stroke before stopping and the expiratory valve will open. This arrangement avoids any risk of an uncontrolled speed during the first inflation. The patient circuit consists of an inlet tube, inlet non-return valve bellows unit, outlet non-return valve, port to patient and exhaust port. All of these parts can be autoclaved and are mounted within a single unit which can be detached from the ventilator without tools within a few seconds. The patient circuit is completed by attaching a pressure relief valve normally set at 50 cmH_2O, inspiratory and expiratory hoses and a Y-piece. For intensive care use a bacterial filter may be connected to the gas inlet or the ventilator can be operated from an air–oxygen mixer unit. A 4 lb size (*c*. 970 litre) CO_2 cylinder will run the ventilator for several hours.

Sugg and Pry-Roberts (1976) describe the Penlon Oxford Ventilator, while Pybus and Kerr (1978) describe a simple system for administering intermittent mandatory ventilation with the Oxford Ventilator.

The Nuffield Anaesthesia Ventilator (previously known as the Pneupac A.P. – Adams and Henville, 1977) is a compact, gas-powered, pneumatic logic ventilator primarily intended for use with a coaxial circuit (Henville and Adams, 1976). It incorporates a detachable patient valve. When this valve is removed, the control module may be employed to cycle a high-pressure gas source for jet ventilation through the open airway during laryngoscopy or bronchoscopy (Gillick, 1976; Pybus, O'Connor and Henville, 1978).

Specific ventilators

From what has been said, it is now possible to describe a particular ventilator in terms of its mode of action and cycling mechanism. The Barnet Ventilator (Rochford *et al.*, 1958) is a time-cycled minute volume divider having optional patient triggering. It is a flow generator. The Howells ventilator (Howells, 1960) is a volume-cycled minute volume divider and is a flow generator, a powerful spring providing the high pressure. It has only two controls, a volume selector and an inspiratory time control. An optional negative phase is available. The Manley Ventilator is a minute volume divider which is volume-cycled up to a limiting pressure (Manley, 1961). It is a pressure generator and provides an optional negative phase. A development of this ventilator is the Manley Pulmovent. It has a maximum inspiratory pressure of 70 cmH_2O with a tidal volume range of 150 to 1200 ml and a ventilatory frequency of 10 to 60 per minute giving a minute volume range of 2–20 litres. The inspiratory flow rate can be varied from 10–180 litres per minute and a negative pressure of up to -10 cmH_2O can be applied during expiration. In the Manley Pulmovent, an automatic pressure regulation system has replaced the sliding weight which was used in the original Manley ventilator to load the bellows which contained the tidal volume. The entire expiratory circuit of the Manley Pulmovent is externally mounted to facilitate autoclaving. It also has the facility to pump the expired gases clear of the ward or operating room in order to prevent pollution. The gases can be pumped to distances of up to 10 metres through a 25 mm bore pipe. Both the Howells and the Manley are gas-powered from the normal 5 lbf in^{-2} (345 kN m^{-2}) gas outlet of the older type of British anaesthesia machines.

Mapleson (1962) discusses the pressure—volume relationships found in both pressure and flow generators, whilst Hill (1966) describes developments in the design of electronically controlled ventilators. Beaver (1962) discusses the management of acute respiratory failure, and the use of an optional negative phase during expiration, and Burchell (1957) describes a modification of the original Beaver ventilator (Beaver, 1953) to give a negative phase. Howells (1960) gives a general account of the considerations involved in choosing a ventilator. The problems involved in the use of automatic ventilators with infants and children are dealt with by Mushin, Mapleson and Lunn (1962). Campbell and Brown (1963) describe a simple R—C circuit analogue of the lung which is useful in evaluating ventilator performance. In a later paper (Campbell and Brown, 1966), they use linear components to describe the lung and chest wall compliance since these stay reasonably linear throughout the greater part of the clinical range but now use non-linear elements to represent the pressure—air flow relationships of the human bronchial tree.

A great deal of information concerning the design of ventilators is contained in British Standard 3806: 1964, 'Breathing machines for medical use'. Price *et al.* (1954) discuss the results of measurements of blood pH, P_{CO_2}, arterial blood pressure, central venous pressure and mean mask pressure on patients ventilated with eight types of ventilator. A clear account of the physiology of intermittent positive pressure ventilation is that of De Kock (1966). Norlander (1964) discuss the functional analysis of the force and power developed by ventilators. Collis and Bushman (1966) give a detailed comparison of the characteristics of ten popular ventilators.

Miniature ventilators

Apart from the sophisticated multi-purpose types of ventilator, there is a need for a simple oxygen-powered ventilator for use as a resuscitator in hospital wards, ambulances, dental surgeries and similar situations. Burchell (1967) describes a simple machine designed for these applications. It is a time-cycled, constant-flow generator with only a single control which allows adjustment of the inflationary period to be made to suit the patient's tidal volume requirements. A pressure relief valve can be set to blow off in the range 30 to 60 cmH_2O. For use during anaesthesia with nitrous oxide, a bag-in-a-bottle arrangement would have to be provided. The dimensions of the ventilator are 7 × 3¼ × 2 inches (178 × 83 × 51 mm). A smaller ventilator which can be held in the palm of one hand is that described by Cohen (1966). The output of gases from the anaesthetic machine is fed into a reservoir bag and when the pressure has built up to a predetermined value, the ventilator releases a magnetically controlled valve to discharge the contents of the bag into the patient's lungs. When the bag pressure has fallen to a pre-set value, the magnetic valve closes, the bag refills and the patient expires passively to the atmosphere. Obviously such a simple system must have its limits but it scores on the grounds of portability.

Neonatal and paediatric ventilators

When a sufficiently small tidal volume is available at a suitable ventilatory rate, a standard adult automatic lung ventilator is often used in conjunction with a small volume, low compliance inspiratory and expiratory hose. The Manley Pulmovent can be fitted with an optional paediatric inspiratory flow control to provide lower flow rates suitable for small children. Special infant ventilators are available such as the Vickers Neovent Model 90. This is a time-cycled minute volume divider which can be operated from the a.c. mains supply, or a 12 V d.c. supply and is also fitted with an internal rechargeable battery. It is thus suitable for use during the emergency transportation of an infant. The Neovent can be operated from an oxygen pipeline, a source of compressed air or an oxygen—air mixture. The expiration time is variable from 0.2 to 2.0 seconds and the inspiration time is variable from 0.2 seconds to the expiration time. The minute volume range is 2 to 10 litres per minute and an adjustable, calibrated, relief valve can be set to limit the pressure applied to the infant to 10—150 cmH_2O. The dimensions of the Neovent are 280 × 180 × 170 mm so that it can be mounted on a shelf above an incubator. A humidifier is available for the Neovent. In some models of paediatric ventilators, a ventilatory rate control is provided. A typical range for this would be 15 to 50 breaths per minute.

Disinfecting ventilators

In most modern ventilators the whole of the channel in contact with the patient's gas is designed to be easily removed for autoclaving as is the humidifier. Sometimes, however, the construction is such that the use of ethylene oxide gas or formalin vapour is necessary rather than autoclaving (Sykes, 1964) or a chemical antimicrobial.

Ventilators can constitute a cross-infection hazard. Apart from the risk that the interior of the ventilator's piping may become contaminated, the expired gases may carry micro-organisms into the room.

High efficiency pleated membrane bacterial filters may be fitted to both the inspiratory and expiratory sections of the ventilator. The filters are disposable and tested to British Standard Specification BS 3928 for 0.001 per cent penetration with a sodium chloride test cloud with a mean particle size of 0.5 micrometres. The expiratory filter is heated to prevent condensation and is replaced at least for every patient. The inspiratory filter prevents airborne contamination from entering the patient system and should be replaced at approximately two monthly intervals. A filter would also be placed in the air line feeding a nebulizer. Mitchell and Gamble (1973) discuss the performance of a siliconized bacterial filter for ventilators. Loeser (1978) found that several American bacterial filters became obstructed when exposed to a sufficient quantity of water following either direct application of water or exposure to humidity.

References

ADAMS, A.P. and HENVILLE, J.D. (1977). A new generation of anaesthetic ventilators. The Pneupac and Penlon A.P. *Anaesthesia* **32**, 34–40

ADAMSON, J.P., LEWIS, L., LEANDRO, S. and STEIN, J.D. (1959). Application of abdominal pressure for artificial respiration. *J. Am. med. Ass.* **169**, 1613

BEAVER, R.A. (1953). Pneumoflator for treatment of respiratory paralysis. *Lancet* **1**, 977

BEAVER, R.A.(1962). Acute respiratory failure. *Lond. Clin. med. J.* **3**, 2

BEAVER, R.A.(1963a). Pneumoflator for treatment of respiratory paralysis. *Lancet* **1**, 977

BEAVER, R.A. (1963b). A simple pneumoflator. *Br. med. J.* **1**, 1375

BOWER, A.G., BONNET, V.R., DILLON, J.B. and AXELROD, B.(1950). Investigation on the care and treatment of poliomyelitis patients. *Ann. west. Med. Surg.* **4**, 561

BURCH, G.E. (1965). Study of water and heat loss from respiratory tract in man. *Archs intern. Med.* **74**, 308

BURCHELL, G.B. (1957). Modified Beaver respirator. *Br. J. Anaesth.* **29**, 183

BURCHELL, G.B. (1967). The Minepac emergency ventilator. *Anaesthesia* **22**, 647

BUSHMAN, J.A. and ROBINSON, S. (1968). A 'single' ventilator hose. *Br. J. Anaesth.* **40**, 796

CAMPBELL, D. and BROWN, J. (1963). The electrical analogue of the lung. *Br. J. Anaesth.* **35**, 684

CAMPBELL, D. and BROWN, J. (1966). The electrical analogues for lung function. In *Biomechanics and Related Bio-engineering Topics*, p. 459. (Ed. by R.M. Kenedi). Oxford; Pergamon Press

CHASE, H.F., KILMORE, M.A. and TROTTA, R. (1961). Respiratory water loss via anaesthetic systems: mask breathing. *Anesthesiology* **22**, 205

CHASE, H.F., TROTTA, R. and KILMORE, M.A. (1962). Simple methods for humidifying non-rebreathing anesthetic gas systems. *Anesthesiology* **41**, 249

COHEN, A.D. (1966). The Minivent respirator. *Anaesthesia* **21**, 563

COLLIER, C.R. and AFFELDT, J.E. (1954). Ventilatory efficiency of the cuirass respirator in totally paralysed chronic poliomyelitis patients. *J. appl. Physiol.* **6**, 531

COLLIS, J.M. and BUSHMAN, J.A. (1966). An assessment of 10 lung ventilators. *Wld med. Electronics,* May, 134

COMROE, H.J., FORSTER, E.R., DUBOIS, A.B., BRISCOE, W.A. and CARLSEN, A.B. (1962). *The Lung.* Chicago; Year Book Publishers

CINWAY, A. (1971). A guide to fluidics. London; Macdonald

De KOCK, M.A. (1966). The physiology of intermittent positive pressure breathing. *S. Afr. med. J.* **43**, Supplement

DRINKER, P. and McKHANN, C.F. (1929). The use of a new apparatus for the prolonged administration of artificial respiration. *J. Am. med. Ass.* **92**, 1658

DUFFIN, J. (1977). Fluidics and pneumatics: principles and applications in anaesthesia. *Can. Anaesth. Soc. J.* **24**, 126

EGAN, D.F. (1973). *Fundamentals of Respiratory Therapy.* 2nd edn, St. Louis; C.V. Mosby Co.

GEEVALGHESE, K.P., ALDRETE, J.A. and PATEL, T.C. (1976). Inspired air temperature with immersion heater humidifiers. *Anesth. Analg.* **55**, 331–334

GILLICK, J.S. (1976). The inflation-catheter technique of ventilation during laryngoscopy. *Can. Anaesth. Soc. J.* **23**, 534–544

GREGORY, G.A., KITTERMAN, J.A., PHIBBS, R.H., TOOLEY, W.H. and

HAMILTON, W.K.(1971). Treatment of the idiopathic respiratory-distress syndrome with continuous positive airway pressure. *New Engl. J. Med.* **43**, 1330

HAN, Y.H. and LOWE, J. (1961). Humidification of inspired air. *Anesthesiology* **22**, 135

HENVILLE, J.D. and ADAMS, A.P. (1976). A coaxial breathing circuit and scavenging valve. *Anaesthesia* **31**, 257–258

HILL, D.W.(1966). Recent developments in the design of electronically controlled ventilators. *Anaesthesist* **15**, 234

HILL, D.W. and MOORE, V. (1965). The action of adiabatic effects on the compliance of an artificial thorax. *Br. J. Anaesth.* **37**, 19

HILLYER, K.W. and JOHNSTON, R.R. (1978). Unsuspected dilution of anaesthetic gases detected by an oxygen analyser. *Anesth. Analg.* **57**, 491–492

HOWELLS, T.H. (1960). A new mechanical ventilator. *Br. J. Anaesth.* **32**, 438

HOWELLS, T.H. (1963). Choosing a pulmonary ventilator. *Br. J. Anaesth.* **35**, 272

JAIN, V.K. (1974). Optimal respirator settings in assisted respiration. *Med. biol. Engng* **12**, 425

JOHNSTON, R.P., DONOVAN, D.J. and MacDONNEL, K.F. (1974). PEEP during assisted respiration. *Anesthesiology* **40**, 308

KELLEHER, W.H.(1961). A new pattern of 'iron lung' for the prevention and treatment of airway complications in paralytic disease. *Lancet* **2**, 1113

KLAIN, M. and SMITH, R.B. (1976). Fluidic Technology. *Anaesthesia* **31**, 750–757

LAMONT, H. and FAIRLEY, H.B. (1965). A pressure sensitive ventilator alarm. *Anesthesiology* **26**, 359

LAWLER, P.G.P. and NUNN, J.F. (1977). Intermittent Mandatory Ventilation. *Anaesthesia* **32**, 138

LEWIS, F.J., DELLER, S. and QUINN, M. (1972). Continuous patient monitoring with a small digital computer. *Computers. Biomed. Res.* **5**, 411–428

LOESER, E.A. (1978). Water-induced resistance in disposeable respirator-circuit bacterial filters. *Anesth. Analg.* **57**, 269–271

MANLEY, R.W. (1961). A new mechanical ventilator. *Anaesthesia* **16**, 317

MANSON, H.J., ROSS, D.G. and DUNDAS, C.R. (1979). A paediatric ventilator with a fluidic control system. *Br. J. Anaesth.* **51**, 249–251

MAPLESON, W.W. (1962). The effect of changes of lung characteristics on the functioning of automatic ventilators. *Anaesthesia* **17**, 300

MITCHELL, N.J. and GAMBLE, D.R. (1973). Evaluation of the new 'Williams' anaesthetic filter. *Br. Med. J.* **2**, 653–654

MUSHIN, W.W., MAPLESON, W.W. and LUNN, J.N, (1962). Problems of automatic ventilation in infants and children. *Br. J. Anaesth.* **34**, 514

MUSHIN, W.W., RENDELL-BAKER, L., THOMPSON, P.W. and MAPLESON, W.W. (1969). *Automatic Ventilation of the Lungs.* 2nd Edn. Oxford; Blackwell

NORLANDER, O.P. (1964). Functional analysis of force and power of mechanical ventilators. *Acta anaesth. scand.* **8**, 57

OSBORN, J.J., BEAUMONT, J.O., RAISON, J.C.A., RUSSELL, J. and GERBODE, F. (1969). Measurement and monitoring of acutely ill patients by digital computer. *Surgery* **64**, 1057–1070

PARKER, G.A. (1967). Some applications of fluidics in medical engineering. *Bio-med. Engng* **2**, 436

PESLIN, R.L. (1969). The physical properties of ventilators in the inspiratory phase. *Anesthesiology* **30**, 315

PRICE, H.L., COOPER, F.H. and DRIPPS, R.D. (1954). Some respiratory and circulatory effects of mechanical ventilation. *J. appl. Physiol.* **6**, 517

PYBUS, D.A. and KERR, J.H. (1978). A simple system for administering intermittent mandatory ventilation (IMV) with the Oxford Ventilator. *Br. J. Anaesth.* **50**, 271–274

PYBUS, D.A., O'CONNOR, A.F. and HENVILLE, J.D. (1978). Anaesthesia for laryngoscopy: A technique using the Nuffield Anaesthetic Ventilator. *Br. J. Anaesth.* **50**, 501–504

ROBINSON, J.S. (1978). Respiratory Care and the Principles of Ventilation. In *The medical management of the acutely ill.* (Ed. by G.C. Hanson and P.L. Wright). London; Academic Press

ROBINSON, J.S., COX, C.A., BUSHMAN, J. and INGLIS, T. (1969). A pressure-cycled ventilator with multiple functional behaviour. *Br. J. Anaesth.* **41**, 455

ROCHFORD, J., WELCH, R.F. and WINKS, D.P. (1958). An electronic time cycled respirator. *Br. J. Anaesth.* **30**, 123

RUSSELL, W.R., SCHUSTER, E., SMITH, A.C. and SPALDING, J.M.K. (1956). Radcliffe respiration pumps. *Lancet* **1**, 539

SHEPARD, R.H., CAMPBELL, E.J.M., MARTIN, M.B. and ENNS, T. (1957). Factors affecting the pulmonary deadspace as determined by single breath analysis. *J. appl. Physiol.* **11**, 241

STRAUS, H.H. and MEYER, J. (1965). An evaluation of a fluid amplifier face mask respirator. Harry Diamond Laboratory Symposium, Washington, U.S.A. **3**, 309

SUGG, B.R. and PRYS-ROBERTS, C. (1976). The Penlon Oxford Ventilator. *Anaesthesia* **31**, 1234–1244

SYKES, M.K. (1964). Sterilizing mechanical ventilators. *Br. Med. J.* **1**, 561

SYKES, M.K. and LUMLEY, J. (1969). The effect of varying inspiratory: expiratory ratios on gas exchange during anaesthesia for open-heart surgery. *Br. J. Anaesth.* **41**, 374

THEILADE, D. (1978). Nasal CPAP treatment of the Respiratory Distress Syndrome. *Intensive Care Med.* **4**, 149–153

TRINKLE, J.K. (1971). A simple modification of existing respirators to provide constant positive-pressure breathing. *J. thorac. cardiovasc. Surg.* **61**, 617

VINCE, J.R. and BROWN, C.C. (1965). The application of fluid jet devices to a medical respirator. 1st Cranfield Fluidics Conf. F4–45

WALD, A.A., MURPHY, T.W. and MAZZIA, V.D. B. (1968). A theoretical study of controlled ventilation. *I.E.E.E. Trans. Biomed. Engng* **BME-15**, 237

WATSON, W.F. (1962). Some observations on dynamic lung compliance during intermittent positive pressure respiration. *Br. J. Anaesth.* **34**, 153

WATSON, W.F., SMITH, A.C. and SPALDING, J.M.K. (1962). Transmural central venous pressure during intermittent positive pressure respiration. *Br. J. Anaesth.* **34**, 278

WOODWARD, K.E., MUW, G., JOYCE, J., STRAUS, H.H. and BARLA, T.G. (1964). *Four fluid amplifier-controlled medical devices.* Washington, U.S.A.; Harry Diamond Laboratory Symposium

WRIGHT, B.M. (1958). A new nebulizer. *Lancet* **2**, 24

5 Properties of liquids, gases and vapours

Density

The pressure exerted by a column of liquid or gas depends on the density of the substance forming the column and on the value of gravity. Density links the volume and mass of a particular substance and is defined as the mass of a unit volume of the substance. In the SI system, density is expressed in kilograms per cubic metre (kg m^{-3}), although grams per cubic centimetre is allowable. The density of water is 1000 kg m^{-3} at 4 °C, while that of mercury is 13 600 kg m^{-3} at 20 °C. Density is temperature dependent, and strictly speaking, a value quoted for density must always be accompanied by the value of the temperature at which it was measured.

Although static columns of liquid are much used for measuring clinical pressures, as in a sphygmomanometer for blood pressure or a saline manometer for central venous pressure, anaesthetists are more concerned with the role of density and other factors in governing the motion and the measurement of flowing gases and liquids. These considerations are of importance in the study both of haemodynamics and respiratory mechanics.

Viscosity

While it is not true that respiratory passages and blood vessels consist of non-distensible pipes, this simplication is of assistance in describing the various patterns of fluid flow which are encountered. Fluid will flow from a region of higher pressure to one of lower pressure, the rate of flow depending on the pressure difference and the resistance to flow existing between the regions considered. For a given pressure drop developed across a given pipe, the volume of fluid (gas or liquid) flowing through the pipe per unit time depends on the *viscosity* of the fluid. This can be defined most simply as the resistance of the fluid to flow. A freely flowing liquid such as water has a low viscosity in contrast to a thick oil. The resistance to flow depends upon the inter-molecular forces operating within the liquid. In a viscous fluid the velocity of adjacent layers of the fluid will differ. Slip will occur between adjacent layers as a result of the shear force acting between them against the intermolecular forces. The viscosity of a fluid can now be defined as the resistance which the fluid exhibits to the flow of one layer over another, or more exactly as the ratio of shear stress to shear strain. The layers in contact with the walls of the pipe are assumed to be at rest, and the linear velocity of the fluid along the direction of flow increases from zero at the walls to a maximum at the axis. Under

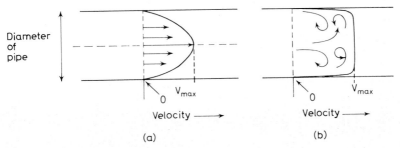

Figure 5.1.(a) Parabolic flow profile in laminar flow; (b) flat flow profile in turbulent flow

these conditions of streamline flow, if the velocity of the fluid is plotted against the distance measured from the axis, a parabolic velocity or flow profile is obtained (*Figure 5.1a*). When a new gas or liquid is introduced into the tube, the boundary between the old and new will move down the pipe with a parabolic profile.

Newton's law of viscous flow

Absolute or dynamic viscosity can be defined in quantitative terms from the simple model of *Figure 5.2*. Consider two parallel layers in the fluid, each of area A, situated at distances X and $X+x$ from one wall. The separation x is small compared with X. Let the corresponding velocities of the planes be V and $V+v$. Due to the internal friction in the fluid, as the layers slide relative to one another, a tangential shear force will exist between them. The shear stress on the fluid causing relative movement of the layers is equal to F/A where F is the tangential force acting. The rate of shear of a particular layer, also

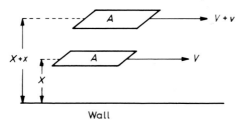

Figure 5.2

called the velocity gradient, is given by v/x, and has dimensions of s^{-1}. In *Figure 5.2*, let $v = 50$ cm s^{-1} and $x = 1$ cm. The velocity gradient between the two planes is then $(50$ cm s$^{-1})/1$ cm $= 50$ s^{-1}. Newton's law of viscous flow states that the rate of shear produced is directly proportional to the shear stress, i.e. $F = \eta A v / x$. The shear stress has dimensions of newtons per square metre. It only applies for streamline flow, that is, when the layers of fluid slide smoothly over each other, and not for turbulent flow. The quantity η is termed the coefficient of viscosity of the fluid. For a Newtonian fluid, the viscosity is independent of the magnitude of the shear stress and shear rate.

Laminar or streamline flow

Under the influence of moderate pressure gradients, the individual molecules of the fluid progress down the pipe in concentric cylindrical layers. The phenomenon is known as a *laminar* or *streamline* pattern of flow. Under these conditions, the volume of fluid (cubic metres) passing a given point in the pipe per second is related to the dimensions of the pipe by the well known Hagen–Poiseuille equation

$$\dot{Q} = \frac{\pi (P_1 - P_2) r^4}{8 \eta l}$$

where $\dot{Q}$ is the volume flowrate in m^{3}s^{-1}, P_1 is the inlet pressure and P_2 is the outlet pressure (both in N m^{-2}), r is the radius of the pipe in metres and η is the coefficient of viscosity of the fluid in millipascal seconds (mPa s) or centipoises, l is the length of the pipe in metres.

What is the volume flowrate in cubic metres per second through a pipe of length 0.1 metres and radius 1 millimetre (0.001 m) for a fluid of viscosity 3.6 mPa s when the pressure drop across the pipe is 10 000 Pa (N m^{-2})?

$$\dot{Q} = \frac{\pi \times 10\,000 \times (0.001)^4}{8 \times 3.6 \times 10^{-3} \times 0.1}$$

$$= 1.091 \times 10^{-5} \text{ m}^3\text{s}^{-1} = 10.91 \text{ cm}^3\text{s}^{-1}$$

It is evident that for a given fluid pressure drop and length of pipe, the quantity of fluid that can be passed per unit time will be dependent mainly on the radius since this occurs in the Poiseuille equation raised to the fourth power. Thus doubling the radius will increase the volume flow by a factor of $2^4 = 16$. It is for this reason that the lumen of endotracheal tubes and connectors should be kept as large as possible, and kinking avoided. Assuming laminar flow conditions, it is possible to apply a form of hydraulic or pneumatic Ohm's law, i.e. driving pressure/flow = resistance. The resistance offered by a pipe under these conditions is $P/\dot{Q} = kl/r^4$ where $P = (P_1 - P_2)$ and k is a constant for the fluid concerned. Hence, for sick patients breathing spontaneously with a weak respiratory effort, the choice of the length and lumen of any breathing circuit tubes should be aimed at reducing the circuit resistance to a minimum.

The achievement of laminar flow conditions is of importance in a pneumotachograph head. This is a resistance to gas flow so designed that the pressure drop developed across it is linearly related to the volume flow of gas through it (Fry *et al.*, 1957; Hill, 1959). Some designs use a 400-mesh gauze as the resistive element, while the well known design of Professor Fleisch of Lausanne can be considered to be a large number of small-bore pipes in parallel (*Figure 5.3*). The flow in each is then small enough to be streamline. Since the pressure drop depends on the viscosity of the gas used, a pneumotachograph must be calibrated for each gas mixture used (Hobbes, 1967). The problems of calibration are more marked when a pneumotachograph is used to monitor the oxygen uptake of a patient (Osborn *et al.*, 1969). Smith (1964) discusses the use of a pneumotachograph with a wide range of nitrous oxide–oxygen mixtures. Douma and Wammes (1978) have also investigated the sensitivity of a Fleisch II pneumotachograph with room

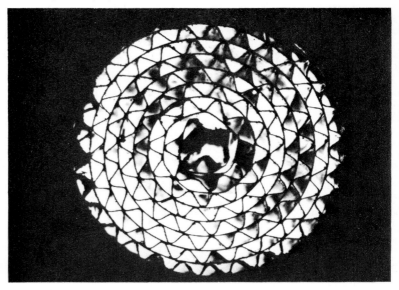

Figure 5.3. Cross-section of a Fleisch pneumotachograph head

air at the same temperature (24 °C) in the forward and reverse directions and with a 17 °C difference between the forward and reverse flow. If the sensitivity in the two directions was different it would cause a drift in the integrated output during respiratory investigations. A small sensitivity difference was detected with gas at the same temperature and this was not changed by the introduction of a 17 °C difference. During alternate inspiration and expiration, the static calibration at the mean temperature of the gas coming from both directions can be used.

Turbulent flow

From Poiseuille's equation, it is seen that the volume of fluid passing through a pipe per unit time is directly proportional to the pressure drop existing across the pipe, provided that the pattern of flow remains streamline. Increasing the value of the pressure drop across the tube above a certain limit will ultimately cause the orderly motion of the streamlines to break down. Localized turbulence starts to set in with the fluid swirling around in eddies. These can be triggered off by rough patches on the walls, sharp bends, branches or changes in diameter.

These local eddies tend to die out downstream when the flow pattern reverts to laminar conditions. At still greater pressure gradients across the pipe, the flow becomes fully turbulent. Whereas in laminar flow the flow profile is parabolic in shape, in fully turbulent flow the flow profile is almost flat (*Figure 5.1b*). That is to say, a marked velocity gradient exists close to the walls, while across the bulk of the pipe diameter the flow is maximum and constant. Turbulent flow is a less efficient manner of transporting the fluid molecules, since in order to produce a given increase in the volume flow, a greater increase in the pressure drop is now required than would have been the case with laminar flow. Particularly with spontaneously breathing patients, turbulence in connecting tubes is to be avoided if possible, since it will increase the work cost of breathing.

Relationship between flow and pressure

When the flow pattern is laminar, the flow through a pipe is directly proportional to the pressure across the pipe, i.e. $P=AF$ where F is the volume flow rate and A is a constant. When the flow is fully turbulent, the volume flow is nearly proportional to the square root of the pressure drop across the pipe, i.e. $P=BF^2$. When both laminar and turbulent conditions exist, these equations can be combined to give $P=AF+BF^2$. In a study in gas flow in post-mortem human air passages, Rohrer (1915) used the equation $P=0.79F+0.81F^2$. Fry *et al.* (1954) used $P=1.5F+0.71F^2$ in normal subjects and found both constants increased in patients with emphysema. A more general form $P=CF^n$ is found to hold over a wide range of flows. Cooper (1961) used $P=2.4F^{1.3}$. Of course $n=1$ for laminar flow and $n=2$ for fully turbulent flow. Taking logarithms of both sides of the equation, $\log P=\log C+n\log F$. The departure from laminar flow can be seen when the slope of the straight-line graph deviates from unity.

Critical velocity

Between the fully streamline and fully turbulent conditions of flow there exists a transitional region. The velocity V_c at which fully turbulent flow sets in is known as the *critical velocity*. It can be shown that for a Newtonian fluid $V_c = k\eta/\rho d$ where k is a non-dimensional constant known as Reynolds number, d is the tube diameter, η is the viscosity of the fluid and ρ is its density. The equation can be re-written in the form

$$V_c = \frac{k}{d}\left(\frac{\eta}{\rho}\right)$$

The ratio η/ρ is known as the kinematic viscosity of the fluid concerned. It is a measure of the 'flow' property of the fluid involving both shear characteristics (absolute viscosity) and fluid inertia (mass density) hence the name 'kinematic viscosity'. The dimensional formula for kinematic viscosity is $L^2 T^{-1}$. The SI unit of kinematic viscosity is the metre squared per second ($m^2 s^{-1}$). The CGS unit of kinematic viscosity is the stokes (St) where one stokes is equal to one square centimetre per second. The centistokes (0.01 stokes) is also allowable and 1 cSt= $10^{-6} m^2 s^{-1}$. The kinematic viscosity of a liquid can be determined by means of a capillary viscometer (Harkness, 1971). The kinematic viscosity of whole blood at 38 °C is approximately 3.8 centistokes.

For both blood and water, the onset of turbulence occurs at a Reynolds number of approximately 2000 (McDonald, 1974). For $k = 2000$, $d = 1$ cm and $\eta/\rho = 3.8 \times 10^{-2}$ St, $V_c = 76$ cm s^{-1}. For a cylindrical vessel the corresponding volume flowrate is 59.7 cm^3 s^{-1}.

The kinematic viscosity for oxygen is approximately twice that for nitrous oxide, so that for a given dimension of tube and a given pressure drop, it is to be expected that the flow for nitrous oxide would become turbulent at a considerably lower volume flow rate than would be the case for oxygen. McIlroy *et al.* (1955) showed how, by the use of gas mixtures having equal kinematic viscosities, it is possible to measure the tissue viscous resistance of a subject's lungs. At low fluid velocities, when the motion is streamline, the volume flow is directly proportional to the pressure drop. When the velocity is increased above the critical value, the volume flow increases less rapidly with increasing pressure. It soon becomes independent of the viscosity of the fluid, and dependent mainly on its density. When fully turbulent, the volume flow is nearly proportional to the square root of the pressure, i.e. the pressure is proportional to the square of the flow. The pressure is now used to overcome the turbulent motion, and in communicating kinetic energy to the fluid. (See also Glauser *et al.* (1969).)

Changes in the velocity profile occurring in a blood vessel can have an effect on the calibration of catheter-tip type electromagnetic flow probes (Mills, 1968). Mills found that the sensitivity of his flow probe increased by 13 per cent when the probe was in a laminar turbulent flow. Mills suggests that the probe averages the velocity over a small distance from itself. He also found that the result of angling the probe axis relative to the flow axis was less than expected, being less than 2 per cent variation at an angle of 30°. This seems to be due to the fact that the velocity stream lines follow the probe for a distance before breaking away, thus reducing the dependence on angle.

Examples of turbulent flow are to be found in both the respiratory and cardiovascular systems. The sound heard through a stethoscope in a healthy person during quiet breathing constitutes the normal respiratory murmur. The inspiratory murmur is a soft blowing sound at a frequency averaging 350 Hz (Graves and Graves, 1964). It is related to turbulence as air flows from the small air passages into the alveoli. It is heard only because it takes place so close to the stethoscope. Turbulent flow can occur at low gas velocities in the tracheobronchial tree due to its hundreds of thousands of branchings, and irregularities in the nature of the surfaces arising from the presence of mucus, exudate or foreign bodies. Under these conditions the flow is partly laminar and partly turbulent, the pressure differential and volume flow being related by $P=AF+BF^2$. Mead (1961) found that only at resting flow rates of 6 l min^{-1} can Reynolds numbers of less than 2000 be obtained in most of the tracheobronchial tree so that under normal conditions one would expect turbulent flow to be the predominant mode of gas transport. McDonald (1974) summarizes the finding of numerous workers on the possibilities of turbulence arising in the cardiovascular system. He points out that the absence of a murmur is no indication that the flow is in fact laminar, since fully developed turbulence can occur without any detectable sound. The high value of Reynolds number at peak systolic ejection suggests that the flow should be unstable for at least part of the cardiac cycle. It would be expected that turbulent flow in the circulation would occur at the root of the aorta and possibly at the heart valves where it may be responsible for the sound of murmurs. However, Bellhouse *et al.* (1968) mention that there has been no evidence produced from flow probes in the ascending aorta of a transition from laminar to turbulent flow. They state that the apparent absence of turbulence may be due to an inadequate frequency response of the flow probe, or the flow may have been truly laminar. Dintenfass (1971) makes the point that turbulence in the circulation must be much more rare than is commonly believed. The particular structure of blood does not yield itself easily to turbulent flow.

Turbulent flow conditions may arise from the rapid flow of blood through dilated vessels if the force and speed of the blood passing is sufficient. It may be possible to hear sounds usually referred to as 'bruits', the bruit generally pulsing in time with the heart beat. Vascular bruits arising from the local turbulence may also be produced by such things as sudden changes in the smoothness of the vessel wall or diameter, when a vessel branches.

Disturbances in the flow pattern arising from branching in a vessel have been considered by Knox (1962). Using branches of the single side-arm type he determined pressure recoveries after the bifurcation. The recovery length is defined as the distance downstream from the branch required for the pressure gradient to again become linear. The recovery length was found to be greater for side-arms than for main stems. Helps and McDonald (1954a, b) investigated venous flow patterns both *in vivo* and in a glass model and found that at Reynolds numbers less than 1000, dye injected had a parabolic profile in the tributary, but at the junction of the branch, a circulating movement developed. McDonald (1952) used the dye injection technique to show that marked flow disturbances were present at the aortic bifurcation in a rabbit at Reynolds numbers less than 1000. Stehbens (1959) simulated arterial bifurcations and the curvature of the carotid artery with glass models and found critical Reynolds numbers ranging from 306 to 1473. Krovetz (1965) found secondary turbulence at the bifurcation even though the upstream flow was well within the laminar range. The critical upstream Reynolds number for the onset of secondary flow in branches ranged from 58 to 79 per cent of the critical Reynolds number for the onset of turbulence in a straight tube. A pronounced secondary flow and significant mixing was found immediately distal to the bifurcation. Most of the mixing occurs close to the inner walls of the branches and little near the outer walls of the branches. The regions along the outer walls in branches thus represent an area of boundary-layer separation and local stasis.

Localized turbulence can be responsible for the erosion of arterial walls and the deposition of debris in stagnant flow regions can lead to the build-up of plaques. Kjeldsen *et al.* (1968) have confirmed that portions of blood vessel wall which are deprived of an adequate oxygen supply will receive an enhanced supply of cholesterol. Dintenfass (1971) states that the rigid arteriosclerotic vessel wall transmits the full force of the pulse wave without the normal damping action of the usual elastic vessel. This increases the systolic arterial pressure which, in turn, stimulates the deposition of collagen in the vessel wall and increases its strength and rigidity. Dintenfass makes the point that rheological changes in the vessel wall will lead to (1) formation of eddies or turbulence; (2) an enhanced aggregation of platelets, especially in stenotic regions; and (3) an initiation of clotting as a result of changes in the surface structure of the wall. The role of local turbulence and venturi effects in arteries in relation to thrombus formation is brought out by Kingsley *et al.* (1967). Two possible physical mechanisms have been proposed to explain the favouring of sites of branching in the arterial system by atherosclerotic disease. The plaque could either form by a deposition of material from the blood in a region of local flow stasis, or indirectly following damage to the arterial wall at points of locally increased shear followed by the fibroplastic proliferation and deposition of mucoid ground substances (Enos *et al.*, 1955). The first mechanism could be expected to start along the outer walls of branches, while the wall damage mechanism would be expected to start along the inner walls. A number of papers such as those of Fox and Hugh (1966), and Imparato *et al.* (1961) suggest wall damage as the initiating factor. Fry (1968) reports that a shear stress of about 300–460 dynes per cm^2 (30–46 N m^{-2}) maintained for as little as one hour is sufficient to produce histological changes in the endothelial cells of the arterial wall in dogs. Such values are likely to occur during peak flow in vessels such as the femoral artery in humans.

A clear account of the distribution of turbulence and disturbed flow patterns is given by McDonald (1974). It is interesting to see that whereas in the capillary circulation of the dog values of 0.001 have been measured for Reynolds number, in the human thoracic inferior vena cava it can have the range 1320–1980 and in the human ascending aorta 5000–12 000. El-Masry, Frierstein and Round (1978) have investigated four models of the aortic birfurcation, iliac bifurcation and a renal artery branch at volume flow rates giving Reynolds numbers in the range 1000–4000. The separated flows seen displayed streamlines forming an open vortex system with flows entering and leaving. These regions, which occur only at distinct combinations of flow rate and flow division may be key centres where platelet aggregations may form, release constituents and cause vessel damage.

The concept of peripheral resistance

Poiseuille's equation can be rearranged to give $(P_1 - P_2) = (8 \eta l \dot{Q})/\pi r^4$ where P_1 is the inlet pressure to a system of pipes in which the flow pattern is streamline, P_2 is the exit pressure and $\dot{Q}$ is the volume flow rate through the system per minute. By writing $\eta l / \pi r^4 = R$, the hydraulic resistance of the system, the equation becomes a form of hydraulic Ohm's law. The length of any vascular channel is virtually constant and so, to an approximation, is the blood viscosity. Thus the hydraulic resistance is largely determined by the radii of the smallest diameter pipes. This reasoning can be applied to the cardiovascular system where the resistance of the arterioles represents the largest proportion of the total resistance. Considering the complete vascular bed of a limb, the total fluid resistance consists of the resistances in series of the arteries, the arterioles, the capillaries and the veins. For a mean arterial blood pressure of 100 mmHg, there will be a pressure drop of about 60 mmHg in the arterioles. The total resistance is largely concentrated in the periphery with the arterioles, but the resistance of other portions of the vascular bed is not negligible. The pressure difference across the cardio-vascular system is approximately mean aortic pressure minus mean right atrial pressure and the volume flow of blood per minute is the cardiac output. Thus (mean aortic pressure) $-$ (mean right atrial pressure)= (cardiac output×total peripheral resistance). It may be possible in fit patients to neglect the mean right atrial pressure in comparison with the mean aortic pressure. The peripheral resistance can be expressed in terms of mmHg ml^{-1} per minute. A unit of peripheral resistance (P.R.U.) can be defined as 1 mmHg ml^{-1} per minute. For a cardiac output of 5 litres per minute and a mean aortic pressure of 100 mmHg, the peripheral resistance is 100/5000=0.02 P.R.U. Even with a low blood pressure, a good cardiac output can be maintained if the resistance is sufficiently low. The total systemic resistance of the vascular system is a crude concept and may not reflect changes occurring in regional blood flows such as renal, skin and muscle flows. In the CGS system, pressure is expressed as dynes cm^{-2}, so that peripheral resistance (pressure/volume flow per second) becomes dyn s cm^{-5}. In the SI system, pressure is in newtons metre^{-2}, so that if a volume flow is in cubic metres per second, then peripheral resistance is expressed in newton seconds metre^{-5}. In practice it is more convenient in the SI system to express peripheral resistance in terms of kN m^{-2} cm^{-3} s. The reason why it is convenient to use kN m^{-2} can be seen by considering a blood pressure of 100 mmHg. The equivalent weight per cm^2 is 10 × 13.6 grams weight, where 13.6 g cm^{-3} is the density of mercury. In dynes this becomes 10 × 13.6 × 981 which is 1.36 × 0.981 N cm^{-2} = 1.33 N cm^{-2} = 13.33 kN m^{-2}. Since 1 dyn cm^{-2} = 10^{-1}N m^{-2} a vascular resistance given in

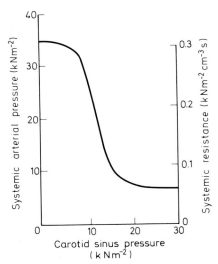

Figure 5.4. Interdependence of systemic arterial pressure, carotid sinus pressure and systemic resistance, all expressed in SI units

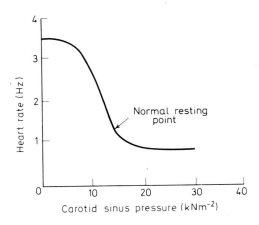

Figure 5.5. Relationship between heart rate expressed in hertz and carotid sinus pressure

dyn s cm^{-5} can be converted to kN m^{-2} cm^{-3} s by multiplying by 10^{-4}. For a cardiac output of 10 litres per minute in man, the vascular resistance might be about 800 dyn s cm^{-5}. This is equivalent to 0.08

kN m^{-2}cm^{-3}s. In *Figure 5.4* is illustrated the interdependence of systemic arterial pressure, carotid sinus pressure and systemic resistance all expressed in the relevant SI units. The relationship between heart rate expressed in hertz rather than beats per minute and carotid sinus pressure is shown in *Figure 5.5*.

Units of viscosity

As has already been demonstrated by means of dimensional analysis, the dimensions of absolute or dynamic viscosity are $ML^{-1}T^{-1}$. This expression can be rearranged to yield $(MLT^{-2})(L^{-2})T$. The product of mass × acceleration (MLT^{-2}) represents a force so that the dimensions of viscosity are those of a (force per unit area) × seconds. Hence the units of viscosity in the SI system are pascal seconds (Pa s). A more convenient unit is the mPa s (e.g. the viscosity of water at 20 °C is 1 mPa s). Blood is a non-Newtonian fluid and its viscosity depends on the shear rate.

The values of viscosity are measured with an instrument known as a viscometer. A capillary viscometer (Bate, 1977) has the advantage that it corresponds to the physiological situation of blood flowing through vessels, neglecting the visco-elastic properties of the vessels and pulsatile flow. In the cone-plate viscometer (Wells *et al.*, 1961) each measurement is made at a constant shear rate, but it is not easy to project the result to the physiological situation. The main disadvantage of the capillary viscometer lies in the range of shear rates present, from zero at the centre of the tube to a maximum at the wall, since the viscosity of whole blood is shear-dependent. Dintenfass *et al.* (1966) quote the following values for the blood viscosities (*Table 5.1*). Shear rates in the human aorta are likely to lie in the range 50 s^{-1} to 100 s^{-1} and Whitmore (1967) found that within this range blood behaves as a nearly Newtonian fluid with an average viscosity of 3.6 mPa s. The blood of

TABLE 5.1. Blood viscosities

Shear rate (s^{-1})	*Whole blood viscosity* (mPa s)	
	Normal women	*Normal men*
0.01	1190	990
0.1	222	210
1.0	41	45
7.2	13	15
29	7.0	9.5
118	4.8	5.6

women has normally a somewhat lower viscosity than that of men, and that of children a lower viscosity than that of adults.

In the CGS system, the unit of viscosity was the Poise (P), equal to 1 dyne centimetre^{-2} second. Now, 1 mPa s = (1/1000) newton metre^{-2} second = (1/100) dyne centimetre^{-2} second. Hence 1mPa s = 1 cP (centipoise, the common CGS unit). A calibration fluid for a capillary viscometer is quoted as having a viscosity of 5.4 cP at 25 °C, i.e., 5.4 mPa s.

The anomalous viscosity of blood

Newton's law of viscous flow states that the shear rate is directly proportional to the shear stress, so that a plot of shear stress against shear rate would be a straight line passing through the origin in the case of a Newtonian fluid such as water. The viscosity is independent of the shear rate while the flow remains laminar. Such a fluid is homogenous, but whole blood is not (Haynes and Burton, 1959). This is apparent from *Figure 5.6* which introduces the concept of the yield stress. A definite initial value of the yield stress must be applied before the blood will flow. However, if whole blood is defibrinated, or washed red cells are suspended in saline solution, an almost Newtonian behaviour is observed (Replogle *et al.,* 1967). The fibrinogen and erythrocytes together produce intercellular bonding, multicellular aggregation and the anomalous flow behaviour of whole blood (Greenbaum, 1969).

Replogle *et al.* (1967) showed that red cell aggregation is reversible. It is a maximum when the flow is zero, the aggregates breaking up as the flow rate is increased. At slow flows much of the shear stress is used to dissipate the aggregates, while at the higher flows most of the shear stress is available to generate the flow velocity. Replogle *et al.* (1967) plotted the square root of the shear stress against the square root of the shear rate and extrapolated back to zero shear rate in order to determine the yield stress. This represents the force required to disrupt aggregates of red cells in stagnant blood. It is positive if the plasma fibrinogen concentration is greater than 140 mg per 100 ml and depends on both the plasma fibrinogen concentration and the haematocrit. The yield stress is responsible for a significant portion of the peripheral resistance when the flow is low and it is not affected by anticoagulants (Greenbaum, 1969).

Gordon and Ravin (1978) state that the rheological behaviour of whole blood is determined by two variables, non-Newtonian viscosity and yield stress. At rest blood forms a three-dimensional network wherein red blood cells are interconnected by negatively charged fibrinogen molecules. A certain minimum stress is required to start this network in motion and this is the yield stress.

The Casson equation (Casson, 1959) can be used to describe the relationship between shear stress and shear rate for blood flow (Merrill, 1969). Casson's equation is: (shear stress)$^{1/2}$ = k_o + k_1 (shear rate). When the shear rate is zero, the yield stress = k_o^2.

In the case of whole blood, deviations from a simple Newtonian behaviour arise in two ways, (1) due to the fact that at low shear rates the viscosity increases, and (2) in small-calibre vessels, the apparent viscosity at all rates of shear is lower than that found in larger vessels (Haynes, 1960; Fahraeus and Lindqvist, 1931; Merrill *et al.,* 1963, 1965). It is seen that the viscosity of whole blood is dependent not only upon the volume concentration of the red cells, but also upon the mechanical factors which operate upon the blood during flow. This is illustrated by the fact that Wells (1967) reports in normal man a blood viscosity value of approximately 5 mPa s above the aortic valve, whereas in the postcapillary venules it will have risen to a value of the order of 50 mPa s. Greenbaum (1969) states that the shear rate in the aorta of man has been estimated to be approximately 100 s^{-1}, while in the arteriolar bed it is about 10 s^{-1}, and in parts of the microcirculation only about 0.01 s^{-1}. These shear rates correspond with viscosity values of 6, 10 and 800 mPa s.

Blood is a thixotropic fluid. Dintenfass (1971) states that a thixotropic system is one in which the viscosity depends on both the time and the shear rate and decreases with increasing rate of shear. Above a critical rate of shear, the viscosity remains constant and is independent of any further increase in the shear rate. It is the basic characteristic of a thixotropic system that when its viscosity is plotted against the shear rate on a log–log scale the plot consists of two straight lines which intersect at the critical shear rate. Dintenfass has found that the thixotropy of human blood is due to at least two or three mechanisms – a contribution due to the aggregation of red cells, contributions of the interior and of the membrane of the red cell, and a possible contribution of the plasma. He also found that blood viscosity measured *in vitro* at low shear rates is 4–5 and sometimes as much as 10 times greater for patients with myocardial infarction or arterial thrombosis than that of healthy subjects.

During haemorrhagic shock, when low blood flow rates can occur, the situation may be exacerbated by the increase in blood viscosity which occurs due to a partial settling out of the cells. If the apparent viscosity of blood depends only upon the shearing force, then it should be independent of the radius of the vessel. In practice, this is so if the radius of the vessel is approximately 100 times greater than the red cell diameter. However, in a 20 μm diameter vessel such as an arteriole, the effective viscosity of the blood is reduced to about two-thirds of the value as measured in a viscometer. The red cells tend to congregate along the axis of the vessel, leaving a layer of plasma lying along the walls. This effect in capillaries having diameters of between approximately 100 and 1000 μm is known as the Fahraeus–Lindqvist phenomenon after the work of Fahraeus and Lindqvist (1931).

Since the plasma has a lower viscosity than the red cells, a greater flow results than would be expected from the value of the *in vitro* viscosity (Hershey and Cho, 1966). The axial drift of the red cells during flow through a narrow tube has been discussed by Bayliss (1959), and the effect of this on the electrical conductivity of flowing blood by Liebman *et al.* (1962). This is a factor in the determination of regional blood flows by the method of electrical impedance plethys-mography.

A detailed account of the anomalous viscosity and rheology of blood is that of Bayliss (1962). Rheology is the study of the properties of a material which affect the way in which it flows. Dintenfass *et al.* (1966) described a trolley-mounted cone-in-cone viscometer which could be used at the bedside in order to obtain data on the viscosity of freshly shed blood, for example in studies on anti-coagulant therapy.

At the start of this chapter, it was mentioned that if Newton's law of viscous flow is obeyed, then the shear rate produced is directly proportional to the applied shear stress. The constant of proportion-ality is related to the viscosity. For a given shear rate, the higher the viscosity of the fluid, the higher will have to be the applied shear stress. For a Newtonian fluid, the viscosity should be independent of the shear stress. A departure from Newtonian behaviour will be revealed by a non-linearity of the plot of shear stress against shear rate. These points are well illustrated in *Figure 5.6* which shows the non-Newtonian behaviour of various bloods at low shear stresses and the increase in viscosity with increasing haematocrit and fibrinogen levels. The effect of increasing the haematocrit on the viscosity of blood has been studied *in vivo* by Agarwal *et al.* (1970). In the majority of their dogs they

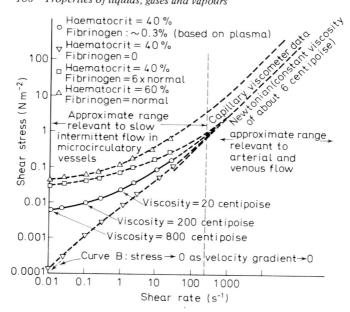

Figure 5.6. A double logarithmic plot of shear stress against shear rate for bloods having various haematocrits and fibrinogen levels. This reveals the dependence of viscosity on shear stress for a non-Newtonian fluid and the effects of haematocrit and fibrinogen level on the viscosity. (From Replogle *et al.* (1967) by permission of the authors and the American Heart Association)

found an exponential relationship between the pulmonary vascular resistance and the haematocrit at a given left atrial pressure. With a left atrial pressure of 5 to 20 mmHg they reported a relative viscosity of blood to plasma of 2.34 with a haematocrit of 45 per cent. Nygaard *et al.* (1935) discuss the relationship between blood viscosity and the haematocrit. The role played by viscosity in determining regional blood flows is discussed by Schenk *et al.* (1964).

The effects of administering low-viscosity dextran to patients in a state of shock are discussed by Carey *et al.* (1965) and by Meiselman *et al.* (1967). Since the dextran is used as a plasma expander, by replenishing the fluid volume lost by patients in shock, it will assist in raising the central venous pressure. Meiselman *et al.* (1967) point out that plasma expanders have as their basic purpose the development of an appropriate 'colloidal' osmotic pressure in a saline solution so that such solutions will at least remain temporarily within the circulating system when infused into patients suffering from a depleted intravascular volume. On this basis, the lowest molecular weight colloids produce the greatest effect per unit concentration. The effect is not reliable in practice because diuresis rapidly removes colloid species having molecular weights significantly less than albumin (67 000). Haldemann *et al.* (1979) indicated that the general effect of the various colloids on the blood volume depends primarily on the molecular size of the colloids. Gelatine has a relatively short duration of action, hydroxyethyl starch a much longer one, and dextran occupies an intermediate position. Haldemann *et al.* (1979) studied the effect of an infusion of 800 ml 3 per cent dextran Ringer's lactate in two groups of young surgical patients who had no significant blood loss during surgery. One group was normovolaemic and the other was made hypovolaemic by the rapid withdrawal of 600 ml of blood. There was a restoration of the initial blood volume within 48 hours for the normovolaemic patients and a maintenance of the restituted volume in the hypovolaemic patients.

Gelin and Ingelman (1961) discuss the use of Rheomacrodex, a dextran fraction with an average molecular weight of approximately 40 000, for the rheological treatment of impaired capillary flow. They showed that in a particular patient with bile peritonitis, the infusion of 500 ml of 15 per cent Rheomacrodex reduced the whole-blood viscosity by approximately one-third. In patients having intravascular aggregation of blood cells and an impaired capillary flow, the infusion of the dextran solution increased the fluidity of the blood and improved both the capillary flow and the peripheral circulation. However, Meiselman *et al.* (1967) showed that dextrans of molecular weights of 40 000 and above increased both the yield stress of blood and the low shear rate viscosity compared with the values obtained with controls of equal haematocrit and plasma protein concentration made with a plain isotonic saline solution. They stated that the flow improvement noted after the infusion of dextran solutions must result from a change in the haematocrit and plasma protein concentration arising from the dilution. Long *et al.* (1961) discussed the use of plasma expanders in an extra-corporeal circulation. Reemtsma and Creech (1962) studied the viscosity of blood, plasma and plasma substitutes. Sykes *et al.* (1967) showed that there was no significant difference in base loss or lactate or pyruvate concentrations between perfusions conducted with whole prime blood and those in which blood diluted with low molecular weight dextran (with or without the addition of dextrose-saline) had been used.

Cullen and Eger (1970) found in dogs that the replacement of shed blood with cell-free solutions such as dextran resulted in an increased cardiac output in order to compensate for the lowered oxygen content of the diluted blood. Chapler *et al.* (1972) found that the mechanisms for the increased cardiac output were an increased cardiac sympathetic drive and a lowered left ventricular outflow impedance.

The flow of fluids through orifices

In a pipe or tube, the length is large compared with the radius. This is in contrast to an orifice where the length is less than the radius. The radius of an orifice is small and the flow pattern of fluid through it is always partly turbulent. The rate of flow is now dependent on the density of the fluid rather than on its viscosity. The lower the density, the less is the pressure drop required across the orifice to sustain a given rate of fluid flow. For this reason, a helium-oxygen mixture is sometimes administered to patients suffering from respiratory obstruction, since this mixture can be respired with less effort than air or pure oxygen. A good account of the principles of helium therapy is given by Egan (1973) who makes the point that a mixture of 70 per cent helium, 30 per cent oxygen by volume is probably the most generally useful mixture. Egan states that the use of helium—oxygen is specifically indicated for the patient with diffuse airway obstruction, especially when due to bronchospasm as in status asthmaticus or following instrumentation or other traumatic bronchial irritation.

The critical orifice

An interesting case arises in that of the so-called *critical orifice*. If the pressure on the downstream side of a thin, sharp-walled, orifice is less than 58 per cent of the absolute pressure on the upstream side then the gas passing through the orifice attains the velocity of sound in a gas given by

$$v = \sqrt{\left(\frac{\gamma P}{\rho}\right)}$$

where γ is the ratio of the specific heats of the gas at constant pressure and constant volume for the gas concerned, P is the pressure at the orifice in N m^{-2}, and ρ is the density of the gas in kg m^{-3} and v is in m s^{-1}. Since the velocity of gas through a critical orifice limits at the velocity of sound, if the cross-sectional area of the orifice is A m^2, the volume flow rate which passes is

$$V = A \sqrt{\left(\frac{\gamma P}{\rho}\right)}$$

A simple carbon dioxide analyser based on this principle is that of Mead and Collier (1959) (*Figure 5.7*). The use of a critical orifice ensures that

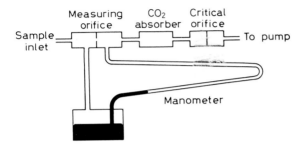

Figure 5.7. Critical orifice carbon dioxide analyser

gas leaves the CO_2 absorber at a constant volume flow rate. This gas consists of the balance of the mixture after the CO_2 has been removed. The pressure drop developed across the inlet's non-critical orifice depends on the rate at which gas enters the system, and this in turn depends on the rate of absorption of carbon dioxide. The inclined manometer can thus be calibrated in terms of the carbon dioxide concentration present in the sampled gas stream.

Factors affecting the calibration of rotameter gas flowmeters

Rotameter-type flowmeters are widely used both mounted on anaesthetic machines and in the laboratory, for the measurement of the volume flow rates of gases. Their construction is illustrated in *Figure 5.8*. It consists basically of a lightweight bobbin, often made of aluminium, and an accurately tapered glass tube. The tube is formed by shrinking the glass down on to a mandrel. The pressure of the gas flowing upwards supports the weight of the bobbin. The bobbin may have flutes cut into it. The action of the gas flowing through these flutes causes the bobbin to rotate and thus minimize friction between

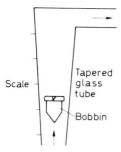

Figure 5.8. Rotameter gas flowmeter

the bobbin and the tube wall. When the flow through the tube is increased, the float is caused to take up a new position higher up the tube, and this action increases the area of the annulus lying between the bobbin and the wall of the tube. At low flow rates, when the gap between the bobbin and tube is small, the restriction is approximately tubular. At the higher flows the width of the gap increases and is greater than the length. Hence, at low flows the calibration is more affected by the gas viscosity, whereas at the higher flows the density is more important. These facts are illustrated by the use of a cyclopropane rotameter to measure carbon dioxide. The two gases have similar densities, but different viscosities. Particularly at the lower flow rates for the rotameter tube concerned, there will be a marked discrepancy between the true volume flow of carbon dioxide and the value indicated on the cyclopropane flowmeter. The indicated value is higher than the true value, approximately double at the lower end and decreasing at the upper end of the scale. Chadwick (1974) discusses a situation where a patient received a hypoxic gas mixture as a result of a cyclopropane rotameter tube being substituted for an oxygen rotameter tube. When the indicated flow was 5 litres of oxygen per minute, the cyclopropane rotameter was only passing 400 ml per minute in fact.

For these reasons, it is desirable to check the calibration of a rotameter experimentally if it is not used with the gas for which it was intended. For flows of up to a few hundred millilitres/minute, a soap film flowmeter can be used as an inexpensive reference, the flow causes the film to rise up a calibrated burette, and the time taken for it to traverse a given volume is recorded. For higher volume flows, a spirometer or dry gas meter are suitable (Adams *et al.,* 1967). Eger and Epstein (1964) discuss the various ways in which an error can arise in the reading of a rotameter flowmeter forming part of an anaesthetic machine. They recommend that the oxygen rotameter should be sited nearest to the patient. In this way, an escape of the gas mixture via a leak in another rotameter tube housing will not diminish the amount of oxygen fed per minute to the patient. Another form of gas flow-meter which may be encountered in anaesthetic practice is the type using a steel ball which is caused by the flow to rise up a tapered glass tube (Ewing, 1925). In some versions the tube is vertical, whilst in others it slopes.

Luminous panels are now available which can be clipped on to the rear of the flowmeter tubes to provide an illumination of the scales when the anaesthetic machine is used in a darkened operating room. They are activated by the radioactive emission of weak beta particles from sealed sources of radioactive hydrogen (tritium)

Dial mixing devices for gases

Anaesthetists commonly require to administer to an anaesthetic circuit a known mixture of oxygen and nitrous oxide at a certain minute volume. This is usually accomplished by means of a needle valve and flowmeter for each gas. Some degree of thought is required to obtain both the desired concentration and the minute volume and there is the possibility of a hypoxic mixture resulting if the emptying of the oxygen cylinder passes unnoticed in the absence of a suitable warning device. These considerations have led to the development of mixing units such as the Quantiflex monitored dial mixer by Cyprane Ltd. The unit is provided with separate mixture and total flow rate controls plus two monitoring ball-in-tube flowmeters. The performance of the Quantiflex has been examined by Heath, Anderson and Nunn (1973). They found that the two controls had a negligible interaction and that the delivered oxygen concentration was sufficiently close to the mixture control setting for safety requirements over a wide range of conditions including variations in gas input and output pressures. Within ±20 per cent of the specified input pressure (4 atmospheres gauge) the delivered oxygen concentrations ranged from 3 per cent below to 4 per cent above the mixture control setting. Concentrations of up to 5 per cent above the setting were given with a combination of a low (2 litres per minute) total gas flow rate and the output resistance provided by a Manley ventilator and a Fluotec Mark 3 vaporizer in series. Under no circumstances did Heath and his colleagues find that the Quantiflex delivered an oxygen concentration which was less than the mixture control setting by a clinically significant margin. The basic principle of the mixer is given in *Figure 5.9*. The mixture control valve which sets the relative proportions of the two gases is a differential needle valve. After leaving the needle valves, the individual gas streams pass

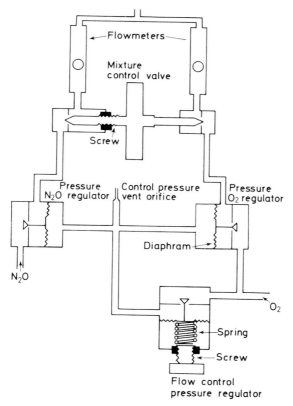

Figure 5.9. Simplified circuit diagram of the Quantiflex to show principles of operation. (From Heath, Anderson and Nunn, 1973)

through a flowmeter before being mixed in order to permit each flow to be visually monitored. The needle valves are fed from a pair of pressure regulators which deliver each gas at the same pressure which is determined by the flow control pressure regulator. This exerts its action by altering the reference pressure applied to the diaphragms of the two supply regulators. A higher reference pressure increases the inlet pressure to each needle valve and thus the gas flow through it. In order that the flow control pressure may be reduced when it is desired to reduce the total gas flow, a bleed orifice is provided in the flow control pressure line. The reference pressure is obtained from the oxygen supply in order that if this runs out, the nitrous oxide valve will be automatically closed. On the other hand, if the nitrous oxide supply becomes exhausted, the oxygen output continues. The control pressure vent actually bleeds into the oxygen outlet of the mixture control valve rather than to atmosphere and two nitrous oxide reducing valves are provided in series as an additional precaution against the release of nitrous oxide in the case of an oxygen supply failure. The mixture control is graduated in steps of 10 per cent oxygen concentration and each flowmeter is scaled from 0–10 litres per minute. The Quantiflex, designed to work with output pressures up to 17 cmH$_2$O, is shown in *Figure 5.10.*

The Dräger company have produced the Oxymix device for mixing air and oxygen for intensive therapy applications. It can provide either preset 100 per cent oxygen or air (21 per cent oxygen), or an infinite adjustment of the mixture between 30 and 90 per cent oxygen. No

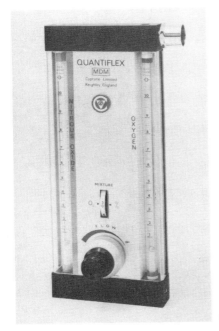

Figure 5.10. The Quantiflex gas mixing device. (By courtesy of Cyprane Ltd)

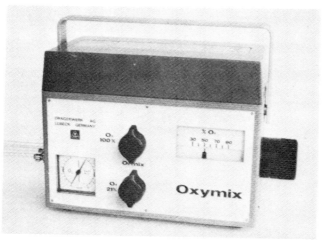

Figure 5.11. The Oxymix gas mixer. (By courtesy of Drägerwerk AG, Lübeck)

flowmeters are provided, *Figure 5.11*. A flow range of 0 to 30 litres per minute is available when the Oxymix is used with a ventilator having an inspiratory/expiratory period ratio of 1:2. If one of the two gas supplies fails, the gas supply is then automatically maintained with whichever supply is still available. A dual pressure gauge is provided to monitor the individual gas supply pressures.

Injectors

An injector is a gas-powered device for producing suction. Quite considerable negative pressures can be produced by this means. Hill (1966b) mentions the use of an injector powered from an oxygen cylinder, and mounted on an electronically controlled automatic lung ventilator. The injector is capable of producing a negative pressure of 600 mmHg for use with suction catheters. The suction from an injector may also be employed to entrain an additional stream of gas for mixing with the driving stream of the injector. Gas from an injector may also be employed to entrain an additional stream of gas for mixing with the driving stream of the injector. Nunn (1961) used an injector drawing one litre per minute from an oxygen cylinder to entrain sufficient air to ensure that the final mixture available to the patient contained 30

per cent v/v of oxygen. The compact Cyclator ventilator produced by
B.O.C. is powered by an oxygen supply from a cylinder or pipeline.
This driving gas passes through a two-stage injector to entrain the anaes-
thetic gas mixture. This design will be discussed further.

The basic action of an injector can be seen by considering a pipe
fitted with a restriction, and through which flows a stream of gas
(*Figure 5.12*). If the volume flow rate is the same throughout the pipe,

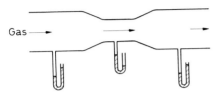

Figure 5.12. Basic action of an entrainer

then the linear velocity must be greater throughout the restriction.
Experiment shows that the lateral pressure in the pipe is lowest where
the velocity is greatest. By making the tube open out in the shape of a
narrow-angle cone immediately after the restriction, the gas is thus able
to regain almost the pressure which it had before the restriction. This
arrangement is known as a *venturi tube*. A side-arm is fitted to the
restriction through which suction is available as in a suction injector. In
a well-designed injector, a considerable subatmospheric pressure can be
generated. In this simple design the increased kinetic energy of the gas
together with frictional losses results in a loss of potential (pressure)

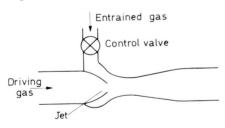

Figure 5.13. Simple injector

energy. In *Figure 5.13* the restriction has been replaced by a jet, and an
entrainment tube provided adjacent to the jet. The conical portion
increases the entrainment efficiency by reducing wasteful turbulence,
and converting as much as possible of the kinetic energy back into
potential energy. The entrainment ratio of a well-designed injector is

relatively independent of the volume flow rate of the driving gas, and is set by the size of the orifice of the entrainment tube. This may be a needle valve or a series of different sized holes in a circular plate. The latter system is used to select various concentrations of oxygen for supply to an oxygen tent.

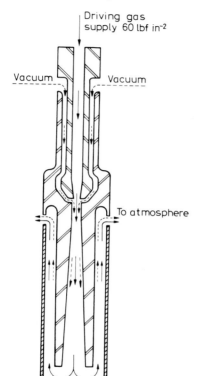

Figure 5.14. Suction injector suitable for use during anaesthesia. With a driving gas pressure of 60 lbf in^{-2} (413 kN m^{-2}) the following (maximum) performance can be expected: vacuum, 0.5 mHg; entrained air, 13.4 l/min. (By courtesy of British Oxygen Co. Ltd)

An injector designed to produce suction for use by the anaesthetist is illustrated in *Figure 5.14*. It develops a negative pressure of 7.2 metres of water when supplied with 28 litres of oxygen per minute from a 60 lbf in^{-2} (413.7 kN m^{-2}) supply. A typical injector having two stages in series is used in the Cyclator ventilator; it has a total entrainment ratio of only 3 to 1 (*Figure 5.15*), but is little affected by the build-up of back pressure (*Figure 5.16*). The variation of the output gas mixture composition over the normal range of lung inflation pressures is only of the order of plus or minus 2 per cent. This is less

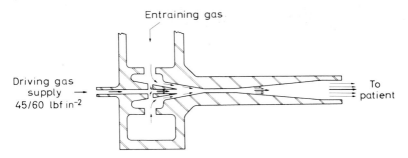

Figure 5.15. Typical two-stage injector producing high-efficiency entraining values. (By courtesy of British Oxygen Co. Ltd)

than the variation in mixture composition consequent upon the use of the usual bank of rotameters. The percentage of driving gas in the output mixture will fall by 3 per cent v/v from its nominal 25 per cent v/v when air or oxygen is entrained, the 25 per cent being set up when entraining pure nitrous oxide. The result of entraining pure helium is to reduce the concentration of driving gas in the output mixture from a nominal 25 per cent v/v to 15 per cent v/v. These effects arise from the changes occurring in the viscosity of the gas mixture.

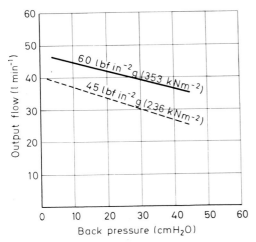

Figure 5.16. The variation of the output flow from an air-driven two-stage injector entraining air against an increasing back pressure. (By courtesy of British Oxygen Co. Ltd)

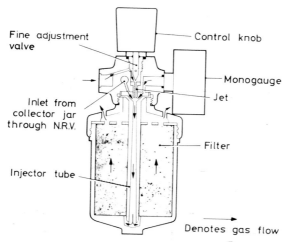

Figure 5.17. Cross-section of injector-type suction unit for use with a pipeline supply of air or oxygen. (By courtesy of British Oxygen Co. Ltd)

An injector can also provide the intermittent suction required for sucking-out patients in an intensive care unit. *Figure 5.17* shows the cross-section of a suction unit which can be run from a 60 lbf in^{-2}g oxygen or compressed air pipeline. The input to the suction unit from the collector jar is via a non-return valve to prevent the ingress of fluid. A suction of 200 mmHg is produced from an oxygen or air consumption of 17 litres per minute. The volume of air entrained is then 24 litres per minute.

Surface tension

The attractive force existing between molecules gives rise, in liquids, to a phenomenon known as *surface tension*. In the bulk of the liquid, a molecule is surrounded by others on all sides, and the attractive forces between neighbouring molecules will tend to cancel. However, a molecule situated at the surface will receive a net inward force from those below it in the liquid. The number of molecules per unit volume in the vapour is obviously much less than that for the liquid. The fact that a liquid surface will contract spontaneously shows that there is free energy associated with it, and that work must be done to extend the surface. The surface of a liquid acts at all times as though it had a thin membrane stretched over it, and for any specified volume of matter a sphere has a smaller surface area than any other geometrical figure. Hence droplets of water and soap bubbles assume a spherical shape as they fall though the air. When a surface pulling with a tension of S newtons per metre is extended by one metre, the work done is S $N \cdot m^{-2}$. A joule is one metre newton, so that the SI units for surface tension are newtons per metre and the dimensions are $M.T^{-2}$. In the CGS system, surface tension is expressed in dynes per cm. In SI units it is more convenient to use millinewtons per metre and 1 dyn $cm^{-1} =$ 1 mN m^{-1}. Surface tension is defined as the force of contraction across a line of unit length, the line and the force being perpendicular to each other, and both lying in the plane of the liquid surface. The surface tension of water at $20\,°C$ is 75 dyn cm^{-1} (75 mN m^{-1}). The surface tension of blood serum at $37\,°C$ is 57–58 mN m^{-1}.

It is shown in standard physics textbooks that the pressure existing inside a bubble is given by $2S/r$ N m^{-2}, where S is the surface tension of the liquid coating the bubble, and r is the radius of the bubble in metres. The pressure inside the bubble, holding it in shape, is raised above atmospheric by the compressive tension of the film. This force can be high when the radius of the bubble is small, resulting in a stable bubble. The formation of such persistent droplets may cause trouble when it is desired to vaporize a liquid such as halothane in order to produce accurate concentrations of halothane vapour. For example, the saturated vapour pressure of halothane cooled to $-30\,°C$ is 16.8 mmHg. Assuming a barometric pressure of 760 mmHg, this will correspond to a halothane concentration of 2.2 per cent v/v. However, a rather higher value is commonly measured due to the carry-over and subsequent evaporation of droplets of liquid. This effect can be eliminated by passing the gas and vapour issuing from the vaporizing vessel through a condensing coil immersed in the coolant bath in order to trap out any droplets.

Surface tension and the lungs

Surface tension plays an important part in the contraction of the lungs. It is responsible for the high opening pressure of collapsed alveoli and is partly responsible for the retractive force of expanded alveoli. The alveoli can be considered as a large number of bubbles, each communi-cating with the lung volume via a duct. If the surface tension of the alveolar lining remained constant, the pressure in the smaller alveoli would be higher than that in the larger alveoli. This would lead to an unstable situation, with the smaller alveoli tending to discharge into the larger ones. Brown, Johnson and Clements (1959), Clements *et al.* (1961), and Pattle (1955; 1967) have shown that the surface tension of the alveolar lining fluid is not constant, but decreases markedly on compression resulting from deflation. With changes of surface area of less than 50 per cent, the lung surface tension approaches a limiting value of $10-15$ mN m^{-1}. On re-expansion of the surface, an upper limiting tension of $40-50$ mN m^{-1} is approached. When the compression is such that the surface area is reduced by more than 50 per cent, considerable hysteresis occurs, indicating a major alteration of the surface. The diminution in the surface tension which occurs with a reduction in area is thought to be due to the action of a lipo-protein or substance which is known as the 'anti-atelectatic substance' or 'surfactant'. It forms a thin insoluble film, about 5 nm thick, floating on the surface of the alveolar fluid. The surfactant acts by forming a monomolecular layer at the interface between the fluid lining and the air in the alveoli. This prevents the formation of a water–air interface which would have a surface tension $7-14$ times greater than the surfactant–air interface. In the absence of a surfactant, lung expansion is almost impossible, so that the presence of a surfactant to reduce the action of surface tension is important. It has been proved that surfactant is absent or diminished in the respiratory distress syndrome of the newborn known as hyaline membrane disease (Avery and Mead, 1969). These workers found that extracts of the lungs of adults and of normal infants over 1.22 kg in weight usually had a minimum surface tension of less than 10 mN m^{-1} whilst those of infants and fetuses less than 1.15 kg in weight and those who had died of hyaline membrane disease always had a minimum surface tension in excess of 20 mN m^{-1}. A reduction of surfactant may also occur in the stiff-lung syndrome which sometimes follows cardiac surgery (Tooley *et al.,* 1961). Greenfield *et al.* (1964) show that prolonged intermittent positive pressure ventilation at normal pressure and volume did not alter the action of the surfactant, and did not produce atelectasis in their study on dogs. Mead and Collier (1959) in dogs reported a slow increase in compliance and a slow collapse of the lungs of dogs ventilated with a Starling pump, and that the use of a large tidal volume at about every 10 minutes would prevent the steady fall in compliance which otherwise occurred. The facility of producing a sigh at pre-set intervals is incorporated in a number of automatic lung ventilators. Pattle (1965) explains this on the grounds that the forced inflation increases the lung internal surface area and raises the surface tension above a critical level at which it is possible for more material to be recruited to the lining film, thus reversing the effects of slow desorption. Greenfield *et al.* (1964) also found that a continuous over-inflation of the lung resulted in depletion of the surfactant and gross atelectasis. Chernick *et al.* (1966) show that the effect of a chronic ligation of one pulmonary artery in dogs is to markedly reduce the production of surfactant in that lung, for the first two weeks.

Chemical composition of the lung surfactant

Colacicco *et al.* (1973) have investigated the chemical characterization of the protein and lipid-protein fractions of lung washings from rabbit lungs as an aid to the identifiction of the surfactant. Bubbles obtained from the lung have a lining of lipid, mainly lecithin with some protein (Pattle and Thomas, 1961; Klaus, Clements and Havel, 1961). The turnover time is of the order of some hours (Young and Tiernay, 1972). Prior to birth, liquid flows from the lung into the amniotic fluid and from estimations of the phospholipids of surfactant in the fluid, it is hoped to be able to predict the presence of the respiratory distress syndrome (Gluck and Kulovich, 1973). Pender (1973) points out that a number of investigators think that the lecithin concentration or the lecithin—sphingomyelin ratio in the amniotic fluid are reliable indicators of both lung maturity and the likelihood of respiratory distress syndrome. Pender quotes evidence which does not bear this fact out. He feels that infants with respiratory distress syndrome may have an adequate supply of surfactant but its continuing synthesis may be inadequate or it may be prevented from reaching the alveolar spaces. He suggests that a lack of pulmonary reserve may be more important than a lack of surfactant.

The type II cells of the lung contain lamellated osmiophilic bodies which are usually 0.5 to 1.0 μm in diameter. That these are the source of the surfactant has been confirmed by Gil and Reiss (1973). Improved methods for the electron microscopy of the bodies have been described by Schock, Pattle and Creasey (1973). Pender (1970) feels that a decrease in surfactant in the respiratory distress syndrome may well be secondary to atelectasis rather than the cause of it. This is because if the alveoli are collapsed, as by adhesive atelectasis due to aspiration of blood, then the surfactant cannot reach the alveolar spaces.

Surfactometers suitable for the measurement of the surface tension of surfactant solutions have been described by Wilbur (1969) and Williams, Rhoades and Adams (1971).

Stanley *et al.* (1975) confirmed that the surface tension of the upper airway secretions correlates closely with the severity of pulmonary diseases and that the measurement of this surface tension may be a simple, clinically applicable, method of assessing alveolar surfactant function.

Diffusion of gases

Gas molecules will move, by a process known as diffusion, from a place where there is a higher partial pressure of the gas concerned, to one where there is a lower partial pressure. This is a molecular process, and should not be confused with processes such as convection in which a movement occurs of the gas in bulk. By diffusion, gas molecules can move through the pores of a porous membrane to equalize the partial pressures on either side. It is now widely accepted that oxygen passes from the alveoli into the pulmonary capillary blood by a passive process of diffusion. Another example of the process occurs with diffusion respiration. This was reported in the dog by Draper and Whitehead (1944) who found that under certain conditions blood will be normally oxygenated from the lungs in the absence of respiratory movements and rhythmical pressure changes in the lungs. Draper and Whitehead (1949) explain the phenomenon as follows; the marked affinity of oxygen for haemoglobin causes the amount of oxygen removed from the alveoli during apnoea to exceed the amount of carbon dioxide that simultaneously leaves the blood. The net result is to reduce the pressure in the alveoli to below atmospheric, thus giving rise to a continuous inward flow of the dead-space gas and the external atmosphere. Essential conditions for diffusion respiration are a high percentage of oxygen in the lungs and in the dead-space, a free airway and an adequate circulation. The technique of diffusion respiration has been applied to man by Enghoff, Holmdahl and Risholm (1951), Payne (1962) and others.

The work of Kylstra and Tissing (1964) and Kylstra (1965) has shown that a form of diffusion respiration can occur when a lung is filled with a liquid instead of gas. Working at the University of Leiden, Kylstra has kept a mouse alive for eighteen hours immersed in an oxygenated, isotonic salt solution, at a pressure of 8 ata. Under these conditions, the mammalian lung was able to function as a gill. The work has now been extended to dogs. The balanced salt solution at 20 °C must contain 0.1 per cent of tris(hydroxymethylamino)-methane, (THAM), in order to minimize hypercapnic acidosis. The dogs taken to 5 ata could live again without any adverse effects after having breathed fluid for prolonged periods of time. Carbon dioxide elimination is deficient during spontaneous respiration under these circumstances. This may be due to inadequate alveolar ventilation as a result of the resistance to flow through the airways of the fluid. Even with artifical ventilation (Kylstra, 1965), carbon dioxide elimination was still generally deficient.

The quantitative treatment of diffusion is based upon Fick's law of diffusion which is analogous to Ohm's law for the conduction of electricity. Fick's law states that the rate of diffusion is proportional to the concentration gradient, that is, to the change of concentration per unit length in the direction of diffusion. In considering the diffusion of a particular component of a gas mixture between two regions, it is clear that it is the difference in partial pressures, not total pressures, which is important. The diffusion process results from a random motion of the molecules and will be temperature dependent. Gas molecules can pass in either direction, but do so at a rate proportional to the partial pressure of the region which they are leaving. The net rate of transfer is the difference between the number of molecules passing per unit time in each direction. This will be proportional to the difference in the partial pressures between the two regions. When a porous membrane separates two enclosures, initially having different partial pressures for a certain gas, the diffusion will eventually produce a state of equilibrium. When the partial pressures on either side of the membrane have equalized, molecules will still pass continuously through the membrane in equal numbers per unit time, but the net transfer will be zero.

An important case arises in the diffusion of oxygen and carbon dioxide across the alveolar membrane. Carbon dioxide diffuses rapidly, with the result that equilibration is normally reached for carbon dioxide between the alveolar air and capillary blood. Oxygen may not always achieve equilibrium, and this fact is reflected in the diffusion capacity for oxygen. The respiratory gases have to cross not only the lung epithelium and the capillary wall, but must diffuse through the layer of moisture lining the alveoli, the interstitial fluid between the alveolar membrane and the capillary membrane, the plasma and the red cell membrane. The various rates of diffusion involved all contribute to the value of the diffusing capacity. Carbon dioxide is much more water soluble than oxygen, and this helps to increase its rate of diffusion.

Fick's law may be written in the form

$$dQ = -kS\frac{dc}{dx}\,dt$$

where dQ is the volume of oxygen diffusing across the alveolar membrane in a time interval dt, k is the diffusion constant for oxygen and the alveolar membrane, S is the effective area of membrane through which the oxygen diffuses, and dc/dx is the concentration gradient across the membrane of thickness dx. For a thin membrane $dc/dx = (c_1 - c_2)/x$ and thus $dQ = -kS(c_1 - c_2)\,dt/x$. By means of the Bunsen solubility coefficient for oxygen, the concentrations c_1 and c_2 can be related to the gas tensions p_1 and p_2 existing on either side of the membrane, i.e., $c_1 = ap_1/B$ and $c_2 = ap_2/B$ where a is the Bunsen solubility coefficient, B is the barometric pressure and p_1 and p_2 are the gas tensions. Fick's law equation becomes

$$\frac{dQ}{dt} = -kSa(p_1 - p_2)/B$$

or

$$\frac{dQ}{dt} = -D(p_1 - p_2)$$

where D is known as the diffusion capacity of the lungs. Diffusing capacity is analogous in electrical terms to conductance (the reciprocal of resistance), thus diffusing capacity = (net rate of gas transfer in ml per min)/(partial pressure gradient in mmHg). Diffusing capacity is expressed in ml min^{-1} mmHg^{-1}. The diffusing capacity for oxygen is defined as oxygen uptake/(alveolar P_{O_2} − mean pulmonary capillary P_{O_2}). The diffusing capacity is the volume of oxygen (STPD) per minute which diffuses through the whole lung when a given mean partial pressure difference exists between the alveolar air and the capillary blood of the lung. The alveolar P_{O_2} can be estimated with reasonable accuracy, but serious problems exist in determining the mean pulmonary P_{O_2} (Nunn, 1969). A typical value of the oxygen diffusing capacity would be 21 ml O_2 min^{-1} mmHg^{-1} in a normal adult subject at rest, the corresponding value for CO_2 being some 20 times greater.

When a gas is diffusing through a membrane into an aqueous solution the diffusing capacity is considered to be proportional to the solubility of the gas concerned. A high value of the solubility implies that for a given gas tension more molecules are present in the liquid. It does not mean that the gas passes through the membrane more easily. The diffusing capacity for N_2O should be of the order 20 times more than the corresponding value for oxygen for a particular gas–water interface. The resistance to diffusion of a particular gas will be directly proportional to the area separating the two regions concerned and inversely proportional to the distance separating them. The diffusing path in the lungs must extend from the gas side of the alveolar membrane to the interior of the red cells.

Graham's law of diffusion states that the rate of diffusion of gases through certain membranes is inversely proportional to the square root of their molecular weight. The molecular weight of oxygen is 32, and that of carbon dioxide is 44. The square roots of their molecular weights are in the ratio of 1.2:1, so that oxygen will diffuse faster by a factor of 20 per cent through a dry porous membrane than will carbon dioxide. In practice the nature of the membrane exerts an important influence on the rate of diffusion. For example, carbon dioxide diffuses more rapidly than oxygen through a rubber-lined Douglas bag (Mills, 1952). The losses of carbon dioxide from the Douglas bag due to diffusion are in the range 0.22 to 0.45 per cent v/v per hour.

The permeability of plastic membranes for oxygen, nitrogen and carbon dioxide is important in the choice of materials for the construction of storage bags for gases and for artificial lungs. The design of a diffusion chamber for measuring the permeability of large plastic sheets is described by Galletti *et al.* (1966). These workers found that Dow-Corning 'Silastic' (a silicone rubber) is about 40 times as permeable to oxygen, 81 times more permeable to carbon dioxide, 44 times more permeable to nitrogen, and 4.1 times more permeable to helium than Dupont 'Teflon' (tetrafluoroethylene) membranes of equal thickness. It was found that these membranes did obey Fick's law. However, the experimental results did not agree with a theory of diffuison through pores, since the order of decreasing permeability did not follow the order of increasing molecular diameter. The solubility of the gases in the plastic materials is an important factor in the transfer of gas across the plastic membrane. A comprehensive list of permeabilities for common plastics and gases is given by Lebovitz (1966). Baker and Doerr (1959) stress the importance of water in affecting the concentration of mixtures stored in plastic bags. The water may be present in the original mixture or already adsorbed on the walls of the bag.

W.L. Robb of the American General Electric Company has kept a hamster alive in a compartment having walls made of silicone rubber and suspended inside a tank of oxygenated water. The animal's respiratory requirements were met by the diffusion of oxygen into the chamber and the diffusion of carbon dioxide out of the chamber. Bodell (1965) describes an artificial gill made of Silastic rubber which can sustain an adult rat for 25 hours. Kolobow and Bowman (1963) discuss the construction and evaluation of an alveolar membrane artificial heart-lung using Silastic. Silicone rubber is also a good, inert, material for encapsulating implanted electronic circuits such as cardiac pacemakers and bladder stimulators. Its use for such purposes is discussed by Boone (1966).

The solubility of gases in liquids

Experimentally, it is found that the amount of a given gas which dissolves in a given liquid is directly proportional to the pressure of the gas. This fact is known as Henry's law (Henry, 1803). The amount of gas which goes into solution depends upon the temperature of the liquid. The higher the temperature of the liquid, the less the amount which goes into solution. At a given temperature, when no more gas dissolves in the liquid, the liquid is said to be fully saturated at that temperature and with the gas in question. When a state of equilibrium has been attained the gas in solution exerts the same 'tension' as the partial pressure of the gas concerned above the liquid. For example, in the well known tonometric technique, blood is equilibrated in a tonometer with a flowing stream of gas containing partial pressures of oxygen and carbon dioxide. The tensions of these gases in the blood then equal the respective partial pressures in the gas phase, and the blood in the tonometer can be used to calibrate blood–gas electrode systems. The design of tonometers is discussed by Thornton and Nunn (1960), Torres (1963), Kelman, Coleman and Nunn (1966) and Adams and Morgan-Hughes (1967).

Current practice is to use a polarographic electrode to measure oxygen tension in blood, and a carbon dioxide electrode to measure the carbon dioxide tension of blood (Severinghaus and Bradley, 1958; Severinghaus, 1962; Fatt, 1964; and Lübbers, 1966). Gotch *et al.* (1966) describe the use of electrodes for the measurement of P_{O_2}, P_{CO_2}, pH, and sodium and potassium ion concentrations. Previous to the development of direct-reading electrode systems the Riley bubble method of Riley, Campbell and Shepard (1957) could be used for the determination of oxygen and carbon dioxide tensions in blood. A small bubble is introduced into the blood sample contained in a syringe, the volume of the bubble being of the order of 1 per cent of that of the blood. The gases in the blood and bubble come into equilibrium, and the composition of the bubble can then be determined as a volume percentage by means of a Scholander micro-gas analyser (Scholander, 1947). From a knowledge of the dry barometric pressure, the percentage concentrations by volume of the gases can be converted into their corresponding tensions. As an example, the oxygen tension of water equilibrated with air at a barometric pressure of 760 mmHg is given by

$$\frac{(760-47) \times 20.95}{100} = 149 \text{ mmHg}$$

The saturated vapour pressure of water at 37 °C is 47 mmHg. Strang (1961) has employed a mass spectrometer to analyse the compositon of the bubble used in Riley's method in studies with neonates, and Bowes (1964) used a gas chromatograph to determine blood nitrous tensions by means of a bubble equilibration technique.

Solubility coefficients

The extent to which a given gas will dissolve in a given liquid can be expressed in terms of its solubility coefficient. The Bunsen solubility coefficient (α) is defined as the volume of gas, reduced to 0 °C and one atmosphere pressure dissolved by unit volume of solvent at the temperature of the experiment, under a partial pressure of the gas of one atmosphere. Power (1968) has measured the Bunsen solubility coefficients of oxygen and carbon dioxide in water, saline, blood and pulmonary and placental tissue. The method used was to equilibrate the sample in a tonometer with oxygen and carbon dioxide. Measured at 37 °C, the Bunsen coefficient for oxygen is 0.0238 ml/ml $\times$ atm in water, the corresponding value for CO_2 being 0.0189, the ratio $\alpha O_2/\alpha CO_2$ being 1.26. In the case of blood, αO_2 was 0.0230 and αCO_2 was 0.0189, the ratio $\alpha O_2/\alpha CO_2$ being 1.22. The Bunsen coefficient at

37 °C is given by $\alpha = C \times 760 / [F(P_B - 47)]$ where F is the fractional concentration of the dry gas concerned in the equilibrium gas mixture, P_B is the barometric pressure in mmHg and C is the volume of gas at STPD dissolved in 1 ml of sample.

The *Ostwald solubility coefficient* (λ) is defined as the volume of gas, measured under the temperature and pressure at which the gas dissolves, taken up by unit volume of the liquid. If v is the actual volume of dissolved gas measured at the experimental temperature of T Kelvin and at the partial pressure of the gas of p atmospheres, then assuming that the gas laws are obeyed, $v = v_0(p_0/p \times T/273)$, where v_0 is the volume of gas dissolved at 0 °C (273 K) and p_0 is the partial pressure at 0 °C. If V is the volume of liquid which has dissolved v ml of gas, then by definition, $\lambda = v/V$ and $\alpha = v_0/V$ so that $\lambda = \alpha(T/273)$ or $\lambda = \alpha(1 + 0.00367t)$ where t is in degrees Centigrade. It can be seen that the Ostwald solubility coefficient is in fact independent of the partial pressure if the gas laws are obeyed. By Henry's law, if the partial pressure of the gas is trebled, three times the number of molecules will dissolve in the liquid. However, by Boyle's law, the product pressure $\times$ volume remains constant so that the volume decreases to one third, that is, the product remains at its original value. It is only the fact that the Bunsen coefficient is in terms of a volume at 0 °C that produces a difference between the Ostwald and Bunsen coefficients.

The Bunsen solubility coefficient is the customary method of expressing solubilities in the International Critical Tables. Thus Orcutt and Seevers (1937) and Larson, Eger and Severinghaus (1962), concerned with the solubilities of anaesthetic gases, measure Ostwald coefficients and then convert them to Bunsen coefficients.

Steward *et al.* (1973) make the point that in the field of anaesthesia, and particularly in the study of the uptake and distribution of anaesthetic agents, the most convenient coefficient is undoubtedly the Ostwald solubility coefficient or the numerically equal tissue–gas partition coefficient. Steward *et al.* (1973) searched the literature and found reports of some 600 coefficients for the solubilities of 18 chosen agents, including nitrogen, krypton and xenon as well as the conventional current anaesthetics in water, saline, olive oil and the blood and tissues of various species. The reported values were then mostly corrected to Ostwald solubility coefficients at 37 °C and presented by Steward *et al.* in the form of a table (*Table 5.2*) with coded information on the number of determinations on which each coefficient was based, and the concentration at which it was determined. Steward *et al.* also

TABLE 5.2. Preferred values of Ostwald solubility coefficients at 37 °C (from Steward et al., 1973)

Anaesthetic	Water	Blood	Grey matter	White matter	Heart	Kidney	Liver	Lung	Muscle	Fat tissue†	Oil**
Chloroform	4.0	8	16	24	8*	11	17*	7*	12*	280	400
Cyclopropane	0.21	0.55	0.8*	2*	1*	0.4*	0.6	—	0.4	8	11.5
Diethyl ether	13	12	12	13	12	10	11*	15*	10	50	65
Divinyl ether	1.4	2.6	3*	4*	—	2*	3*	—	2*	40	60
Enflurane	0.78*	1.9*	—	—	—	—	—	—	—	70	98*
Ethyl chloride	1.2	2*	—	—	—	—	—	—	—	—	—
Ethylene	0.090	0.15	—	—	—	—	—	—	—	0.95	1.27
Fluroxene	0.85	1.4	1.6	2.4	—	1.3*	2.0	—	2	34	48
Forane	0.62	1.4	—	—	—	—	—	—	—	68	97
Halopropane	—	5.5	—	—	—	—	—	—	—	225	320
Halothane	0.80	2.4	5.0	8	7*	3.5	6.0	—	6	155	220
Krypton	0.051	0.06	—	—	—	—	—	—	—	0.33	0.46
Methoxyflurane	4.5	11	20	30	—	20*	25*	—	20	670	950
Nitrogen	0.014	0.015	—	—	—	—	—	—	—	0.054	0.07
Nitrous oxide	0.47	0.47	0.50	0.50	0.52	0.4*	0.43	0.47	0.4*	1.1	1.4
Teflurane	0.32*	0.60*	1.08*	1.15*	—	—	1.02*	—	2.26*	20	29*
Trichloroethylene	1.7*	9	15*	30*	—	10*	20*	—	12*	600	900
Xenon	0.085	0.14	0.13	0.23	—	0.10*	0.10	—	0.10	1.3	1.8

Solubility coefficients for saline may be taken as 94 per cent and for CSF as 95 per cent of that for water – probably for all agents.

*Value dependent on human data from one group of workers only or on animal data.

† Based mainly on olive oil and human fat extract.

**Calculated from coefficients for human blood and oil.

include a table of preferred values for man, a table of MAC values and an exposition of the relationships between various solubility and partition coefficients.

The value of the Ostwald solubility coefficient decreases with increasing temperature of the medium, the relationship being linear. Those agents with a large negative temperature coefficient also have a high value of solubility coefficient. Allott _et al._ (1973) list the temperature coefficients of the Ostwald solubility coefficient for a number of anaesthetic agents with respect to water, oil and biological media. Munson _et al._ (1978) found that the act of eating increased the values of the blood solubility coefficients for some anaesthetic agents in man by 17–34 per cent. This occurred for enflurane, halothane, isoflurane and methoxyflurane but not for nitrous oxide. The rates of rise of the end-tidal enflurane, halothane and methoxyflurane concentrations after eating were 7–8 per cent below the control values prior to eating and the rates of anaesthetic uptake increased by 20–23 per cent.

In tables of the solubilities of gases in water, the solubility coefficients are listed in terms of the number of millilitres of the gas measured at 0 °C and 760 mmHg which will dissolve in 1 ml of water at the temperature stated and when the pressure of the gas minus that of the water vapour is 760 mmHg. Thus 0.88 ml of CO_2 will dissolve in 1 ml of water of 20 °C and 760 mmHg. Convenient numbers are obtained by considering the volume of gas which will dissolve in 100 ml of water. This procedure gives the following solubility coefficients at 20 °C; carbon dioxide 88, nitrogen 1.6, nitrous oxide 63, oxygen 3. Since both the volume of the dissolved gas and the volume of the liquid in which it has dissolved are expressed in millilitres, their ratio which is the solubility coefficient is dimensionless.

The high solubility of nitrous oxide makes it necessary to use saturated caustic solution in a Haldane apparatus when oxygen and carbon dioxide measurements have to be made in the presence of nitrous oxide (Nunn, 1958). The volume of gas in millilitres dissolving in 100 ml of a liquid can be expressed in millilitres of gas at STPD per 100 ml of liquid, that is, volumes per cent. By dividing by the pressure of the gas, further standardization is possible — volumes per cent per mmHg. In the case of carbon dioxide dissolved in blood, the units of millimoles of CO_2 per litre per mmHg are often used. For CO_2 in blood at 37 °C, the solubility is 0.03 $mmol^{-1}$ $mmHg^{-1}$.

The oxygen content, capacity and saturation of blood

The physical solution of oxygen in plasma depends on the partial pressure of the gas and the temperature. At 38 °C, 0.023 ml of oxygen dissolves in a millilitre of blood when the partial pressure is 760 mmHg or one atmosphere. That is, the amount of oxygen in simple physical solution is $0.023 \times (P_{O_2}/760)$ ml per ml. This value for the dissolved oxygen multiplied by 100 gives the dissolved oxygen content in ml per 100 ml of blood. The solubility figure is quoted in terms of whole blood, although the solution occurs into the plasma.

As an example, it is required to know how many volumes per cent of oxygen are dissolved in blood equilibrated with a gas mixture containing 15 per cent v/v of oxygen at a barometric pressure of 760 mmHg and a temperature of 38 °C. At this temperature the partial pressure of water vapour is 47 mmHg. Dry gas pressure=(760–47) =713 mmHg, P_{O_2}=713 × 15/100=107 mmHg. The volume of oxygen dissolved per ml of blood is $0.023 \times 107/760 = 0.00324$ ml per ml, and thus the amount of dissolved oxygen is 0.324 volume per cent.

The total oxygen content carried in the blood consists of both physically dissolved oxygen and oxygen in chemical combination with haemoglobin. Each gram of haemoglobin can combine with 1.34 ml of oxygen. If the haemoglobin concentration of the blood sample referred to previously is 15 g HbO_2 per 100 ml, the volume per cent of the combined oxygen is 15 × 1.34=20.1. The total oxygen content of the blood is now 20.1+0.34=20.44 volumes per cent.

When blood is equilibrated with room air at 20 °C, the haemoglobin is fully converted to oxyhaemoglobin. This is due to the alkalinity arising from the lack of CO_2 and the effect of the low (room) temperature on the oxygen dissociation curve. The oxygen content under these conditions is known as the oxygen capacity and this corresponds to an oxygen saturation of 100 per cent. The oxygen saturation relates the amount of oxyhaemoglobin to the total haemoglobin in a given blood sample. The percentage saturation can be calculated from a knowledge of the oxygen content and capacity of the blood sample concerned, thus at 38 °C, percentage saturation

$$= \frac{\text{(oxygen content–dissolved oxygen) at 38 °C}}{\text{(oxygen capacity–dissolved oxygen) at 20 °C}}$$

$$= \frac{\text{(oxygen content–}P_{O_2} \times 0.023)}{\text{(oxygen capacity–}P_{O_2} \times 0.034)}$$

where the solubility coefficients for oxygen in blood at 20 °C and 38 °C are respectively 0.034 and 0.023 ml gas per ml liquid at 760 mmHg pressure.

The oxygen content or capacity of a blood sample can be measured using a Van Slyke apparatus (Van Slyke and Neill, 1924), spectrophotometry (Wade *et al.*, 1953) or gas chromatography (Hill, 1966a; Davies, 1970).

The partition of carbon dioxide in plasma

Carbon dioxide produced by the tissues diffuses into the plasma, the major proportion being buffered by the erythrocytes, some dissolved carbon dioxide forms carbamino compounds with plasma proteins while the remainder is in equilibrium with carbonic acid. In plasma the concentration of CO_2 is about one thousand times that of carbonic acid. Of the CO_2 diffusing into the erythrocytes, some remains as dissolved CO_2, a significant fraction combines with haemoglobin and the largest fraction is hydrated to form carbonic acid. Most of this is ionized to form hydrogen ions and bicarbonate ions.

Considering the plasma alone, the solubility coefficient for CO_2 in plasma at 38 °C is 0.51, so that if the P_{CO_2} is 40 mmHg, then the volume per cent of dissolved CO_2 at a barometric pressure of 760 mmHg is $(40/(760-47)) \times 100 \times 0.51 = 2.86$. By analysis it was found that the total volume per cent of CO_2 in the plasma was 55.5. The difference between the total carbon dioxide content and the dissolved carbon dioxide content equals the bicarbonate concentration, that is, 52.6 volume per cent. The solubility coefficient for whole blood at 38 °C for CO_2 is 0.49. It is also possible to express CO_2 contents in terms of millimoles per litre. If the content is X volume per cent, this is the same as $10X$ ml per litre. One mole of CO_2 at 0 °C and 760 mmHg occupies a volume of 22 260 ml. Hence $10X$ ml per litre = $10X/22\ 260$ moles per litre = $10X/2.226$ millimoles per litre. Volumes per cent divided by 2.226 equals millimoles per litre. The total volume per cent of 55.5 for the CO_2 in the plasma previously mentioned is equal to 24.9 millimoles per litre.

The partition of carbon dioxide in whole blood

In the case of whole blood, the P_{CO_2} is the same for both plasma and erythrocytes, but the concentrations of dissolved CO_2 and bicarbonate will be different in the two phases. The total amount of CO_2 in whole blood will equal the sum of that in the plasma and that in the cells. If V_c is the fractional volume of the cells in the blood sample and V_p is the fractional volume of the plasma, then $V_c/V_p = H$ where H is the haematocrit. If $T_{CO_{2c}}$ is the total number of millimoles of CO_2 per litre of erythrocytes, then in one litre of whole blood there will be V_c × $T_{CO_{2c}}$ millimoles of CO_2 in the erythrocytes. Similarly for the plasma there will be $V_p \times T_{CO_{2p}}$ millimoles. The total CO_2 in the blood is then given by $T_{CO_{2b}} = V_c T_{CO_{2c}} + V_p T_{CO_{2p}}$. The concentration of the dissolved CO_2 for the erythrocytes can be calculated from a knowledge of the P_{CO_2} (which is the same as that for the plasma) and the solubility coefficient. At 38 °C, for the erythrocytes it is 0.025 when the P_{CO_2} is in mmHg and the dissolved CO_2 (CO_{2cd}) is in millimoles per litre. Thus $CO_{2cd} = P_{CO_2} \times 0.025$. The difference between the total CO_2 ($T_{CO_{2c}}$) and the dissolved CO_2 (CO_{2cd}) gives the carbon dioxide carried as bicarbonate ions and carbamino-CO_2. For the blood sample previously discussed which had a P_{CO_2} of 40 mmHg and a total CO_2 in the plasma of 23.7 millimoles per litre, the measured whole-blood total CO_2 was 18.2 millimoles per litre corresponding to 40.6 volume per cent. If the haematocrit is 0.45, the total CO_2 in the erythrocytes $T_{CO_{2c}}$ is 11.6 millimoles per litre and the dissolved CO_2 in the erythrocytes CO_{2cd} is 1 millimole per litre. The amount of CO_2 carried as bicarbonate ions and carbamino-CO_2 is 11.6−1=10.6 millimoles per litre. A more detailed discussion of the carriage of both oxygen and carbon dioxide in the blood is given by Davenport (1969).

Solubility considerations of hyperbaric oxygen therapy

The compositon of alveolar air when breathing air or oxygen at a pressure of one atmosphere absolute (1 ata) or oxygen at a pressure of two atmospheres absolute is given in *Table 5.3*. At one atmosphere

TABLE 5.3

Inspired Gas	Alveolar PO_2	Alveolar PCO_2	Alveolar PN_2	Alveolar PH_2O	Total Pressure (mmHg)
1 ata air	100	40	573	47	760
1 ata oxygen	673	40	0	47	760
2 ata oxygen	1433	40	0	47	1520

breathing air, the haemoglobin is 97 per cent saturated, the amount of oxygen dissolved in the plasma is 0.3 ml/100 ml, and the total oxygen content (dissolved plus combined) is 20 ml per 100 ml of blood. When pure oxygen at one atmosphere is breathed, the partial pressure of oxygen in the alveoli rises from 100 to 673 mmHg, an increase of 6.7

times. As a result, the dissolved oxygen rises to 2 ml/100 ml. The haemoglobin becomes fully saturated, and the additional amount of oxygen now carried in the blood as a result of breathing pure oxygen is 2.5 ml/100 ml of blood. The total percentage increase of oxygen carried in the blood is only about 10 per cent of the original 20 volumes per cent. However, the increase in Po_2 from 100 to 673 mmHg will greatly assist oxygenation of the tissues, since this occurs by a diffusion process and depends on the tension gradient between the blood supply and the tissue concerned. When the oxygen pressure is increased to two atmospheres absolute, the dissolved oxygen increases in proportion to the pressure, rising to 4.3 ml/100 ml of blood. The pressure increase from one to two atmospheres gives rise to an extra 2.3 ml of oxygen per 100 ml of blood, i.e. a total of 4.8 ml/100ml of blood above that carried when air is breathed at normal atmospheric pressure. Smith *et al.* (1963) found, in dogs, that the use of oxygen at two atmospheres absolute increased the duration of 'safe' circulatory arrest from 5 to 8 minutes at normal temperature, and from 20 to 30 minutes at 28 °C during hypothermia.

The solubility of volatile anaesthetics in water or blood

The solubility of an anaesthetic agent in blood is important, since the magnitude of the solubility governs the rate of induction of anaesthesia. For an agent having a small solubility, the tension in the blood will rise rapidly and the brain is soon presented with an appreciable tension of the agent. On the other hand, for an agent having a high solubility in blood, the tension will rise slowly. It follows that cyclopropane which is relatively insoluble produces a rapid induction, whereas both ether and chloroform which are markedly soluble produce a slow induction of anaesthesia. In general, the situation is more complicated and allowance must be made for the potency of the agent and losses of the

TABLE 5.4. Ostwald solubility coefficients at 37 ± 0.5 °C and 760 mmHg

Agent	Water/Gas	Blood/Gas	Oil/Gas
Cyclopropane	0.204	0.415	11.2
Nitrous oxide	0.435	0.468	1.4
Halothane	0.74	2.3	224
Trichloroethylene	1.55	9.15	—
Chloroform	3.8	10.3	265
Diethyl ether	15.61	15.2	50.2

agent to the anaesthetic circuit components. *Table 5.4* taken from Larson, Eger and Severinghaus (1962), compares the Ostwald solubility coefficients of some gaseous and volatile anaesthetic agents at 37 °C and 760 mmHg. The solubility of oxygen in blood is discussed by Hedley-Whyte and Laver (1964) and by Power (1968). The solubility of nitrous oxide in water and in canine blood has been measured by Sy and Hasbrouck (1964), and by Ostiguy and Becklake (1966). The use of a gas chromatograph to measure the solubility of nitrous oxide is described by Borgstedt and Gillies (1965). Eger and Larson (1964) give values for the solubilities of anaesthetics in blood and tissues and discuss their significance.

Partition or distribution coefficients

The partition coefficient of a substance between two phases is defined as the ratio of the amount of the substance present in equal volumes of the two phases at a stated temperature, independent of pressure, when the two phases are in equilibrium. Thus a partition coefficient will indicate how a substance will distribute itself between two phases in contact, e.g. between gas and water, gas and blood or fat and blood. Payne, Hill and King (1966) used a partition coefficient of 2060 1^{-1} at 34 °C for the distribution of ethyl alcohol between arterial blood and breath. This contrasts with the value of 2.3 for halothane (Bourne, 1964).

A tissue—blood coefficient may be obtained by dividing the tissue—gas coefficient by the blood—gas coefficient, i.e. $T/B = (T/G)/(B/G)$. Thus for halothane using the data of Steward *et al.* (1973), the fat—blood coefficient = (fat/vapour)(blood/vapour) = $155/2.4 = 64.6$.

Lowe (1972) points out that blood—gas partition coefficients may be measured within a few minutes by simultaneously and separately equilibrating a drop of water and a drop of blood with any fixed anaesthetic concentration of vapour at a known temperature. The vapour content of a one microlitre sample of each is then determined by means of a calibrated flame ionization detector gas chromatograph and $B/G = (B/W)/(G/W)$.

Using this approach, Lowe has also obtained values for tissue—gas partition coefficients. Homogenates of the tissues are prepared in known amounts of water and the anaesthetic dissolved in the added water is subtracted in order to obtain the tissue solubility. For example, if a known weight of minced tissue is homogenized with four times its weight of distilled water and the homogenate-anaesthetic vapour partition coefficient (H/G) measured, the tissue–vapour partition coefficient (T/G) can be calculated from $T/G = 5H/G -4W/G$ where W/G is the known water–vapour partition coefficient. Lowe states that it is generally possible to calculate the solubility or partition coefficient of a volatile anaesthetic agent in a given tissue as the sum of the individual partition coefficients for that agent in each of the lipids comprising the tissue.

The blood–gas partition coefficient of a given volatile anaesthetic agent varies from person to person and its value depends on the haematocrit, the water and lipid content and the protein composition of the individual's blood. Lowe (1972) gives the following relationships for approximating blood–gas partition coefficients:

Methoxyflurane = 6.5 + 0.095 × Haematocrit
Halothane   = 1.37 + 0.021 × Haematocrit

In a group of 75 patients, Lowe found that the pre-anaesthetic methoxyflurane and halothane partition coefficients varied between 8.0 and 13.5 and 1.7 and 2.5 respectively.

In the case of liquid–gas partition coefficients, the concentration of the substance in the gas phase and in the liquid phase are expressed in the same units, so that their ratio is dimensionless. When the concentrations are both in terms of the content per unit volume then the liquid–gas partition coefficient is numerically equal to the Ostwald solubility coefficient for that substance. For liquid–liquid partition coefficients such as tissue–blood there is less agreement over units of concentration (Steward *et al.*, 1973). Usually, both concentrations are in terms of units of substance content per unit volume. The resulting tissue–blood coefficient may then be referred to as a conventional volume–volume partition coefficient and is equal to the ratio of either the Ostwald or the Bunsen solubility coefficients of the tissue and of the blood. Thus the muscle–blood partition coefficient for halothane would be $6/2.4 = 2.5$, whereas the halothane fat–blood partition coefficient is $155/2.4 = 64.6$.

Suppose that the concentraton of halothane in a blood sample is X mg/100 ml of blood. Then 1 ml of blood contains $X = 10^{-5}$ g of liquid halothane. Assuming that 1 gram-molecular weight (197 g) of halothane occupies 22.4 litres at STPD it will occupy

$$(22.4 \times 760)/(BP -47) \times 310/273 \text{ litres}$$

at BTPS (37 °C) where *BP* is the barometric pressure. Then $X \times 10^{-5}$ g of halothane will occupy *V* litres where

$$V = (22.4/197) \times (760/BP-47) \times (310/273)X \times 10^{-5}$$

Considering the gas phase in equilibrium with the blood at 37 °C, then 1 ml of gas will contain *L* litres of halothane vapour where $L=F/1000$ and *F* is the fractional concentration of halothane present in the gas. The partition coefficient λ is given by $\lambda=V/L$. Hence,

$$F=1000 \times v/\lambda=1000 \times (22.4/197) \times (760/BP-47) \times (310/273) \times X/\lambda$$

This expression can be used to determine the blood halothane concentration in mg/100 ml when blood is tonometered at 37 °C with a gas containing $F \times 100$ per cent v/v of halothane vapour.

The dependence of solubility coefficients upon the gas concentration and the concept of MAC (minimum alveolar concentration) for a volatile anaesthetic agent

If Henry's law was strictly obeyed, the solubility coefficients would be independent of the concentration of the substance concerned in the gas phase. Lowe (1972) points out that the partition coefficients of ether and cyclopropane vary with the gas concentration. For this reason, Steward *et al.* (1973) in their comprehensive list of solubility coefficients for inhaled anaesthetic agents quote, wherever possible, the gas concentration at which the particular coefficient was measured. For compactness in the table, Steward *et al.* distinguish only three concentration ranges; greater than clinical, clinical and less than clinical. The clinical range is defined by them as being between 0.5 and 2 MAC. The concept of MAC was introduced by Saidman and Eger (1964) as the minimum alveolar concentration of a particular inhalational agent required to prevent movement in response to a surgical incision for 50 per cent of the group of patients studied. For halothane, Saidman and Eger found the MAC to be 0.75 per cent v/v. The MAC required for a volatile anaesthetic agent may be reduced by the use of premedication, barbiturate induction and the addition of nitrous oxide. Saidman and Eger (1964) found that the addition of nitrous oxide without narcotic premedication allowed a reduction to be made in the alveolar halothane concentration to 0.29 per cent v/v. Steward *et al.* (1973)'s MAC values are given in *Table 5.5*. In dogs, Eger, Saidman and Brandstater (1965) found that the MAC values fell linearly with a decrease in body temperature. For an average temperature of 39.3 °C, the MAC was 0.98

TABLE 5.5

Substance	MAC (% v/v)
Chloroform	0.5
Cyclopropane	9.2
Diethyl ether	3.0
Enflurane	1.7
Halothane	0.75
Methoxyflurane	0.16
Trichloroethylene	0.2
Nitrous oxide	101

per cent halothane whereas for 27.9 °C it had decreased to 0.47 per cent.

Lowe (1972) takes a value of 1.3 MAC as being a suitable maintenance level for anaesthesia, i.e. 0.975 per cent alveolar concentration. Eger *et al.* (1965) found that the values of MAC for various agents correlated with the solubility of each agent in olive oil, and this correlation has been extended to other lipids (human fat, cephalin and the lipids of grey and white brain matter) by Lowe and Hagler (1971). The more lipid soluble an agent, the lower is the arterial concentration required to produce anaesthesia. Saidman and Eger (1964) assumed that the alveolar gas or vapour was in equilibrium with arterial blood and with the brain and that the tension of the agent in the brain was proportional to the depth of anaesthesia. Maintaining the alveolar concentration (rather than the inspired concentration) constant provided an indirect method of establishing a steady state in the brain. The alveolar concentration at 1 MAC multiplied by the oil-gas solubility coefficient for the particular agent should be approximately the same for most volatile anaesthetic agents.

As has been mentioned, during hypothermia or hyperthermia, the value of the MAC for a certain agent must be altered accordingly as the body temperature changes. Lowe (1972) mentions that cardiac output, oxygen consumption and carbon dioxide output will decrease by a factor of approximately 2 for each 10 °C fall in body temperature. In calculating the dose of an inhaled anaesthetic agent, it is necessary to take into account both cardiac output and MAC changes with body temperature. Raising or lowering the body temperature does not alter the amount of an agent required to obtain anaesthesia and the product $1.3 \times MAC \times \lambda$ remains constant. At lower body temperatures, the reduced cardiac output and organ blood flow will lengthen the organ time constants and prolong the induction.

Gregory *et al.* (1969) have shown that the MAC for halothane also reduces with increasing age of the patient. This fact is attributed to an alteration in the lipid composition of the brain which results in an increase in anaesthetic brain solubility (brain solubility × MAC = constant) with increasing age. The MAC of other agents should fall with age in a similar manner.

The solubility of volatile anaesthetics in oil

The solubility of volatile anaesthetic agents in oil governs the uptake and elimination of the agents by the fat deposits of the body. It has also been shown that there is a correlation between the potency of an anaesthetic agent and its solubility in oil (Meyer and Hemmi, 1935). This correlation is in agreement with the work of Ferguson (1939) who showed that the narcotic concentration of an agent is related to its saturated vapour pressure. Meyer and Hemmi related isonarcosis to equimolar concentrations of the various agents in lipid membranes. Lowe (1972) makes the point that the principle of isonarcosis at iso-concentration implies that at equipotent anaesthetic concentrations, the brain lipid or fat will dissolve equal amounts of each agent. Conversely at equipotent alveolar concentrations (9.2 per cent cyclopropane, 0.75 per cent halothane, 0.16 per cent methoxyflurane) the body lipid or fat cannot dissolve more of one agent than another. Consider an alveolar concentration of 1.3 MAC (0.208 per cent v/v) of methoxyflurane. Taking a blood—gas partition coefficient of 11, the arterial blood concentration is 2.288 per cent. Taking a blood—brain partition coefficient of 2.5 the brain concentration at equilibrium is 5.72 per cent. For a brain volume of 2100 ml, the saturated brain will contain a total of 120.1 ml of methoxyflurane vapour. For 1.3 MAC (0.975 per cent v/v) of halothane, the blood—gas partition coefficient of 2.4 gives a blood level of 2.34 per cent. The blood—brain partition coefficient of 2.3 gives a brain level of 5.38 per cent. The brain volume of 2100 ml now contains 113 ml of halothane vapour. Nunn (1960) discusses the solubility of chloroform in oleyl alcohol, and shows that the uptake of chloroform vapour by oil is not comparable with its uptake by water. At tensions corresponding to the saturated vapour pressure, a marked deviation from Henry's law occurs, the solubility coefficient now rising towards infinity. At the lower values of tension, chloroform appears to have a finite solubility coefficient. Nunn shows that the solubility coefficient of volatile anaesthetic agents in oil can be evaluated by means of Raoult's law. This law states that in a solution of two liquids, the vapour pressure of each constituent is proportional to the number of moles of the substance present in unit volume of solution. For a pure liquid, the vapour pressure will be the saturated vapour pressure of the pure component concerned at the temperature of the mixture. Thus it follows that for a mixture, $p = p_o X$, where p is the vapour pressure exerted by one component of the mixture, p_o is the saturated vapour pressure of the pure component concerned at the temperature of the mixture, and X is the mole fraction of the component concerned in the mixture. The mole fraction of any constituent in a mixture is defined as the number of moles (gram molecules) of the constituent divided by the total number of all moles in the mixture. It is easier to use volume fractions provided that allowance is made where necessary for the fact that equal numbers of molecules of different liquids occupy different volumes even under identical conditions of temperature and pressure. This is in contrast to gases which obey Avogadro's hypothesis that equal volumes of gases at the same temperature and pressure contain equal numbers of molecules. The number of molecules contained in 1 cm^3 of an ideal gas is known as Lodschmit's number (2.678×10^{19}). When the anaesthetic vapour is in equilibrium with an anaesthetic–oil mixture, the partial pressure in the vapour phase will equal the tension of the anaesthetic in the mixture. Thus

$$ pa = p_o \cdot \frac{V_a}{(F.V_a + V_{oil})} $$

where p_a is the partial pressure of the anaesthetic vapour, V_{oil} is the volume of oil in the mixture, p_o is the saturated vapour pressure of the pure anaesthetic at the temperature concerned, and F is the mole volume of oil divided by the mole volume of the anaesthetic. The mole volumes are obtained by multiplying the relevant mole-fractions and densities. If the ratio V_a/V_{oil} is known, then the volume of the anaesthetic agent which can be taken up by unit volume of oil can be calculated. There is considerable experimental evidence to show that the solubility of volatile anaesthetics does obey Raoult's law over clinical ranges of concentration.

The properties of vapours

The inhalational anaesthetic agents and water are substances which are commonly encountered in the vapour phase by anaesthetists. The term 'vapour' is generally reserved for the gaseous state of a substance which at room temperature and pressure is a liquid. This classification gives ether, chloroform and halothane as vapours, but nitrous oxide and cyclopropane as gases since the latter substances can only be liquefied in cylinders under pressure. Oxygen is obviously a gas since it boils at $-183\,°C$ at atmospheric pressure. In practice it is found that one gram-molecular weight of a volatile anaesthetic liquid will vaporize to yield 22.4 litres of vapour at a temperature of $0\,°C$ and a pressure of 760 mmHg, i.e. a similar volume to that occupied by one gram-molecule of a gas under these conditions. Thus 197.4 g of liquid halothane or 74.1 g of liquid diethyl ether will vaporize to yield 22.414 litres of vapour at STP. By means of Charles' law, it is possible to calculate the volume at other temperatures since the 22.414 litres at $0\,°C$ becomes $22.414 \times (T/273)$ where T is the ambient temperature in kelvins on the absolute scale. At $20\,°C$ (293 K) 197.4 g of liquid halothane will vaporize into 24.056 litres so that each 1 ml of vapour contains 8.21 mg of halothane. At $37\,°C$ (310 K) the volume is 25.452 litres and each 1 ml of vapour then contains 7.76 mg of halothane. At $0\,°C$, 1 g of liquid halothane will produce 113.5 ml of vapour, whereas at $20\,°C$ and $37\,°C$ it will produce 121.9 and 128.9 ml respectively. Some techniques of administering volatile anaesthetic agents into a closed circle anaesthetic system use a manually- (Wolfson, 1962) or power-driven syringe (Lowe, 1972) to deliver known amounts of halothane to the circuit over definite periods of time. In this case it is convenient to know how many millilitres of vapour will be produced by 1 ml of the liquid agent rather than by 1 g. This is obtained from the ratio (liquid density)/(vapour density). Density is defined as the mass per unit volume at a specified temperature and is usually expressed in grams per cc. In this case it is more convenient to work in mg per ml. At $20\,°C$, the density of liquid halothane is 1.86 g per cm^3 = 1.86 g per ml and the vapour density of halothane at $20\,°C$ is 8.21 mg per ml. Thus 1 ml of liquid halothane at $20\,°C$ produces $1860/8.21 = 226.6$ ml of vapour. The properties of some volatile anaesthetic agents are given in *Table 5.5*.

By Charles' law, the volume of a gas is directly proportional to its absolute temperature. Thus 22.4 litres at $0\,°C$ and 760 mmHg becomes 22.4 (293/273) = 24.04 litres at $20\,°C$ and 25.44 litres at $37\,°C$. Hence at $0\,°C$, 1 ml of halothane vapour will contain 8.81 mg of halothane, the corresponding figures for $20\,°C$ and $37\,°C$ being 8.21 mg and 7.76 mg, respectively. A 1 per cent v/v mixture of halothane at $0\,°C$ and 760 mmHg contains by definition 1 ml of halothane vapour per 100 ml of

TABLE 5.5

Agent	Chloroform	Diethyl ether	Ethrane	Fluroxene	Forane	Halothane	Methoxy-flurane	Trichloro-ethylene
Formula	$CHCl_3$	$C_4H_{10}O$	$C_3H_2OClF_5$	$C_4H_5OF_3$	$C_3H_2OClF_5$	$C_2HClBrF_3$	$C_3H_4OCl_2F_2$	C_2HCl_3
Molecular weight	119.4	74.1	184.5	126.0	184.5	197.4	165.0	131.4
mg per ml of vapour at 760 mmHg 0°C	5.33	33.1	7.56	5.62	7.56	8.81	7.36	5.86
20°C	4.96	3.08	7.67	5.24	7.67	8.21	6.86	5.46
37°C	4.69	2.91	7.25	4.95	7.25	7.76	6.48	5.16
at 713 mmHg 37°C	4.40	2.73	6.80	4.64	6.80	7.28	6.08	4.84
Density g/ml at 20°C	1.47	0.72	1.52	1.13	1.49	1.86	1.42	1.46
ml vapour/ml liquid 20°C	296	234	198	216	194	227	207	267
Vapour pressure at 20°C in mmHg	159	442	180	286	250	242	26	58
Latent heat of vaporixation Jg^{-1}	247	360	157	222	151	147	205	239

gas mixture, i.e. 8.81 mg. Warming the mixture to 20 °C will reduce the mass of halothane to 8.81 × (273/293) = 8.21 mg, the mixture still being 1 per cent by volume. At 37 °C, 100 ml of mixture will contain 7.76 mg. If the mixture was saturated with water vapour (partial pressure 47 mmHg at 37 °C), the mass of halothane per 100 ml will be 7.76 × (760 − 47)/760 = 7.28 mg. For an alveolar halothane concentration of 1.3 MAC (0.975 per cent v/v) each 100 ml of alveolar gas at 37 °C will contain 7.28 × 0.975 = 7.10 mg per 100 ml. Since the halothane blood–gas partition coefficient is 2.4 the arterial blood halothane concentration in equilibrium with the alveolar gas is 17.04 mg per 100 ml.

Factors affecting the uptake of anaesthetic gases and vapours

The body can be considered to consist of a number of compartments in parallel (*Figure 5.18*) with each other and with the lungs. Each compartment is considered to have a specific gas or blood supply and able

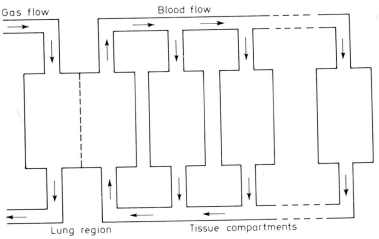

Figure 5.18. Multi-compartment model of the body (after Whelpton, 1969)

to contain a certain quantity of gas. The volume of gas dissolved in the *x*th compartment is

$$V_x = (VT_x \times \lambda T_x + Q \, \lambda_b) f_x$$

where VT_x is the volume of tissues in the xth compartment, λT_x is the tissue–gas partition coefficient, Q_x is the volume of blood in equilibrium with the tissue and f_x is the fractional concentration of the anaesthetic vapour with which the tissue is in equilibrium. λ_b is the blood–tissue partition coefficient. Similarly, the volume of anaesthetic vapour contained in the lungs is

$$V_L = (V_A + V_P \lambda_P + Q_A \lambda_b) f_A$$

where V_A is the mean volume of gas in the alveoli, V_P is the volume of the lung tissue having a tissue-gas partition coefficient of λ_P, Q_A is the volume of blood which is in equilibrium with the gas in the alveoli, λ_b is the blood–gas partition coefficient and f_A is the fractional concentration of anaesthetic agent present in the alveoli.

The rate of uptake of the agent concerned by the whole body is $dV/dt = \dot{V}_A(f_I - f_A)$ where $\dot{V}_A$ is the alveolar ventilation responsible for carrying gas having a fractional anaesthetic concentration f_I into the lungs and gas having an alveolar fractional concentration f_A out of the lungs. For simplicity is is assumed that there is no dead space volume and that the inspired and expired alveolar volumes are equal, i.e. that the uptake of the agent is infinitely slow. This implies that the inspired concentration is infinitely low. In the case of the xth compartment,

$$\frac{dV_x}{dt} = \dot{Q}_x \lambda_b (f_a - f_v)_x$$

where $\dot{Q}_x$ is the blood flow per minute to the xth compartment, f_a and f_v are the respective arterial and venous blood levels of the agent from the xth compartment at equilbrium. It is assumed that the anaesthetic vapour may diffuse freely through the alveolar and capillary walls, i.e. that no alveolar-to-arterial gradient exists for the agent in question. It is also assumed that the tension of the gas vapour in the tissue is the same as that of venous blood draining from the tissue. Thus $f_a = f_A$, and

$$\frac{dV_x}{dt} = \dot{Q}_x \lambda_b (f_a - f_v)_x$$

For a constant blood flow and arterial concentration, the tissue tension in each compartment will rise exponentially, so that the rate of uptake of the agent in each compartment will fall off exponentially with time.

If this simple type of multicompartment model is used to simulate the uptake of halothane, for example by the body, then serious discrepancies will be found between the calculated uptakes and the experimental values (Whelpton, 1969). A good correspondence can be obtained by making allowances for the *concentration effect*, the *second gas effect* and venous admixture.

In Chapter 1, it was shown that if the right heart is suddenly presented with a bolus of M_0 mg of dye, then assuming perfect mixing within the heart and pulmonary circulation the wash-out curve of the dye from the left heart for a constant cardiac output is a simple exponential equation of the form

$$M = M_0 \exp(-\dot{Q}/V)t$$

After the passage of an infinite time, the dye concentration will have decreased to zero. In this case, the heart and pulmonary circulation were considered to be non-absorbing and of a fixed volume V. The indicator present in this volume is washed out by the steady inflow ($\dot{Q}$ the cardiac output) of fresh blood. Consider the case of a vessel of volume V perfused with a steady flow F litres per minute of gas and suppose that a steady concentration C_{in} (ml of vapour per 100 ml of gas) of a volatile anaesthetic agent is added to this gas. If C_{out} is the concentration of agent measured in the output from the vessel, then after the passage of an infinite time the vessel will be saturated with the agent and $C_{out} = C_{in}$. The wash-in equation is

$$C_{out} = C_{in} [1 - \exp(-F/V)t]$$

When we consider the case of the uptake of an anaesthetic vapour by a particular organ, for simplicity we can assume the organ to have a fixed volume V, but it is now necessary to take into account the tissue–blood partition coefficient since the effective volume of the organ for the vapour is $V \times \lambda_{t/b}$. The outflow concentration $C_{out} = C_{\bar{v}}$ the mixed venous blood concentration in ml of vapour per 100 ml of blood leaving the organ; C_{in} becomes C_a the arterial blood concentration in ml of vapour per 100 ml of blood entering the organ and F is the blood flow in litres per minute to the organ, V is the volume of the organ in litres and $\lambda_{t/b}$ is the tissue–blood partition coefficient at body temperature.

The percentage saturation of the organ is $(C_{\bar{v}}/C_a) \times 100$ per cent which is

$$\left\{1 - \exp\left[-F/(V \times \lambda_{t/b})\right]t\right\} \times 100 \text{ per cent}$$

after t minutes of anaesthesia. When the organ is saturated with vapour the capacity of the organ is $10 \times V \times C_a \times \lambda_{t/b}$ ml. Thus after t minutes of anaesthesia the organ content is given by capacity $\times$ percentage saturation. The factor 10 occurs because C_a is quoted in ml of vapour per 100 ml of blood. The time constant of the organ is $V \times \lambda_{t/b} \times F$ minutes.

In order to be able to calculate the uptake of a volatile agent by a particular organ, it is necessary to know the blood flow to the organ, the organ volume and the tissue–blood partition coefficient. Lowe (1972) uses the data in *Table 5.6* for a 100 kg man, and uses the

TABLE 5.6

Organ	Volume (litres)	Percentage of the cardiac output			
Heart	0.4	4			
Brain	2.1	14			
Liver	5.7	29			
Kidneys	0.6	26			
Muscle	42.5	11			
Fat	15	6			
Skin	11	10	Poorly perfused tissue		
Bone	12	10	"	"	"
Connective tissue	4	10	"	"	"

TABLE 5.7

Agent	Blood–Gas	Tissue–Blood					
		Brain	Liver	Kidney	Muscle	Fat	Poorly perfused tissue
Cyclopropane	0.46	3.9	1.3	0.87	0.87	32.6	–
Halothane	2.40	2.3	1.9	1.3	1.3	75	2.0
Methoxyflurane	10	2.5	2.3	3.1	2.0	100	1.0

partition coefficients in *Table 5.7* at 37 °C. Lowe states that the partition coefficients for poorly perfused tissue have not been measured directly but were calculated from the known fat and water content of these tissues, so that at best the figures are estimates. Lowe takes a typical cardiac output of 7 litres per minute for a 100 kg man. Mapleson (1973) also quotes a set of tissue volumes, together with their associated blood flows and tissue–blood partition coefficients. Mapleson does not associate any blood–flow to bone cortex, but introduces quite a large 'peripheral shunt'. For his 'standard man',

Mapleson assumes a total tissue volume of 70 litres, an FRC (functional residual capacity) of 2.5 litres, an alveolar ventilation of 4 litres per minute BTPS and a cardiac output of 6.48 litres per minute. The adaptation of such a model to simulate the uptake of nitrous oxide in man at atmospheric and hyperbaric pressures is given by Mapleson *et al.* (1974).

Suppose that an alveolar concentration of the agent of 1.3 MAC is required to prevent the patient moving. This corresponds with an alveolar halothane concentration of 0.975 per cent, so that the alveoli will contain 0.975 ml of vapour per 100 ml of gas. Multiplying this value by the blood—gas coefficient of 2.4 gives the arterial concentration of 2.34 ml of vapour per 100 ml of blood. Before this amount of vapour can be supplied to the alveoli, the anaesthetic circuit and the functional residual capacity (FRC) of the patient's lungs must first be charged with vapour. Allowance will also have to be made for any vapour absorbed by the hoses of the circuit and any losses from the circuit relief valve if the circuit is not completely closed. For a total circuit and FRC non-absorbing volume of 10 litres, $(10 \times 1000 \times 0.99/100) = 99$ ml of halothane vapour must be supplied in the first minute. Assuming a blood volume of 7 litres and a blood—gas coefficient of 2.4, in the first minute of anaesthesia the blood will absorb $(7 \times 1000 \times 2.4 \times 0.99/100) = 166.3$ ml of halothane vapour.

It is now possible to consider the uptake of halothane by individual organs. For a brain volume of 2100 ml and a brain halothane concentration at equilibrium of 5.38 per cent, the brain capacity is 113 ml of halothane vapour. The percentage saturation of an organ is given by

$$(C_{\bar{v}}/C_a) \times 100 \text{ per cent} = \left\{1 - \exp\left[-F/(V \times \lambda_{t/b})\right] t\right\} \times 100 \text{ per cent}$$

From this equation, the time constant of the brain for the uptake of halothane is

$$(V \times \lambda_{t/b})/F$$

where V is the volume of the brain in litres, $\lambda_{t/b}$ is the blood—brain partition coefficient and F is the brain blood flow in litres per minute. Thus the brain time constant for halothane is

$$(2.1 \times 2.3)/0.98 = 4.9 \text{ minutes,}$$

since the brain blood flow is taken as being 14 per cent of a 7 litres per minute cardiac output.

The brain saturation at the end of the first minute is

$$[1 - \exp(-0.98/2.1 \times 2.3)] \times 100 \text{ per cent} = 18 \text{ per cent}$$

Thus the brain content at the end of the first minute is 18 per cent of 113 ml = 20.3 ml of halothane vapour.

The uptake sequence of halothane by the brain is shown in *Table 5.8.*

TABLE 5.8. Uptake of halothane by the brain

Time in minutes	Uptake	Saturation (%)	Content
1	20.3	18.0	20.3
2	17.0	33.0	37.3
3	13.6	45.0	50.9
4	11.3	55.0	62.2
5	9.0	63.0	71.2
10	3.4	86.0	97.2

After 3 minutes the brain is 45 per cent saturated with halothane; this corresponds with 0.45×1.3 MAC = 0.59 MAC. According to Lowe (1972), the patient could be expected to move at this level of anaesthesia during the surgical incision unless the premedication or the induction dose of sodium pentothal contributed the equivalent of 0.5 MAC. Without this supplement it would be necessary to wait another four minutes until the brain was 75 per cent saturated i.e. 0.75×1.3 MAC = 0.98 MAC.

For the liver $C_a = 2.38$ ml of vapour per 100 ml of blood, $F = 2.03$ litres per minute, $V = 5.7$ litres and $\lambda_{t/b} = 1.9$. The uptake sequence for the liver is shown in *Table 5.9*. The liver capacity is 257.8 ml of halothane vapour, and its time constant is 5.3 minutes.

For muscle, $C_a = 2.38$ ml of vapour per 100 ml of blood, $F = 0.77$ litres per minute, $V = 42.5$ litres and $\lambda_{t/b} = 1.3$. The uptake sequence

TABLE 5.9. Uptake of halothane by the liver

Time in minutes	Uptake	Saturation (%)	Content
1	43.8	17.0	43.8
2	38.7	32.0	82.5
3	28.3	43.0	110.9
4	25.7	53.0	136
5	16.1	59.0	152
10	7.7	85.0	219

TABLE 5.10. Uptake of halothane by muscle

Time in minutes	Uptake	Saturation (%)	Content
1	13.2	1.0	13.2
2	13.2	2.0	26.4
3	13.2	3.0	39.6
4	13.2	4.0	52.8
5	13.2	5.0	66.0
10	13.1	10.0	131.5

of muscle is shown in *Table 5.10*. The muscle capacity is 1315 ml of halothane vapour and its time constant is 71.8 minutes.

For the body fat, $C_a = 2.38$ ml of vapour per 100 ml of blood, $F = 0.42$ litres per minute, $V = 15$ litres and $\lambda_{t/b} = 75$. The uptake sequence of the fat is shown in *Table 5.11*. The fat capacity is 28.78 litres and its time constant is 2679 minutes = 44.6 hours.

TABLE 5.11. Uptake of halothane by fat

Time in minutes	Uptake	Saturation (%)	Content
1	10.7	0.04	10.7
2	8.1	0.07	18.8
3	10.7	0.11	29.5
4	10.7	0.15	40.2
5	10.7	0.19	50.9
10	11.8	0.37	100
20	9.9	0.74	199
60	9.88	2.22	594
120	9.65	4.38	1173
240	9.42	8.6	2303
300	8.93	10.6	2839

Lowe (1972) assumes that the patient's blood concentration of anaesthetic must have fallen to 0.37 MAC for recovery and arousal, i.e. 0.28 per cent halothane. After four hours of anaesthesia, the patient's muscle is virtually saturated and holds 1269 ml of halothane vapour, i.e. approximately 5.6 ml of liquid halothane, assuming that the arterial blood concentration has remained steady at 2.38 ml of vapour per 100 ml of blood. At 0.37 MAC the blood concentration will have fallen to 0.67 ml of vapour per 100 ml of blood. During the period of recovery from the anaesthetic, the average mixed venous blood halothane concentration will be $(2.38 + 0.67)/2 = 1.53$ ml of vapour per 100 ml of blood. For a cardiac output of 7 litres per minute, the average amount of halothane vapour returning to the lungs per minute = 70 × 1.53 = 107 ml. The mean concentration in the alveolar gas will be 1.53/2.4 = 0.64 ml of vapour per 100 ml of gas. For an alveolar ventilation of 5 litres per minute, 32 ml of halothane vapour would be cleared from the lungs per minute. To achieve 0.37 MAC, the halothane content of the muscle would have to fall to 28 per cent of the saturation value, i.e. 914 ml of vapour must be removed. This would take 29 minutes, ignoring uptake by fat. After four hours of halothane anaesthesia, the body fat is absorbing about 21 ml of halothane vapour per minute and the lungs are clearing 32 ml per minute. This would reduce the recovery time to 17 minutes neglecting vapour stored in other organs.

When the uptake for each organ has been calculated for the first minute of anaesthesia, these can be totalled and this amount of halothane plus the amount needed to prime the circuit and the blood must be provided during the first minute, i.e. 99 ml (circuit) + 166.3 ml (blood) + 20.3 ml (brain) + 43.8 ml (liver) + 13.2 ml (muscle) + 10.7 ml (fat) = 353 ml. Subsequently, the rate of delivery of vapour to the patient should be reduced in such a fashion as to match the predicted rate of uptake of the organs. This technique is known as 'programmed' anaesthesia. Lowe (1972) reported that in more than 200 anaesthetics, this approach yielded blood anaesthetic levels within ± 15 per cent of the predicted values. Lowe also found that when the predicted cumulative anaesthetic vapour requirement for each agent was plotted against the square root of time, a linear relationship was obtained.

The concentration and second gas effect

The uptake of an anaesthetic gas or vapour accelerates its own uptake. Assuming that the patient's airway is patent, the gas or vapour which is absorbed is continuously replaced by the gas mixture filling the anaesthetic circuit. This so-called *concentration effect* has been described by Eger (1963a, b); Epstein *et al.* (1964) and Mapleson (1964a). Mapleson (1964b) proposed a mathematical correction to the uptake equations to allow for the concentration effect. Essentially, the action of the absorbed gas or vapour is to produce an equivalent increase in the alveolar ventilation. Agents such as halothane are commonly used in the presence of a large percentage of a second soluble gas such as nitrous oxide. As the second gas dissolves in the tissue and blood of the patient, the concentration of this gas in the alveoli will fall and thus the fractional concentration of the first gas or vapour will rise. The *second gas effect* was described by Epstein *et al.* (1964), Mapleson (1964a) and Stoelting and Eger (1969). Kitahata, Taub and Conte (1971) showed that in decerebrated cats with an equilibrated P_{ACO_2} of 40 mmHg, administration of 80 per cent nitrous oxide produced an increase in P_{ACO_2} of 2.6 mmHg due to the concentrating effect of the rapid absorption of the nitrous oxide. Bojrab and Stoelting (1974) studied the enhanced uptake of oxygen in the presence of nitrous oxide. They found that the arterial oxygen tension during the inhalation of a mixture of (30 per cent O_2 + 70 per cent N_2O) was greater than that measured during the inhalation of a (30 per cent O_2 + 70 per cent N_2) mixture. This is the result of the large rate of N_2O uptake which increases the tracheal inflow of oxygen-containing gas and also concentrates the oxygen in a smaller lung volume. However, Bojrab and Stoelting state that the *second gas effect* cannot be relied upon to produce a clinically significant increase in arterial oxygenation.

When the alveoli are presented with a concentration of 10 per cent N_2O, the initial rate of uptake is given by

$$F_A \times \lambda_{t/b} \times \dot{Q}$$

where $\dot{Q}$, the cardiac output, is in decilitres per minute. For a cardiac output of 7 litres per minute the uptake is $10 \times 0.47 \times 70 = 329$ ml per minute. If the alveolar ventilation was 5 litres per minute prior to giving the nitrous oxide the effective alveolar ventilation is now increased to 5.329 litres per minute. When 70 per cent nitrous oxide is given the alveolar ventilation is increased to $5 + 2.303 = 7.303$ litres per minute. The increased uptake of nitrous oxide at an alveolar concentration of 70 per cent relative to that at 10 per cent has been called the 'augmentation ratio' by Epstein *et al.* (1964). It is equal to

$$F_E/F_I \text{ (70 per cent } N_2O) \div F_E/F_I \text{ (10 per cent } N_2O)$$

where F_I and F_E are the fractional inspired and expired concentrations of the gas or vapour at 10 and 70 per cent N_2O. Lowe (1972) shows that the augmentation ratio is given by

$$F_E/F_I = 1/(1 + \dot{Q}\,\lambda_{b/g}/\dot{V}_A)$$

where $\dot{Q}$ is the cardiac output in litres per minute, $\dot{V}_A$ is the alveolar ventilation in litres per minute and $\lambda_{b/g}$ is the blood–gas partition coefficient. Thus with 10 per cent N_2O,

$$F_E/F_I = \left(1 + \frac{7 \times 0.47}{5.329}\right)^{-1} = 0.62$$

Lowe calculates the augmentation ratio for N_2O alone as 1.09 but for halothane administered with 10 per cent and 70 per cent N_2O respectively it is 1.18. The augmentation ratio for halothane at increasing concentrations of nitrous oxide is known as the *second gas effect* and is greater than the effect of the augmentation ratio of N_2O upon its own absorption. The use of 70 per cent N_2O increases the initial rate of uptake of halothane by a factor of 1.25, since

$$(F_E/F_I) \frac{10 \text{ per cent } N_2O}{\text{Halothane}} = \left(1 + \frac{7 \times 2.3}{5.329}\right)^{-1} = 0.249$$

and

$$(F_E/F_I) \frac{70 \text{ per cent } N_2O}{\text{Halothane}} = \left(1 + \frac{7 \times 2.3}{7.303}\right)^{-1} = 0.312$$

so that

$$0.312/0.249 = 1.25$$

Losses of anaesthetic vapour to the rubber components of the anaesthetic circuit

The concentration of an anaesthetic vapour reaching the patient may be significantly reduced from that delivered by the vaporizer to the circuit as a result of uptake by the the rubber tubing, breathing bag and soda lime absorber. The rubber—gas partition coefficient is defined as the number of millilitres of anaesthetic vapour which are absorbed by each 100 ml of rubber when equilibrated with a 1 per cent concentration of the vapour. For example, each 100 ml of rubber can absorb 120 ml of halothane vapour at 23 °C which equals 0.53 ml approximately of

TABLE 5.12

Agent	Rubber—gas partition coefficient at 23 °C
Nitrous oxide	1.2
Cyclopropane	6.6
Diethyl ether	45
Halothane	120
Chloroform	300
Methoxyflurane	630
Trichloroethylene	830

liquid halothane. Titel and Lowe (1968) give rubber–gas partition coefficients (*Table 5.12*).

Lowe, Titel and Hagler (1971) found that the absorption of an anaesthetic vapour by a breathing circuit was proportional to:

(1) The delivered vapour concentration F_D
(2) The internal surface area A of the circuit
(3) The rubber–gas partition coefficient for the agent concerned
(4) The molecular diffusion coefficient D of the agent in rubber
(5) The square root of time

The capacity of a length of tubing 1 metre long by 20 mm in diameter by 1.5 mm thick (47 cm^3 of rubber) for halothane is 56 ml of vapour. Lowe (1972) states that the circuit losses can be reduced to negligible amounts by the use of polyethylene, polyolefin or polyurethane disposable circuits.

Losses of anaesthetic vapour to the soda lime

As well as the absorption by rubber, in the case of methoxyflurane, there can also be a substantial loss of the agent to the soda lime in the carbon dioxide absorber. Lowe (1972) reports a linear relationship between the partition coefficient for methoxyflurane and soda lime and the logarithm of the water content of the soda lime. For fresh soda lime the partition coefficient had a value of about 7, whereas for completely dry soda lime it was about 200. The time constant of a given volume of soda lime is equal to

$$\left(\frac{\text{volume of soda lime} \times \lambda}{\text{gas flow rate}} \right)$$

For a 500 ml volume of soda lime, a partition coefficient of 200 and a 5 litre per minute gas flow, the time constant is $(0.5 \times 200/5) = 20$ minutes. This means that after 20 minutes the concentration of methoxyflurane leaving the soda lime will only be 63 per cent of that entering it.

In non-rebreathing and semi-closed circle systems it can be seen that apart from the amount of anaesthetic vapour actually taken up by the patient, it will be necessary to provide additional supplies of vapour to replace the losses to the rubber surfaces and the soda lime, the losses of inspiratory gas from the upper airway due to the presence of dead space and the loss of expiratory gases which vent out of the circuit, i.e. amount taken up = (amount delivered − rubber and soda lime loss) − (dead space ventilation + expirate). Lowe (1972) considers the case of a 100 kg man who is ventilated at 5 litres per minute and has a dead space of 15 per cent of the tidal volume. The inspiratory rubber hose has not been previously exposed to halothane and the soda lime is moist. The anaesthetic circuit is chosen to be as efficient as possible. The cardiac output is taken as 7 litres per minute and an FRC of 3 litres is added to the circuit volume. The circuit and lungs can be primed initially by giving 5 litres per minute of 9.5 per cent halothane, reducing this to 3.2 per cent at the end of the first minute, then to 2.8 per cent at the end of the second minute, 2.4 per cent at the end of the fifth minute, 2 per cent at the end of the 10th minute, 1.8 per cent at the end of 20 minutes, 1.5 per cent at the end of 60 minutes and 1.4 per cent at the end of 2 hours.

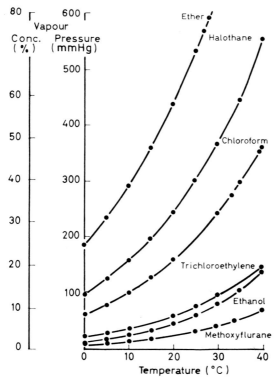

Figure 5.19. Variation of the saturated vapour pressure of various volatile anaesthestic agents with temperature

The variation of saturated vapour pressure with temperature

When a liquid is in contact with its vapour in a closed container, a state of equilibrium is attained where as many molecules leave the liquid by evaporation per second to escape into the vapour phase as rejoin the liquid per second. When this occurs, the vapour above the liquid is said to be fully saturated. The vapour molecules bombard the vessel walls and give rise to a pressure, known as the Saturated Vapour Pressure, (SVP). It is important to remember that the SVP depends only upon the nature of the liquid and its temperature. The effect of pressure can be neglected over the range encountered in anaesthesia. This fact is of importance in explaining the operation of anaesthetic vaporizers under hypobaric and hyperbaric atmosphere conditions.

For a given agent, the graph of SVP against temperature is a smooth curve as shown in *Figure 5.19*. The curve for each agent is characterized by its own Antoine equation (Antoine, 1888) as follows — the values being taken from Rodgers and Hill (1978):

Diethyl ether

$$\log_{10}P = 7.02683 - \frac{1109.577}{t + 233.155}$$

Halothane

$$\log_{10}P = 6.85426 - \frac{1125.046}{t + 222.014}$$

Chloroform

$$\log_{10}P = 6.83695 - \frac{1198.47}{t + 216.436}$$

Trichloroethylene

$$\log_{10}P = 6.83695 - \frac{1198.477}{t + 216.436}$$

Methoxyflurane

$$\log_{10}P = 7.08219 - \frac{1336.580}{t + 213.480}$$

In each case P is in mmHg and t in $^\circ$C.
A slightly different equation for methoxyflurane has been given by Nahrwold *et al.* (1973):

$$\log_{10}P = 7.11693 - \frac{1353.150}{t + 214.944}$$

Rodgers and Hill (1978) give a detailed description of Antoine equations for volatile anaesthetic agents and discuss their use in controlling the concentration of anaesthetic agent delivered to a patient, for example with the use of a copper kettle vaporizer.

The saturated concentration of a volatile anaesthetic agent

The saturated vapour pressure of halothane at 20 °C is 243 mmHg, so that by Dalton's law of partial pressures at a standard barometric pressure of 760 mmHg the saturation concentration is (243/760) × 100 per cent = 32.0 per cent v/v. At a city such as Denver where the altitude is 5000 feet and the barometric pressure has fallen to 635 mmHg, the saturation concentration at 20 °C has increased to (243/635) × 100 per cent = 38.3 per cent v/v.

The relationship between the saturated vapour pressure and the boiling point of a volatile anaesthetic agent

The boiling point of a liquid is that temperature at which the vapour pressure of the liquid is equal to the atmospheric pressure. Hence it will

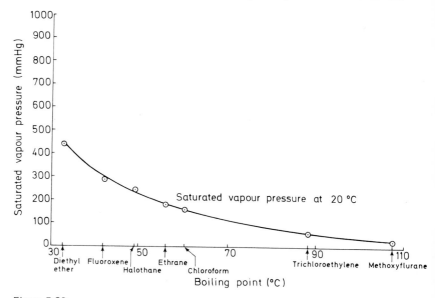

Figure 5.20

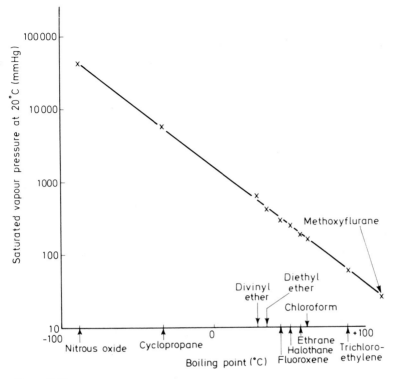

Figure 5.21

decrease with increasing altitude. When the boiling point of the volatile anaesthetic agents is plotted against the corresponding saturated vapour pressure, the vapour pressure decrease exponentially (*Figure 5.20*) but when the logarithm of the vapour pressure is plotted against the boiling point for each agent, a straight line is obtained (*Figure 5.21*).

The relationship between the concentration of a volatile anaesthetic agent expressed in volume per cent and in milligrams per litre

The concentration of a volatile anaesthetic vapour can be expressed in terms of a percentage by volume or on a weight per unit volume basis. Consider one litre of a gas mixture containing C per cent by volume of halothane vapour at $t\ °C$. Then the volume of vapour contained in that one litre equals $(C/100) \times 1000$ ml. Since the molecular weight of halothane (197.4 g) will vaporize into a volume of 22.4 litres at 0 °C and 760 mmHg and this becomes

$$\frac{(273 + t)}{273} \times \frac{760}{P} \times 22.4 \text{ litres}$$

at a temperature of t °C and a pressure of P mmHg, the mass of halothane present under these conditions is

$$\frac{C \times 10 \times 197.4 \times 273 \times P}{22.4 \times (t + 273) \times 760} \text{ mg}$$

By substituting the appropriate molecular weight this expression can be used for any agent. For the case of a one per cent by volume concentration of halothane at 20 °C and one atmosphere (760 mmHg) the mass in one litre of mixture is

$$\frac{1 \times 197.4 \times 273 \times 760}{2.24 \times 293 \times 760} = 82.11 \text{ mg}$$

For the same one per cent concentration at 20 °C but at two atmospheres (1520 mmHg) the mass of halothane in one litre becomes 164.22 mg. Thus, doubling the ambient pressure doubles the mass per unit volume for the same volume concentration. Normally, if a one per cent concentration by volume at one atmosphere is subjected to a further one atmosphere, the saturation volume concentration will be halved since the saturated vapour pressure of the agent can be assumed to remain constant as the temperature is unaltered. Since the volume concentration has halved and the pressure doubled, the mass per unit volume will remain the same. It is for this reason that the clinical performance of anaesthetic vaporizers used under hyperbaric conditions is similar to that found under ordinary atmospheric pressure.

The concentration in mg per 100 ml is related to the concentration C in volumes per cent by

$$\frac{C \times MW \times 273 \times P}{0.224 \times (t + 273) \times 760} \text{ mg/100 ml}$$

where MW is the molecular weight in grams of the agent concerned. This expression can also be used to relate a concentration expressed in terms of parts per million by volume to an equivalent mg/100 ml since 1000 parts per million by volume equals 0.1 per cent by volume.

Thus 100 parts per million of halothane vapour at 20 °C and atmospheric pressure is equivalent to 0.82 mg per litre.

Humidity

For most clinical purposes, it is sufficient to assume that the gas issuing from cylinders is dry. Hill and Newell (1965) measured the water vapour concentration of the gas obtained from a number of cylinders of argon using an electrolytic hygrometer. A typical value for the water content of argon was less than ten parts per million by volume for cylinder pressures greater than 100 lbf in^{-2} (698.4 kN m^{-2}). In the case of oxygen, the water vapour concentration is likely to be of the order of 200 p.p.m. by volume (private communication, British Oxygen Company). Since the saturated vapour pressure of the water depends only upon the temperature, the concentration of water vapour in the cylinder will rise markedly as the gas pressure falls when the cylinder becomes nearly empty.

Expired air is assumed to leave the mouth fully saturated at the temperature of the mouth. The author has observed mouth temperatures of twenty subjects breathing room air at 20 °C through the nose, to be distributed over the range 34–36 °C. When making allowance for the presence of water vapour in gas law calculations a knowledge of the variation of the SVP of water vapour with temperature is required. Typical values are 18 mmHg at 20 °C and 47 mmHg at 37 °C. Assuming a barometric pressure of 760 mmHg, the water vapour concentration in breath saturated at 37 °C would be 6.2 per cent v/v. Since 1 per cent is equivalent to 10 000 parts per million this would be equivalent to 62 000 p.p.m. If sufficient water vapour is added to a closed container of air at 37 °C and 760 mmHg, the pressure will rise to 760 + 47 = 807 mmHg. Ernst and Perez-Zamura (1969) have measured water vapour pressures in blood and tissues. At 37 °C they found values of 47.1 mmHg in distilled water, 45.6 mmHg in physiological saline and 49.6 mmHg in whole blood. Déry (1971) discusses the role of humidity in anaesthesia and has measured the alveolar humidity and temperature in the dog.

Absolute humidity

Absolute humidity is defined in terms of the actual mass of water vapour contained in a given volume of gas at a given temperature and pressure, and is expressed in terms of grams of water vapour per cubic metre. A typical expired air humidity for anaesthetized patients is 23 mg per litre (0.023 kg m^{-3}). It is of importance in specifying the quantity of water which must be evaporated to raise the humidity of an operating room to a particular value.

Relative humidity

Relative humidity is a term frequently encountered when dealing with air conditioning of operating rooms, and also when considering the loss of water by patients during respiration. It indicates the actual amount of water vapour present in a volume of gas, expressed as a percentage of the maximum possible amount obtainable at the specified ambient temperature. For example, a relative humidity of 50 per cent at 20 °C means that there is only one half the water vapour present per unit volume of gas than there would be if the gas was fully saturated at 20 °C. The actual water vapour pressure will be 9 mmHg, i.e. one-half of the saturated vapour pressure which is 18 mmHg at 20 °C. If the relative humidity was 40 per cent at 20 °C, this would fall to 16 per cent if the temperature of the air was raised to 37 °C.

Since alveolar air has a relative humidity of 100 per cent at 37 °C, any inhaled air having a lower humidity will absorb moisture from the respiratory tract. The warming, wetting and filtering of the inspired air takes place in the upper portions of the tract. When this natural air-conditioning system is bypassed by the performance of a tracheostomy, excessive drying of bronchial secretions will arise if the patient breathes dry air for an extended period. For this reason, automatic ventilators designed for long-term use by patients suffering from respiratory insufficiency are fitted with a device known as a humidifier, which adds moisture to the inspired gases.

Dew point

If air is saturated with water vapour at body temperature (37 °C) and then cooled to 20 °C, the saturated water vapour pressure must fall from 47 to 20 mmHg. As a result, the excess water will condense on the surface of piping or valves which are at 20 °C. This accounts for the droplets of water which form on the expiratory valve of a circle anaesthetic system. The *dew point* of the gas is defined as the temperature to which the gas must be lowered in order for water to condense from it. When condensation commences, the partial pressure of the water vapour is equal to the saturated vapour pressure at the temperature. This fact is utilized in Regnault's hygrometer.

Hygrometers

Hygrometers are instruments designed to measure the amount of water vapour contained in a given sample of gas. Many types are calibrated in terms of relative humidity, but others are calibrated in terms of water vapour concentration. In Regnault's hygrometer, a silver tube can be cooled by the evaporation of liquid ether. When the tube has been cooled to the dew point of the surrounding air, a film of condensed moisture forms on the tube. The temperature of the ether, and thus that of the tube, is read on a thermometer when the condensastion is first observed. Suppose that the temperature is 10 °C. The saturated vapour pressure for water at 10 °C is 10 mmHg and at room temperature (20 °C) it is 18 mmHg. Thus the relative humidity of the air on this occasion is $10/18 \times 100 = 56$ per cent.

A type of compact hygrometer frequently encountered in operating rooms and incubators for neonates is the *hair hygrometer*. This operates on the principle that human hair increases in length as the humidity of the surrounding air increases. A simple lever system is employed to magnify the change in length, and to cause a pointer to move across a scale calibrated in percentage relative humidity. Hair hygrometers are limited to the range 15 and 85 per cent relative humidity.

The need for providing reliable control systems for modern air-conditioning schemes has led to the development of a number of humidity transducers. These operate on the principle of measuring the change in resistance or dielectric constant of a suitable element as it absorbs water. Low water vapour contents from a few parts per million up to 3000 parts per million can conveniently be measured by means of an electrolytic hygrometer. This device is very suitable for the measurement of water concentrations in gases drawn from cylinders. Penman (1958) gives a good, compact account of the physics of humidity.

Humidifiers

Anaesthetists are often called upon to supervise the ventilation of patients suffering from a respiratory insufficiency. Automatic ventilators for this application are usually provided with a humidifier. The humidification of the inspired gases prevents an undue drying out of the secretions of the tracheobronchial tree and lungs of the patient, and consequent irritation. This is likely to arise when the air-conditioning properties of the nose are bypassed by an endotracheal tube or tracheostomy (Bendixen *et al.*, 1965). Marshall and Spalding (1953) describe a suitable humidifier for use with long-term automatic ventilation of the lungs. It consists of an electrically heated water bath through which is passed the inspired air. The design is such that the temperature and water content of the gas is practically unaffected by changes in the minute volume of the gas. The size of the water bath renders the arrangement rather bulky but it is widely encountered. This is an active type of humidifier which adds water to the inspired gases in contrast to a passive type which merely conserves the water present. Over recent years considerable improvements have been made in the design of humidifiers of the 'bubbler' type. In addition to a thermostat controlling the temperature of the water in the reservoir tank, a thermistor is mounted in the delivery tube from the humidifier to the patient. This monitors the temperature of the moist gases supplied to the patient and cuts out the bath heater if the temperature exceeds 40 °C. The water bath of the humidifier is now usually made from stainless steel and can be autoclaved.

The size of an active humidifier can be reduced by making use of a pump to add water in an aerosol-like spray to the gases. A fine jet of water is generated by a vibrator pump and caused to strike the wall of a metal tube where it forms a fine mist of water vapour which is entrained by the inspired gas stream. The humidifier uses a maximum of 20 ml of water per hour, and has a reservoir capacity of 500 ml of water. If the water vapour content of the inspired gases without humidification is zero, and that of the expired gases is 6 per cent v/v at 37 °C, this represents a loss of 480 ml of water vapour per minute if the patient's minute volume is 8 litres. At 37 °C, 1 ml of liquid water is equivalent to 1400 ml of water vapour, so that in one hour 20 ml of liquid water are consumed. In order to prevent an excessive condensation of water vapour in the connecting tubes to the patient, the humidifier is built into a head unit which is electrically heated to 40–45 °C, and can be mounted close to the patient's endotracheal tube. A pair of concentric tubes feeds the humidifier gas to the patient, where it arrives at 37 °C. The inner of the pair of concentric tubes carries the expired air, the outer tube carrying the inspired air. The heated head unit also carries mica-disk type inspiratory and expiratory valves together with a volumeter for measuring the tidal and minute volumes, plus an aneroid manometer for measuring the inflation pressure.

A simpler, but less efficient, type of humidifier suitable for use during anaesthesia is the multi-layer gauze type of passive humidifier.

This consists of ten or more gauze screens mounted in a housing, and connected to the patient's endotracheal tube. During expiration, warm moist expired air passes into the relatively cool gauzes. Some of the moisture condenses, and the gauzes become warmed. During inspiration, a proportion of the condensed moisture is evaporated, and the gases reaching the patient are warmed and humidified. Mapleson, Morgan and Hillard (1963) discuss the performance of a ten-gauze humidifier. They show that this arrangement should give an inspired humidity which is 58 per cent of the expired humidity. Unlike the active types of humidifier, the condenser type cannot put back into the inspired air more moisture than is contained in the expired air. However, its compact construction makes it very useful in practice. Smith (1964) describes the construction of a low-resistance condenser humidifier for holding constant the temperature and moisture content of the gases being respired through a pneumotachograph head. The flow resistance of the device was equivalent to a pressure drop of 9 mm of water at a gas flow rate of 60 litres per minute. Shanks and Sara (1973) have investigated the performance of a multiple gauze heat and moisture exchanger at five levels of measured fresh gas humidity. They found that, as predicted theoretically, the unit functioned best when presented with fresh gases having a high water vapour content. When arid fresh gas was employed, the unit did not moisten this sufficiently during inspiration for a prolonged use. However, it was found that the combination of a simple, unheated, humidification system with the standard gauze condenser humidifier produced a microclimate suitable for entry into the trachea during spontaneous or controlled respiration. Quadrupling the number of gauzes in the unit improved both the heat and moisture exchange performance with all but the saturated fresh gases, but considerably increased the weight of the unit. Stevens and Albregt (1966) compare the performance of conventional air-activated humidifiers with a far more efficient ultrasonic humidifier. They used a compact sodium chloride crystal as a humidity transducer placed in the tracheobronchial tree of dogs to measure the actual humidity in the respiratory tract. Ultrasonic humidifiers use a beam of ultrasound at a frequency of several megahertz to agitate the fluid and produce a vapour. The fluid in some models can be in a disposable cup which is placed on the ultrasonic generator. A powerful ultrasonic humidifier can produce copious quantities of mist and care may be required to see that the patient is thereby not caused to drown. Some anaesthetists alternate the use of a bubbler humidifier and an ultrasonic humidifier.

Nebulizers

An aerosol is defined as a suspension of very fine particles of a liquid or a solid in a gas, in general with a range of diameters from 0.005 μm to 50 μm, but in respiratory therapy practice those with a diameter of less than 3 μm are important because then the effect of gravity loses its influence (Egan, 1973). Nebulizers are used with assistors for presenting patients with medication in aerosol form, e.g. bronchodilators and decongestants. Some nebulizers work on a scent spray principle powered by a compressed gas supply whilst others are of the ultrasonic type. Their use is well described by Egan (1973).

References

ADAMS, A.P. and MORGAN-HUGHES, J.O. (1967). Determination of the blood-gas factor of the oxygen electrode using a new tonometer. *Br. J. Anaesth.* **39**, 107

ADAMS, A.P., VICKERS, M.D.A., MUNROE, J.P. and PARKER, C.W. (1967). Dry displacement gas meters. *Br. J. Anaesth.* **39**, 174

AGARWAL, J.R., PALTTO, R. and PALMER, W.H. (1970). Relative viscosity of blood at varying haematocrits in pulmonary circulation. *J. appl. Physiol.* **29**, 866

ALLOTT, P.R., STEWARD, A., FLOOK, VALERIE and MAPLESON, W.W. (1973). Variation with temperature of the solubilities of inhaled anaesthetics in water, oil and biological media. *Br. J. Anaesth.* **45**, 294

ANTOINE, C. (1888a). Tensions des vapeurs: nouvelle relation entre les tensions et les temperatures. *Comptes Rendus* **107**, 681

ANTOINE, C. (1888b). Tensions de diverses vapeurs. *Comptes Rendus* **107**, 836

ANTOINE, C. (1888c). Volumes des vapeurs saturées. *Comptes Rendus* **107**, 1143

AVERY, M.E. and MEAD, J. (1969). Surface properties in relation to atelectasis and hyaline membrane disease. *Am. Med. Ass. J. Dis. Childrn* **97**, 517

BAKER, R.A. and DOERR, R.C. (1959). Methods of sampling and storage of air containing vapours and gases. *Int. J. Air Pollut.* **2**, 142

BATE, H. (1977). Blood viscosity at different shear rates in capillary tubes. *Biorheol.* **14**, 267–275

BAYLISS, L.E. (1959). The axial drift of the red blood cells when blood flows in a narrow tube. *J. Physiol.* **149**, 593

BAYLISS, L.E. (1962). The rheology of blood. In *Handbook of Physiology* Vol. 2, Sect. 2 (Circulation), p. 137. Baltimore; Williams and Wilkins

BELLHOUSE, B.J., SCHULTZ, D.L., KARATZAS, N.B. and LEE, G. de J. (1968). A catheter tip method for the measurement of the pulsatile blood flow velocity in arteries. In *Blood Flow Through Organs and Tissues*, p. 43. (Ed. by W.H. Bain and A.M. Harper). Edinburgh; Livingstone

BENDIXEN, H.H., EGBERT, L.D., HEDLEY-WHYTE, J., LAVER, M.B. and PONTOPPIDON, H. (1965). *Respiratory Care*. St. Louis; Mosby

BODELL, B.R. (1965). An artificial gill. *Am. J. Med. Electron.* **4**, 170

BOJRAB, L. and STOELTING, R.K. (1974). Extent and duration of the nitrous oxide second-gas effect on oxygen. *Anesthesiology* **40**, 201

BOONE, J.L. (1966). Silicone rubber insulation for subdermally implanted devices. *Med. Res. Engng* **5**, 34

BORGSTEDT, H.H. and GILLIES, A.J. (1965). Determination of the solubility of nitrous oxide in water by gas chromatography. *Anesthesiology* **26**, 675

BOURNE, J.G. (1964). Uptake, elimination and potency of inhalational anaesthesia. *Anaesthesia* **19**, 12

BOWES, J.B. (1964). A method of measuring nitrous oxide, nitrogen and oxygen in blood. *Anaesthesia* **19**, 40

BROWN, E.S., JOHNSON, R.P. and CLEMENTS, J.A. (1959). Pulmonary surface tension. *J. appl. Physiol.* **14**, 717

CAREY, J.S., WOODWARD, N.W., MOHR, P.A., SUZUKI, F., BROWN, R.S., BAKER, R.J., and SHOEMAKER, W.C. (1965). Circulatory response to low viscosity dextran in clinical shock. *Surg. Gynec. Obstet.* **121**, 563

CASSON, N. (1959). A flow equation for pigment-oil suspensions of the printing ink type. In *Rheology of disperse systems* (Ed. by C.C. Mills), Chapter 5. Oxford; Pergammon

CHADWICK, D.A. (1974). Transposition of rotameter tubes. *Anesthesiology* **40**, 102

CHAPLER, C.K., HATCHER, J.D. and JENNINGS, D.B. (1972). Cardiovascular effects of propanolol during acute experimental anaemia in dogs. *Can. J. Physiol. Pharmacol.* **50**, 1052

CHERNICK, V., HODSON, W.A. and GREENFIELD, L.J. (1966). Effect of chronic pulmonary artery ligation on pulmonary mechanics and surfactant. *J. appl. Physiol.* **21**, 1315

CLEMENTS, J.A., HUSTEAD, R.F., JOHNSON, R.P. and GRIBETZ, I. (1961). Pulmonary surface tension and alveolar stability. *J. appl. Physiol.* **16**, 444

COLACICCO, G., BUCKELEW, A.R. Jr. and SCALPELLI, E.M. (1973). Protein and lipid-protein fractions of lung washings: chemical characterization. *J. appl. Physiol.* **34**, 743

COMROE, J.H., FORSTER, R.E., DUBOIS, A.B., BRISCOE, W.A. and CARLESEN, E. (1962). *The Lung*, 2nd edn. Chicago; Year Book Publishers

COOPER, E.A. (1961). Behaviour of respiratory apparatus. *Medical Memorandum* **2**, 11. London; National Gas Board

CULLEN, D.J. and EGER, E.I. (1970). The effects of hypoxia and iso-volumic anaemia on the halothane requirement (MAC) of dogs. III. The effects of acute isovolumic anaemia. *Anesthesiology* **32**, 46

DAVENPORT, H.W. (1969). *The ABC of Acid-base Chemistry*, 5th edn. Chicago; University Press

DAVIES, D.D. (1970). A method of gas chromatography for quantitative analysis of blood gases. *Br. J. Anaesth.* **42**, 19

DÉRY, R. (1971). Humidity in Anaesthesia IV. *Can. Anaesth. Soc. J.* **18**, 145–151

DINTENFASS, L. (1971). *Blood Microrheology*. London; Butterworths

DINTENFASS, L., JULIAN, D.G., and MILLER, G.E. (1966). Viscosity of blood in normal subjects and in patients suffering from coronary occlusion and arterial thrombosis. An *in-vitro* rotational cone-in-cone viscometer. *Am. Heart J.* **71**, 587

DORMANDY, J.A. (1974). Medical and engineering problems of blood viscosity. *Biomed. Engng* **9**, 284

DOUMA, J.H. and WAMMES, L.J.A. (1978). The influence of the composition and the state of the gas on a Fleisch pneumotachograph. *Bull. Europ. Physiopath. Resp.* **14**, 68P–70P

DRAPER, W.B. and WHITEHEAD, R.W. (1944). Diffusion respiration in the dog anaesthetized by sodium pentothal. *Anesthesiology* **5**, 262

DRAPER, W.B. and WHITEHEAD, R.W. (1949). The phenomenon of diffusion respiration. *Curr. Res. Anesth. Analg.* **28**, 307

EGAN, D.F. (1973). *Fundamentals of Respiratory Therapy* 2nd edn. Saint Louis; C.V. Mosby

EGER, E.I. (1963a). A mathematical model of uptake and distribution. In *Uptake and Distribution of Anaesthetic Agents* (Ed. by E.M. Papper and R.J. Kitz). New York; McGraw-Hill

EGER, E.I. (1963b). Effect of inspired anaesthetic concentration on the rate of rise of alveolar concentration. *Anesthesiology* **25**, 620

EGER, E.I. II (1964). Uptake of methoxyflurane at constant inspired and constant alveolar concentrations. *Anesthesiology* **25**, 94

EGER, E.I., BRANDSTATER, B., SAIDMAN, L.J., REGAN, M.J., SEVERING-HAUS, J.W. and MUNSON, E.S. (1965). Equipotent alveolar concentrations of methoxyflurane, halothane, diethyl ether, fluroxene, cyclopropane, xenon and nitrous oxide in the dog. *Anesthesiology*

26, 771

EGER, E.I. and EPSTEIN, R.M. (1964). Hazards of anesthetic equipment. *Anesthesiology* **25**, 490

EGER, E.I. and LARSON, C.P. Jun.(1964). Anaesthetic solubility in blood and tissues: Values and significance. *Br. J. Anaesth.* **36**, 140

EGER, E.I., SAIDMAN, L.J. and BRANDSTATER, B. (1965). Temperature dependence of halothane and cyclopropane anaesthesia in dogs: correlation with some theories of anaesthetic action. *Anesthesiology* **26**, 764

EL-MASRY, O.A., FRIERSTEIN, I.A. and ROUND, G.F. (1978). Experimental evaluation of streamline patterns and separated flows in a series of branching vessels with applications to atherosclerosis and thrombosis. *Circ. Res.* **43**, 608–618

ENGHOFF, H., HOLMDAHL, M.H. and RISHOLM, L.(1951). Diffusion respiration in man. *Nature, Lond.* **168**, 830

ENOS, W.F. Jun., BEYER, J.C. and HOLMES, R.H. (1955). Pathogenesis of coronary disease in American soliders killed in Korea. *J. Am. med. Ass.* **158**, 912

EPSTEIN, R.M., RACKAW, H., SALANITRE, E. and WOLF, G.L.(1964). Influence of the concentration effect on the uptake of anesthetic mixtures: the second gas effect. *Anesthesiology* **25**, 364

ERNST, E.A. and PEREZ-ZAMURA, P. (1969). Water vapour in blood and tissues. *Anesthesiology* **31**, 272

EWING, Sir J.A. (1924–25). A ball-and-tube flowmeter. *Proc. R. Soc. Edinb.* **65**, 308

FAHRAEUS, R., and LINDQVIST, T. (1931). The viscosity of blood in narrow capillary tubes. *Am. J. Physiol.* **96**, 562

FATT, I. (1964). Rapid responding carbon dioxide and oxygen electrodes. *J. appl. Physiol.* **19**, 550

FERGUSON, J. (1939). The use of chemical potentials as indices of toxicity. *Proc. R. Soc.* **B127**, 387

FOX, J.A. and HUGH, A.E. (1966). Localisation of atherome: a theory based on boundary layer separation. *Br. Heart J.* **28**, 388

FRY, D.L. (1968). Acute vascular endothelial changes associated with increased blood velocity gradients. *Circulation Res.* **22**, 165

FRY, D.L., EBERT, R.V., STEAD, W.W. and BROWN, C.C. (1954). The mechanism of pulmonary ventilation in normal subjects and in patients with emphysema. *Am. J. Med.* **16**, 80

FRY, D.L., HYATT, R.E., McCALL, C.B. and MALLOS, A. (1957). Evaluation of three types of respiratory flowmeters. *J. appl. Physiol.* **10**, 210

GALLETTI, P.M., SNIDER, M.T. and GILBERT-AIDEN, D. (1966). Gas permeability of plastic membranes for artificial lungs. *Med. Res. Engng* **5**, 13

GELIN, L-E. and INGLEMAN, B. (1961). Rheomacrodex–a new dextran solution for rheological treatment of impaired capillary flow. *Acta chir. scand.* **122**, 294

GIL, J. and REISS, O.K. (1973). Isolation and characterization of lamellar bodies and tubular myelin from rat lung homogenates. *J. Cell. Biol.* **58**, 152

GLAUSER, S.C., GLAUSER, ELINOR M. and RUSY, B.F. (1969). Influence of gas density and viscosity on the work of breathing. *Archs envir. Hlth.* **19**, 654

GLUCK, L. and KULOVICH, M.V. (1973). Lecithin-sphyingomyelin ratios in amniotic fluid in normal and abnormal pregnancy. *Am. J. Obstet. Gynecol.* **115**, 539

GORDON, R.J. and RAVIN, M.B. (1978). Rheology and Anesthesiology. *Anesth. Analg.* **57**, 252–261

GOTCH, F., MEYER, J.S. and EBIHARA, S. (1966). Continous recording of human cerebral blood flow and metabolism. *Med. Res. Engng* **5**, 13

GRAVES, G., and GRAVES, V. (1964). *Medical Sound Recording.* London; Focal Press

GREENBAUM, R. (1969). The blood and transfusion fluids in shock. In *Physiological and Practical Aspects of Shock,* p. 775. Ed. by J. Freeman. Boston; Little, Brown

GREENFIELD, L.J., EBERT, P.A. and BENSON, D.W. (1964). Effect of positive pressure ventilation on surface tension properties of lung extracts. *Anesthesiology* **25**, 312

GREGORY, G.A., EGER, E.I. II and MUNSON, E.S. (1969). The relationship between age and halothane requirements in man. *Anesthesiology* **30**, 488

HALDEMANN, G., SCHAER, H., SPRING, C., FREY, P., GEBAUER, U. and HOSSLI, G. (1979). Effect of dextran on blood volume and interactions with volume regulatory systems. *Intensive Care Med.* **5**, 11–14

HARKNESS, J. (1971). The viscosity of human blood plasma: its measurement in health and disease. *Biomed. Engng* **9**, 284; *Biorheology* **8**, 171

HAYNES, R.H. (1960). Physical basis of the dependence of blood viscosity on tube radius. *Am. J. Physiol.* **198**, 1193

HAYNES, R.H. and BURTON, A.C. (1959). Role of non-newtonian behaviour of blood in haemodynamics. *Am. J. Physiol.* **197**, 943

HEATH, J.R., ANDERSON, M.M. and NUNN, J.F. (1973). Performance of the Quantiflex monitored dial mixer. *Br. J. Anaesth.* **45**, 216

HEDLEY-WHYTE, J. and LAVER, M.B. (1964). O_2 solubility in blood and temperature calibration factors for Po_2. *J. appl. Physiol.* **19**, 901

HELPS, E.P.W. and McDONALD, D.A. (1954a). Observations on laminar flow in veins. *J. Physiol., Lond.* **124**, 631

HELPS, E.P.W. and McDONALD, D.A. (1954b). Streamline flow in veins. *J. Physiol., Lond.* **126**, 56

HENRY, W. (1803). Experiments on the quantity of gases absorbed by water, at different temperatures, and under different pressures. *Phil. Trans. R. Soc.* **93**, 29

HERSHEY, D. and CHO, S.J. (1966). Blood flow in rigid tubes: thickness and slip velocity of plasma film at the wall. *J. appl. Physiol.* **21**, 27

HILL, D.W. (1959). The rapid measurement of respiratory pressures and volumes. *Br. J. Anaesth.* **31**, 352

HILL, D.W. (1966a). Methods of measuring oxygen content of blood. In *Oxygen Measurements in Blood and Tissues*. (Ed. by J.P. Payne and D.W. Hill), p. 63. London; Churchill

HILL, D.W. (1966b). Recent developments in the design of electronically controlled ventilators. *Anaesthetist* **15**, 234

HILL, D.W. and NEWELL, H.A. (1965). Effect of water vapour on the sensitivity of a macro-argon ionisation detector. *Nature, Lond.* **205**, 593

HOBBES, A.F.T. (1967). A comparison of methods of calibrating the pneumotachograph. *Br. J. Anaesth.* **39**, 289

IMPARATO, A.M., LORD, J.W. Jun., TEXON, M. and HELPERN, M. (1961). Experimental atherosclerosis produced by alterations in blood vessel configuration. *Surg. Forum.* **12**, 245

KELMAN, G.R., COLEMAN, A.J. and NUNN, J.F. (1966). A microtonometer used with a capillary glass pH electrode. *J. appl. Physiol.* **21**, 1103

KINGSLEY, B., SEGAL, B.L. and LIKOFF, W. (1967). Principles of hydromechanics: comments on thrombus formation. In *Engineering in the Practice of Medicine*, p. 278. (Ed. by B.L. Segal and D.G. Kilpatrick). Baltimore; Williams and Wilkins

KITAHATA, L.M., TAUB, A. and CONTE, A.J. (1971). The effect of nitrous oxide on alveolar carbon dioxide tensions: a second gas effect. *Anesthesiology* **35**, 607

KJELDSEN, K., WANSTRUP, J. and ASTRUP, P. (1968). Enhancing influence of arterial hypoxia on the development of atheromatosis in cholesterol-fed rabbits. *J. Atheroscler. Res.* **8**, 835

KLAUS, M.H., CLEMENTS, J.A. and HAVEL, R.J. (1961). Composition of surface-active material isolated from beef lung. *Proc. natn. Acad. Sci., U.S.A.* **47**, 1858

KNOX, C.K. Jun. (1962). An experimental investigation of the steady flow of a viscous fluid in circular branched tubes. M.S. Thesis, Minneapolis; University of Minnesota

KOLOBOW, T. and BOWMAN, R.L.(1963). Construction and evaluation of an alveolar membrane artificial heart lung. *Trans. Am. Soc. artif. internal Organs* **9**, 238

KROVETZ, L.J. (1965). The effect of vessel branching on haemodynamic stability. *Physics Med. Biol.* **10**, 417

KYLSTRA, J.A. (1965). Gas exchange in liquid ventilated dogs. In *Hyperbaric Oxygen*, p. 367. (Ed. by I. McA. Ledingham). Edinburgh; Livingstone

KYLSTRA, J.A. and TISSING, M.O. (1964). Fluid breathing. In *Clinical Application of Hyperbaric Oxygen*, p. 371. (Ed. by I. Boerema, W.H. Brummelkamp and N.G. Meijne). Amsterdam; Elsevier

LARSON, C.P., EGER, E.I. and SEVERINGHAUS, J.W.(1962). Ostwald solubility coefficients for anaesthetic gases in various fluids and tissues. *Anesthesiology* **28**, 686

LEBOVITZ, A. (1966). Permeability of polymers to gases, vapours and liquids. *Mod. Plast.* **43**, 139

LIEBMAN, F.M., PEAR, J. and BAGNO, S. (1962). The electrical conductance properties of blood in motion. *Physics Med. Biol.* **7**, 177

LONG, D.M., SANCHEZ, L., VARLO, R.L. and LILLEHEI, C.W. (1961). The use of low molecular weight dextran and serum albumin as plasma extenders in extra-corporeal circulation. *Surgery* **50**, 12

LOWE, H.J. (1972). Dose-regulated penthrane anaesthesia. Chicago; Abbott Laboratories

LOWE, H.J. and HAGLER, K. (1971). Determination of volatile organic anaesthetics in blood, gases, tissues and lipids: partition coefficients. CIBA Symposium on *Gas Chromatography in Biology and Medicine*, p. 86. (Ed. by R. Porter). London; Churchill

LOWE, H.J., TITEL, H.J. and HAGLER, K. (1971). Absorption of anaesthetics by conductive rubber in breathing circuits. *Anesthesiology* **34**, 283

LÜBBERS, D.W. (1966). Methods of measuring oxygen tensions of blood and organ surfaces. In *Oxygen Measurements in Blood and Tissues*, p. 103. (Ed. by J.P. Payne and D.W. Hill.) London; Churchill

MAPLESON, W.W. (1964a). Mathematical aspects of the uptake, distribution and elimination of inhaled gases and vapours. *Br. J. Anaesth.* **36**, 129

MAPLESON, W.W. (1964b). Inert gas exchange theory using an electrical analogue. *J. appl. Physiol.* **19**, 1193

MAPLESON, W.W. (1973). Circulation-time models of the uptake of inhaled anaesthetics and data for quantifying them. *Br. J. Anaesth.* **45**, 319

MAPLESON, W.W., MORGAN, J.G. and HILLARD, E.K. (1963). Assessment of condenser humidifiers with special reference to a multiple gauze model. *Br. med. J.* **1**, 300

MAPLESON, W.W., SMITH, W.D.A., SIEBOLD, K., HARGREAVES, M.D. and

CLARKE, G.M.(1974). Nitrous oxide anaesthesia induced at atmospheric and hyperbaric pressures. Part II: comparison of measured and theoretical pharmacokinetic data. *Br. J. Anaesth.* **46**, 13

MARSHALL, J. and SPALDING, J.M.K. (1953). Humidification in positive-pressure respiration for bulbo-spinal paralysis. *Lancet* **2**, 1022

McDONALD, D.A. (1952). The occurrence of turbulent flow in the rabbit aorta. *J. Physiol., Lond.* **118**, 340

McDONALD, D.A. (1960). *Blood Flow in Arteries.* London; Arnold

McDONALD, D.A. (1974). *Blood Flow in Arteries.* 2nd edn. London; Arnold

McILROY, M.B., MEAD, J., SELVERSTONE, N.J. and RADFORD, E.P.(1955). Measurement of lung tissue resistance using gases of equal kinematic viscosity. *J. appl. Physiol.* **7**, 491

MEAD, J. (1961). Mechanical properties of the lungs. *Physiol. Rev.* **41**, 281

MEAD, J., and COLLIER, C.(1959). Relation of volume history of lungs to respiratory mechanics in anaesthetized dogs. *J. appl. Physiol.* **14**, 669

MEISELMAN, H.J., MERRILL, E.W., SALZMANN, E.W., GILLILAND, E.R. and PELLETIER, G.A.(1967). Effect of dextran on rheology of human blood: low shear viscosity. *J. appl. Physiol.* **22**, 480

MERRILL, E.W. (1969). Rheology of blood. *Physiol. Rev.* **49**, 863–888

MERRILL, E.W., BENIS, A.M., GILLILAND, E.R., SHERWOOD, T.K. and SALTZMAN, E.W.(1965). Pressure-volume relationships of human blood in hollow fibres at low flow rates. *J. appl. Physiol.* **20**, 954

MERRILL, E.W., GILLILAND, E.R., COKELETT, G.R., BRITTON, A., SHIN, H. and WELLS, R.E. (1963). Rheology of blood flow in the microcirculation. *J. appl. Physiol.* **18**, 225

MEYER, K.H., and HEMMI, H. (1935). Beitrage zur Theorie der Narkose III. *Biochem. Z.* **227**, 39

MILLS, C.J. (1968). A catheter tip electromagnetic velocity probe for use in man. In *Blood Flow Through Organs and Tissues*, p. 38. (Ed. by W.H. Bain and A.M. Harper.) Edinburgh; Livingstone

MILLS, J.N. (1952). The use of an infra-red analyser in testing the properties of Douglas bags. *J. Physiol., Lond.* **116**, 22P

MUNSON, E.S., EGER, E.I. II, THAM, M.K. and EMBRO, W.J.(1978). Increase in anaesthetic uptake, excretion and blood solubility in man after eating. *Anesth. Analg.* **57**, 224–231

NAHRWOLD, M.L., ARCHER, P. and COHEN, P.J. (1973). Application of the Antoine-equation to anaesthetic vapour pressure data. *Anesth. Analg.* **52**, 866

NUNN, J.F.(1958). Respiratory measurements in the presence of nitrous oxide. *Br. J. Anaesth.* **30**, 254

NUNN, J.F. (1960). The solubility of volatile anaesthetics in oil. *Br. J. Anaesth.* **32**, 346

NUNN, J.F. (1961). Portable anaesthetic apparatus for use in the Antarctic. *Br. med. J.* **1**, 1139

NUNN, J.F. (1969). *Applied Respiratory Physiology.* London; Butterworths

NYGAARD, K.K., WILDER, M. and BERKSON, J. (1935). The relation between viscosity of the blood and the relative volume of the erythrocytes. *Am. J. Physiol.* **114**, 128

ORCUTT, F.F. and SEEVERS, M.H.(1937). A method for determining the solubility of gases by the Van Slyke manometer apparatus. *J. biol. Chem.* **117**, 501

OSBORN, J.J., BEAUMONT, J.O., RAISON, J.C.A. and ABBOTT, R.P.(1969). Computation for quantitative on-line measurements in an intensive care ward. In *Computers in Bio-medical Research,* **3**, p. 207. (Ed. by R.W. Stacy and B.D. Waxman.) New York; Academic Press

OSTIGUY, G.L. and BECKLAKE, M.R.(1966). Solubility of nitrous oxide in human blood. *J. appl. Physiol.* **21**, 1397

PATTLE, R.E. (1955). Properties, functions and origin of the alveolar lining layer. *Nature, Lond.* **175**, 1125

PATTLE, R.E. (1965). Surface lining of lung alevoli. *Physiol. Rev.* **45**, 48

PATTLE, R.E. (1967). Lung surfactant and its possible reaction to air pollution. *Archs envir. Hlth* **14**, 70

PATTLE, R.E. and THOMAS, L.C. (1961). Lipoprotein compositon of the film lining of the lung. *Nature, Lond.* **189**, 844

PAYNE, J.P. (1962). Apnoeic oxygenation in anaesthetized man. *Acta anaesth. scand.* **6**, 129

PAYNE, J.P., HILL, D.W. and KING, N.W. (1966). Observations on the distribution of alcohol in blood, breath and urine. *Br. med. J.* **1**, 196

PENDER, C.B. (1970). Respiratory distress in the newborn infant due to blood aspiration in infants delivered by cesarean section. *Am. J. Obstet. Gynec.* **106**, 711

PENDER, C.B. (1972). Respiratory distress in multiple births and premature infants. *Am. J. Obstet. Gynec.* **112**, 298

PENDER, C.B. (1973). Respiration distress in the newborn due to aspiration of amniotic fluid and its contents. *Resuscitation* **2**, 157

PENMAN, H.L. (1958). *Humidity.* London; Chapman and Hall

POWER, G.G. (1968). Solubilities of O_2 and CO_2 in blood and pulmonary and placental tissue. *J. appl. Physiol.* **24**, 468

REEMTSMA, K. and CREECH, O. (1962). Viscosity studies of blood, plasma and plasma substitutes. *J. thorac. cardiovasc. Surg.* **44**, 674

REPLOGLE, R.L., MEISELMAN, H.J. and MERRILL, E.W. (1967). Clinical implications of blood rheology studies. *Circulation* **36**, 148

RILEY, R.L., CAMPBELL, E.J.M. and SHEPARD, R.H. (1957). A bubble method for the estimation of P_{CO_2} and P_{O_2} in whole blood. *J. appl. Physiol.* **11**, 245

RODGERS, R.C. and HILL, G.E. (1978). Equations for vapour pressure versus temperature: derivation and use of the Antoine equation on a hand-held programmable calculator. *Br. J. Anaesth.* **50**, 415–424

ROHRER, F. (1915). Der Stromungswiderstand in den menschlichen Atemwegen. *Pflügers Arch. ges. Physiol.* **162**, 225

SAIDMAN, L.J. and EGER, E.I. II. (1964). Effect of nitrous oxide and narcotic premedication on the alveolar concentration of halothane required for anaesthesia. *Anesthesiology* **25**, 302

SCHENK, W.G., DELIN, N.A., DOMANIG, E., HAHNLOSER, P. and HOYT, R.K. (1964). Blood viscosity as a determinant of regional blood flows. *Archs Surg., Lond.* **89**, 783

SCHOCK, C., PATTLE, R.E. and CREASEY, J.M. (1973). Methods for electron microscopy of the lamellated osmiophilic bodies of the lung. *J. Microsc.* **97**, 321

SCHOLANDER, P.F. (1947). Analyser for accurate estimation of respiratory gases in one-half cubic centimetre samples. *J. biol. Chem.* **167**, 235

SEVERINGHAUS, J.W. (1962). Electrodes for blood and gas P_{O_2}, P_{CO_2} and blood pH. *Acta anaesth. scand. Suppl.* **11**, 207

SEVERINGHAUS, J.W. and BRADLEY, A.F. (1958). Electrodes for blood and gas P_{O_2} and P_{CO_2}. *J. appl. Physiol.* **13**, 515

SHANKS, C.A. and SARA, C.A. (1973). Airway heat and humidity during endotracheal intubation I: inspiration of arid atmospheres. *Anaesth. Intens. Care* **1**, 211

SMITH, G., LEDINGHAM, I.McA., NORMAN, J.N., DOUGLAS, T.A., BATES, E.H. and LEE, F.D. (1963). Prolongation of the time of 'safe' circulatory arrest by preliminary hyperbaric oxygenation and body cooling. *Surgery Gynec. Obstet.* **117**, 411

SMITH, W.D.A. (1964). The measurement of uptake of nitrous oxide by pneumotachograpy. 1. Apparatus, methods and accuracy. *Br. J. Anaesth.* **36**, 363

STANLEY, T.H. and ZIKRIS, B.A. (1975). The surface tension of upper airway secretions in patients with and without respiratory disease. *Anesth. Analg.* **54**, 600–602

STEHBENS, W.E. (1959). Turbulence of blood flow. *Q. Jl. exp. Physiol.* **44**, 110

STEVENS, H.R. and ALBREGT, H.B. (1966). Assessment of ultrasonic nebulization. *Anesthesiology* **27**, 648

STEWARD, A., ALLOTT, P.R., COWLES, A.L. and MAPLESON, W.W. (1973). Solubility coefficients for inhaled anaesthetics for water, oil and biological media. *Br. J. Anaesth.* **45**, 282

STOELTING, R.K. and EGER, E.I. II. (1969). An additional explanation for the second gas effect: a concentration effect. *Anesthesiology* **30**, 273

STRANG, L.B. (1961). Blood gas tension measurement using a mass spectrometer. *J. appl. Physiol.* **16**, 562

SY, W.P. and HASBROUCK, J.D. (1964). Solubility of nitrous oxide in water and canine blood. *Anesthesiology* **25**, 59

SYKES, M.K., NEEMATALLAH, F.A. and COOKE, P.M. (1967). The effect of low molecular weight dextran and haemodilution on acid-base balance and lactate and pyruvate levels during cardiopulmonary bypass. *Br. J. Anaesth.* **39**, 94

THORNTON, J.A., and NUNN, J.F.(1960). Accuracy of determination of Pco_2 by the indirect methods. *Guy's Hosp. Rep.* **18**, 203

TITEL, J.H. and LOWE, H.J. (1968). Rubber-gas partition coefficients. *Anesthesiology* **29**, 1215

TOOLEY, W., GARDNER, R., THUNG, G. and FINLEY, T.N. (1961). Factors affecting the surface tension of lung extract. *Fed. Proc.* **20**, 428

TORRES, G. (1963). Validation of oxygen electrode in blood. *J. appl. Physiol.* **18**, 1008

VAN SLYKE, D.D. and NEILL, J.M. (1924). The determination of gases in blood and other solutions by vacuum extraction and manometric measurement. *J. biol. Chem.* **61**, 523

WADE, O.L., BISHOP, J.M., CUMMING, G. and DONALD, K.W. (1953). A method for the rapid estimation of the percentage oxygen saturation and oxygen content of blood. *Br. med. J.* **2**, 902

WELLS, R.E. (1967). The viscosity of blood. In *Engineering in the Practice of Medicine*, p. 273. (Ed. by B.L. Segal and D.G. Kilpatrick.) Baltimore; Williams and Wilkins

WELLS, R.E., DENTON, R. and MERRILL, E.W. (1961). Measurement of viscosity of biological fluids by cone-plate viscometer. *J. Lab. Clin. Med.* **57**, 646–656

WHELPTON, D. (1969). Ph. D. Thesis, Sheffield University

WHITMORE, R.L.(1967). The flow behaviour of blood in circulation. *Nature, Lond.* **215**, 123

WILBUR, R.L. (1969). Instrument for the measurement of surface tensions of aqueous surfactant solutions. *Rev. Sci., Instrum.* **40**, 355

WILLIAMS, R.A., RHOADES, R.A. and ADAMS, W.S. (1971). Modification of a surfactometer for increased versatility. *Med. & biol. Engng* **9**, 729

WOLFSON, B. (1962). Closed circuit by intermittent injection of halothane. *Br. J. Anaesth.* **34**, 733

YOUNG, S.L. and TIERNEY, D.G. (1972). Dipalmitoyl lecithin secretion and metabolism by the rat lung. *Am. J. Physiol.* **222**, 1539

6 The gas laws

Dalton's law of partial pressures

Dalton's law states that the pressure exerted by a mixture of gases, or gases and vapours, enclosed in a given space is equal to the sum of the pressures which each gas or vapour would exert if it alone occupied the same space. From this it follows that the volume percentage of any one of the gases comprising the mixture is given by the ratio of its partial pressure to the total pressure, multiplied by one hundred. Thus, if a cylinder is first evacuated and then filled with one atmosphere absolute of CO_2 and a further three atmospheres of oxygen added, the concentration of CO_2 in the mixture would be 25 per cent by volume. Anaesthetic vapours are administered in such concentrations and at such pressures that Dalton's law of partial pressures can be taken to apply to them. For example, the saturated vapour pressure of halothane at 20 °C is 243 mmHg, so that at an atmospheric pressure of 760 mmHg, this corresponds to a saturation concentration of (243/760) $\times$ 100 per cent = 32 per cent by volume.

By using gas burettes in conjunction with Dalton's law, small quantities of known gas and vapour mixtures can be prepared at pressures near atmospheric. However, at pressures of several hundred pounds per square inch (several hundred kilonewtons per square metre), marked deviations from Boyle's law can occur due to the compressibility of gases such as carbon dioxide and nitrous oxide. This fact is clearly illustrated in *Figure 6.1* where the compressibility for oxygen, Entonox and nitrous oxide is plotted against absolute pressure. Both nitrous oxide and the Entonox mixture are markedly more compressible than

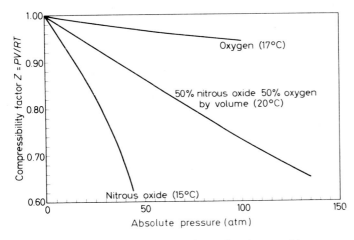

Figure 6.1. Compressibility factor isotherms for nitrous oxide, oxygen and 50/50% by volume mixtures of nitrous oxide and oxygen (Entonox). (By courtesy of British Oxygen Co. Ltd)

oxygen. For this reason it is not possible accurately to calculate the composition of such a mixture on a simple partial pressure basis. It is better to use the Law of Additive Partial Volumes (Hill, 1961). Even at a pressure of 400 lbf in^{-2} (2.758 MN m^{-2}) absolute there is a measurable effect. Consider a cylinder which is first evacuated, and to which is then admitted CO_2 to an absolute pressure of 20 lbf in^{-2} (0.1379 MN m^{-2}). The cylinder is then filled with oxygen up to a final pressure of 400 lbf in^{-2} (2.758 MN m^{-2}) absolute. From Dalton's law, the percentage of CO_2 in the resulting mixture should be 5 per cent by volume. Analysis, using a Lloyd–Haldane gas analyser, showed it to be 4.91 per cent. This result follows since the compressibility of the CO_2 allows more oxygen into the cylinder than would be expected from Dalton's law. Freshly filled cylinders should be thoroughly rolled after filling to ensure adequate mixing of their contents. Bracken, Broughton and Hill (1968) report that mixtures of oxygen and nitrous oxide at pressures of 1000 lbf in^{-2} (6.896 MN m^{-2}) can take up to two weeks to mix without rolling when the oxygen concentration is 80 per cent and the cylinders are stored in a vertical position. The nitrous oxide was admitted first to the cylinder. *Figure 6.2* taken from Broughton (1969) shows the variation with mixture composition of the mixing time for cylinders stored vertically and filled to 1000 lbf in^{-2} (6.896 MN m^{-2}). Storage in a vertical position represents the worst possible case since the cross-sectional area of the interface between the gases across which diffusion must take place is a minimum. With a horizontal position the cross-sectional area is larger and mixing is complete within one to six hours. Persistent rolling will reduce the mixing time to the order of ten to fifteen minutes.

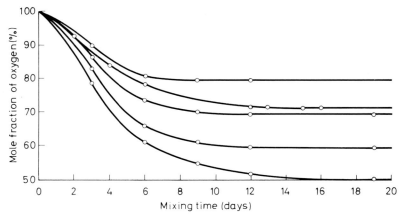

Figure 6.2. Variation with mixture composition of the mixing time for gas cylinders stored vertically. (After Broughton, 1969)

The concept of a partial pressure is of importance in considering the rate of transfer of gases and anaesthetic vapours across the alveolar membrane. At normal atmospheric pressure the partial pressure of oxygen in the alveoli is some 100 mmHg, and in the venous capillaries the oxygen tension is some 40 mmHg. The pressure difference of 60 mmHg causes the diffusion of oxygen to take place across the membrane.

At an altitude of 5000 feet (1524 m) the barometric pressure has fallen to 632 mmHg. The water vapour pressure in the alveoli depends only on body temperature and can be taken as constant at 47 mmHg. The partial pressure of CO_2 in the alveoli remains at 40 mmHg if there is no hyperventilation. The percentage of oxygen in dry, CO_2-free alveolar air is 15 per cent at this altitude, so that the partial pressure of oxygen in the alveoli at an altitude of 5000 ft is 0.15 $[632 - (47 + 40)]$ = 82 mmHg. The pressure difference across the alveolar membrane is now 42 mmHg.

Safar and Tenicela (1964) list physiological data on inhabitants of Peru living at sea level and at an altitude of 14 900 ft (4450 m) (*Table 6.1*).

TABLE 6.1

	Sea level	*15 000 ft (4572 m)*
Mean barometric pressure	760 mmHg	446 mmHg
Ambient PO_2 (dry)	158 mmHg	94 mmHg
Effective alveolar PO_2	96.2 mmHg	46.4 mmHg
Arterial PO_2	87.3 mmHg	44.9 mmHg
Arterial O_2 sat. of Hb.	98.0%	79.6%
Arterial O_2 content	20.7 ml/100 ml	23.0 ml/100 ml
Alveolar PCO_2	39.3 mmHg	30.2 mmHg
Arterial PCO_2	40.1 mmHg	33.0 mmHg
Ventilation	7.77 l/min	9.49 l/min
	BTPS	BTPS

The alveolar PCO_2 has fallen as a result of the hyperventilation, and the reduced value of the alveolar PO_2 has resulted in a lower arterial PO_2 and oxygen saturation.

Boyle's law

This well known gas law was first published by Robert Boyle in 1662. It states that for a given mass of gas, provided that the temperature is kept constant, the volume varies inversely as the pressure. It is important to state that the mass of gas is constant, since then there will always be the same number of molecules irrespective of any changes occurring in the temperature, pressure or volume of the gas. For a given mass of gas and temperature, since the volume is inversely proportional to the pressure, it follows that the product pressure $\times$ volume is a constant. Strictly speaking, Boyle's law applies only to *perfect gases*. In practice, Boyle's law is accurately obeyed for real gases such as oxygen and nitrogen over a wide range of pressures. For example, in the case of oxygen, the value of $P \times V$ at 100 atmospheres is about 95 per cent of that at 1 atmosphere. In practical situations, the temperature is not always constant and this makes it necessary now to consider Charles' law.

Charles' law

This law, due to the Frenchman Jacques Charles, states that for a given mass of gas at a constant pressure, the volume varies directly as the *absolute temperature.* Thus V/T is a constant, where T designates a temperature on the Absolute or Kelvin scale of temperature.

The absolute scale of temperature

On the Celsius (Centigrade) scale of temperature, the temperature of melting ice is taken as 0 °C. On the Absolute scale, 0 °Absolute is the lowest possible temperature that can ever be attained, and corresponds to −273 °C. The intervals corresponding to a degree are the same on both Celsius and Absolute (Kelvin) scales. Thus 0 °C corresponds to 273 °A. There are no negative temperatures on the Absolute scale. In order to convert °C to °A, simply add 273, e.g. 20 °C= 293 °A, now written 293 K.

The expansion of gases

When gases are cooled, their volumes diminish by a fraction approximately equal to 1/273 of the original volume per degree reduction in temperature. According to Charles' law the volume and absolute temperature are linearly related, so that at a temperature of −273 °C the volume of a gas should fall to zero. In practice this does not happen since Charles' law fails and the gas liquefies first. Charles' law can be stated in the form that at a constant pressure, the volume of any gas expands by the same fraction of its volume at 0 °C for every 1 °C rise of temperature. Gay-Lussac's law is related to Charles' law and states that for a given mass of gas kept at a constant volume the pressure increases by the same fraction of its pressure at 0 °C for every 1 °C rise in temperature. Under these circumstances, the pressure will rise by approximately 1/273 of the original pressure per degree rise in temperature.

The equation of state of a perfect gas

An ideal or perfect gas can be regarded as one in which the attraction between the molecules can be regarded as negligible and the volume of the molecules is small compared with the space which they inhabit.

A perfect gas would always obey the laws of Boyle and Charles. These laws can be combined to give the equation of state of a perfect gas which is obeyed by real gases to a good approximation. Thus PV/T is a constant, i.e.

$$\frac{P_1 V_1}{T_1} = \frac{P_2 V_2}{T_2}$$

This equation has many practical applications.

Suppose that the pressure gauge of a 48 ft^3 capacity oxygen cylinder indicates a pressure of 2000 lbf in^{-2} in a laboratory at 20 °C, what would be the reading of the gauge if the cylinder was taken into an operating room at 24 °C? Assume that the volume of the cylinder remains constant. Provided that the units chosen to express pressure, volume and temperature are the same on both sides of the equation, it does not matter what these units are, e.g. N m^{-2} or lbf in^{-2}

$$\frac{2000 \times 48}{273+20} = \frac{P_2 \times 48}{273+24}$$

$$P_2 = \frac{2000 \times 297}{293} = 2027 \text{ lbf in}^{-2}$$

Suppose that a patient expires into a Douglas bag which is then removed into a laboratory at 20 °C and squeezed out through a dry gas meter. From a knowledge of the number of expirations collected and the respiratory frequency, the volume of gas at 20 °C corresponding to the minute volume can be easily calculated. If the minute volume was six litres, what would this volume, which is measured under the conditions of Ambient Temperature and Pressure Saturated (ATPS), become when referred back to the conditions of Body Temperature and Pressure Saturated (BTPS)?

Assume that the patient's body temperature is 37 °C, the saturated vapour pressure of water is 18 mmHg at 20 °C and 47 mmHg at 37 °C and that the barometric pressure is 760 mmHg. In order to work only in terms of gas pressures, the appropriate water vapour pressures must be subtracted from the barometric pressure.

$$\frac{(760-18) \times 6}{273+20} = \frac{(760-47) \times V_2}{273+37}$$

so that

$$V_2 = \frac{742 \times 6 \times 310}{713 \times 293} = 6.61 \text{ litres}$$

What would be the volume of the six litres, measured under atmospheric conditions, when referred to the conditions of Standard Temperature and Pressure Dry (STPD) i.e. 760 mmHg and 0 °C?

$$\frac{(760 - 18) \times 6}{273 + 20} = \frac{760 \times V_3}{273}$$

so that

$$V_3 = \frac{742 \times 6 \times 273}{760 \times 293} = 5.46 \text{ litres}$$

By the use of this equation, it is possible to change gas volumes measured under one set of conditions to those which would obtain under another set of conditions. That this manipulation is often necessary is illustrated by Dittmer and Grebe (1958) who quote BTPS for the conditions under which lung volumes and ventilation are to be quoted, ATPS for maximal inspiratory and expiratory flow rates, and STPD for oxygen consumption and carbon dioxide output.

The equation of state of a perfect gas can be written as $PV=RT$ where R is known as the molar gas constant. Consider one mole of ideal gas, this has a volume of 22.4 litres at one atmosphere and 273.16K, so that $R = 1 \times 22.4/273.16 = 0.082$ litre-atmospheres per degree per mole. This is equivalent to 1.987 joules per degree per mole in SI units.

Van der Waals equation

In order to make allowance for the forces of attraction and repulsion between the molecules, the equation of state for a perfect gas must be modified so that it does represent the behaviour of real gases. Considering a molecule situated towards the centre in the mass of gas, it will be surrounded by molecules equally distributed in all directions. As a result, there will be no net attractive force on that particular molecule. For a molecule near the walls of the container, there will be fewer molecules surrounding it on one side than on the other so that there will be a net inward force acting upon it. The pressure recorded in the vessel arises from the molecular bombardment upon its walls. As a molecule approaches the walls the result is an inwardly-directed force which reduces the measured pressure. Thus a correction term p must be added to the measured pressure P. The inward force acting on an individual molecule is proportional to the total number of molecules present and thus to the gas density d. The number of molecules impinging on the walls at any moment is also proportional to the density so that the total inward force is proportional to d^2. If V is the molar volume of the gas, then d is proportional to $1/V$ so that p is proportional to d^2 and thus to $1/V^2$. Hence $P+p=(P+a/V^2)$, where a is a constant of proportionality. The molecules of a real gas are not infinitely small in size, and this fact acts to reduce the effective volume of the gas. In order to obtain the real volume a correction term b must be subtracted from the measured volume V. The corrected volume is $(V-b)$. The equation of state of a perfect gas is thus modified to $(P+a/V^2)(V-b) = RT$. This is the Van der Waals equation of state. The dimensions of a are

$$\frac{\text{litres}^2 \times \text{atmospheres}}{\text{moles}^2}$$

and those of b are litres $\times 10^2$/mole when the pressure P is in atmospheres. In SI units with the pressure in N m^{-2} the units of a would be m$^3 \times$ N m$^{-2} \times$ moles^{-2}. The correction terms a and b are a measure of the attractive forces between the molecules and the volume of the molecules, respectively.

Wulf and Featherstone (1957) point out that all reactions or interactions between any atoms or molecules depend on these fundamental properties. They show that a list of substances arranged in order of their Van der Waals b constants shows a good correlation between the a and b constants and the anaesthetic potencies of the substances.

Isothermals

Boyle's law states that for a given mass of gas, at a constant temperature, the product pressure $\times$ volume is a constant. In mathematical

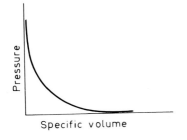

Figure 6.3. Boyle's law relationship for a perfect gas at a constant temperature

264

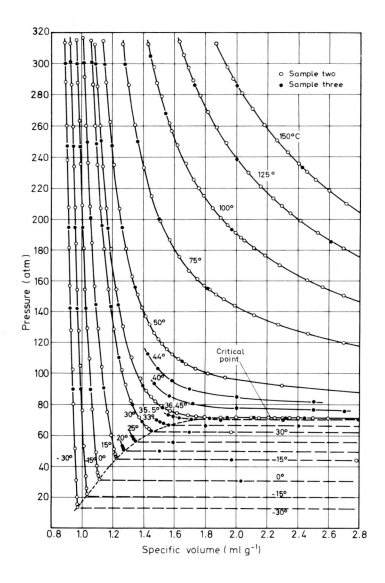

Figure 6.4. Isotherms for nitrous oxide. (After Couch and Kobe, 1961)

terms, the equation $P \times V =$ constant is the equation to a *rectangular hyperbola*. The curve is of the form of *Figure 6.3*. The value of the constant depends on the temperature. Hence a series of smooth curves is obtained for different temperatures as shown in the upper part of *Figure 6.4* for nitrous oxide (Couch and Kobe, 1961). Above a certain temperature, known as the *critical temperature*, the volume diminishes smoothly as the pressure is increased. However, below this temperature, the curves start to exhibit a flat portion or 'plateau'. Over this portion, liquefaction of the gas occurs, and the pressure remains constant during this change of state. When all the nitrous oxide has been liquefied, a small decrease in volume is associated with a large increase in pressure since the liquid phase is much less compressible than the gas phase. Above its critical temperature, a substance cannot exist as a liquid however much pressure is applied. During condensation the nitrous oxide behaves like a vapour. There is no sharp difference between the terms 'gas' and 'vapour', although the term vapour is usually taken to refer to the gaseous state of a substance which at room temperature and pressure is a liquid. Thus nitrous oxide can exist as a liquid in a cylinder under pressure at room temperature, but only under increased pressure. In contrast, ether can be in liquid form at room temperature and pressure.

The critical temperature of nitrous oxide is 36.5 °C, and just below this temperature, it has a pressure of 74 atmospheres (1088 lbf in^{-2}, 7.502 MN m^{-2}). At 20 °C, a pressure of 51 atmospheres (749 lbf in^{-2}, 5.165 MN m^{-2}) is required to liquefy nitrous oxide. The curves in *Figure 6.4* are known as *isothermals*, and a similar set can be drawn for carbon dioxide. The critical temperature for carbon dioxide is 31.1 °C. At 20 °C, the pressure in a cylinder containing some liquid carbon dioxide is 56 atmospheres (825 lbf in^{-2}, 5.689 MN m^{-2}). Cyclopropane has a critical temperature of 125 °C and a full cylinder of cyclopropane also contains both liquid and gas. At 20 °C, the pressure in a cylinder containing both liquid and gaseous cyclopropane is 6.3 atmospheres (78 lbf in^{-2}, 0.538 MN m^{-2}).

The withdrawal of gas from a nitrous oxide cylinder

A 'full' nitrous oxide cylinder contains both liquid and gaseous nitrous oxide if the ambient temperature is below the critical temperature of nitrous oxide 36.5 °C (98 °F). At 20 °C, the saturated vapour pressure of nitrous oxide is 51 atmospheres (749 lbf in^{-2}, 5.165 MN m^{-2}), so that this will be the pressure indicated on the cylinder gauge if one is fitted. When gas is withdrawn at temperatures below 36.5 °C, the liquid nitrous oxide boils, replenishing the gas which has been withdrawn. The heat necessary to produce this evaporation comes from the atmosphere of the room, and has to be transferred through the cylinder wall. If the rate of withdrawal is sufficiently high, a frost may form on the bottom of the cylinder. Expansion of the issuing gas at the cylinder valve may cause a marked cooling, and for this reason precautions are taken during manufacture to ensure that the gas is dry. This prevents ice formation from blocking the valve. In practice it is possible for the issuing gas to have a temperature of −60 °C.

The cylinder pressure gauge would indicate a pressure of 749 lbf in^{-2} g (5.165 MN m^{-2}) as long as any liquid nitrous oxide remained in the cylinder and the temperature of the nitrous oxide remained at

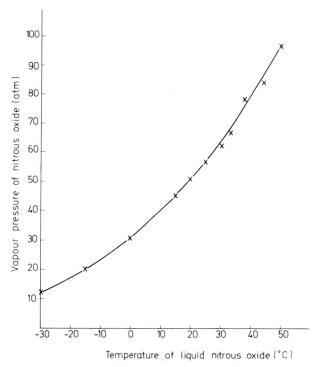

Figure 6.5. The relationship between the saturated vapour pressure of nitrous oxide in contact with the liquid and the temperature of the liquid nitrous oxide

20 °C. As the liquid nitrous oxide is evaporated, the latent heat of vaporization must be removed from it, heat being conducted in via the cylinder wall from the surroundings. In practice, even at flow rates of a few litres per minute, the temperature of the nitrous oxide falls steadily as insufficient heat is transferred through the cylinder. From the data of *Figure 6.4*, it is possible to construct the curve of *Figure 6.5* which shows the vapour pressure of nitrous oxide in contact with its liquid in relation to the temperature of the liquid nitrous oxide. *Figure 6.6* shows the measured pressure taken from the gauge of an 1800 litre

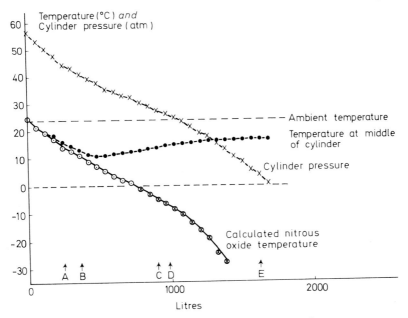

Figure 6.6. The variation in pressure and surface temperature of a nitrous oxide cylinder as gas is withdrawn.
A. Cylinder feels slightly damp. B. Lower three-quarters of cylinder wet. C. Frost forming on lower third of cylinder. D. Marked frost on lower third of cylinder. E. Thick frost on lower sixth of cylinder

nitrous oxide cylinder emptied at a steady flow of 6 litres per minute plotted against the number of litres of gas removed. Using the graph of *Figure 6.5*, the temperature of the liquid nitrous oxide has been calculated for each pressure reading and plotted in *Figure 6.6*. A calibrated thermistor temperature probe was employed to monitor the outside surface temperature of the cylinder wall at the middle of the cylinder. It is interesting to see that the calculated nitrous oxide temperature followed a parallel course to the steady decline in cylinder pressure. Soon after the calculated temperature had fallen below 0 °C, a frost was observed on the lower one-third of the cylinder and this became marked as the temperature fell further. The wall temperature fell from ambient by about 14 °C and then started to increase. As the amount of cold liquid nitrous oxide present in the cylinder decreased, the amount of frost decreased and the cooling effect on the middle portion of the cylinder wall also decreased. The fall in pressure becomes steeper towards the end as the temperature starts to drop more rapidly owing to the smaller thermal capacity of the small amount of liquid nitrous oxide left. Over a considerable range, there is a roughly linear relationship between the quantity of gas remaining and the indicated pressure in the cylinder. This only applies when the cylinder is steadily emptied. If the flow is stopped and the cylinder allowed to warm, the pressure indicated on the gauge will rise. If reliance was placed on the pressure readings, the cylinder would apparently contain more nitrous oxide than it actually did. If the anaesthetic machine had been out of use for a sufficient length of time for the nitrous oxide cylinder to warm, it might well be used subsequently by another anaesthetist who could be unfamiliar with the amount of nitrous oxide which had been used on the previous occasion. For this reason, caution must be exercised in relating the pressure indicated on a nitrous oxide pressure gauge to the cylinder contents. A more accurate method is to weigh the cylinder in order to check its contents. A 200-gallon nitrous oxide cylinder of nominal water capacity 82 fluid ounces (2000 cm^3) when containing only gaseous nitrous oxide at a pressure of 749 lbf in^{-2} (5.165 MN m^{-2}) will contain 36.2 gallons (164.6 litres) of gas reduced to one atmosphere and 15.5 °C, and thus will permit withdrawal at a rate of 8 litres per minute for 20 minutes. Throughout this time, the pressure gauge will fall steadily to zero. For a 100-gallon (454.6 litres) nitrous oxide cylinder, the volume of gas left is halved to 18.1 gallons (82.3 litres) (personal communication, British Oxygen Company).

In hot climates, where the ambient temperature is above 36.5 °C, (98 °F), the cylinder will always contain only gaseous nitrous oxide. At 37 °C, the pressure in the cylinder would be 1125 lbf in^{-2} (7.757 MN m^{-2}) and this would fall steadily as gas is withdrawn.

The nitrous oxide cylinder pressure gauges of current Boyle anaesthetic machines have calibration marks at 0, 15, 54 and 100 kPa × 100 (0, 218, 783 and 1450 lbf in^{-2}g) with a red band from 0 to 15 kPa ×

100. At 20 °C, the vapour pressure of nitrous oxide is 51.6 kPa $\times$ 100 (749 lbf in^{-2} g) so that at normal room temperatures a full cylinder containing liquid nitrous oxide will have a pressure lying close to the white region of the scale.

Carbon dioxide, cyclopropane and nitrous oxide cylinders are never filled to the point where they contain only liquid. Under these circumstances, any slight increase in the ambient temperature would raise the pressure in the cylinder to dangerously high values, since the liquid is almost incompressible. The degree of filling of a cylinder with (liquid + gas) is expressed in terms of the *filling ratio*. This is defined as

$$\frac{\text{Weight of substance (liquid + gas) in a cylinder}}{\text{Weight of water required to fill the cylinder completely}}$$

Cylinders of nitrous oxide are normally filled to a ratio of 0.75, a 'full' cylinder then containing about 9/10 of liquid, the rest being gas. The only satisfactory means of keeping a check on the contents of carbon dioxide, cyclopropane and nitrous oxide cylinders is by weighing them. Suppose that a gram-molecular weight of N_2O (44 g) occupies a volume of 22.4 litres at STP, then the specific volume of gaseous N_2O is $22.4/44 = 0.509$ litres per gram. Considering a mass of 1 g of N_2O, Charles' law gives that the volume it occupies is directly proportional to the absolute temperature, so that the specific volume at 15 °C is 0.509 $\times$ 288/273 = 0.537 litres per gram. A 100-gallon cylinder contains 455 litres of nitrous oxide (when allowed to expand to the conditions of 760 mmHg) and this has a mass of 455/0.537 grams at 15 °C, i.e. 847 g

TABLE 6.2

Property	Nitrous oxide	Carbon dioxide	Oxygen	Cyclopropane
Chemical formula	N_2O	CO_2	O_2	C_3H_6
Molecular weight	44.02	44.01	32.00	42.08
Density at one atmosphere and 15 °C (60 °F)	0.1169 lb/ft^3 1.872 g/l	0.1170 lb/ft^3 1.867 g/l	0.08441 lb/ft^3 1.352 g/l	0.116 lb/ft^3 1.782 g/l
Boiling point	−89.5 °C (−129.1 °F)	− −	−183 °C (−297.4 °F)	−32.86 °C (−27.15 °F)
Critical temperature	36.5 °C (97.7 °F)	31.0 °C (87.8 °F)	−118.38 °C (−181.1 °F)	124.4 °C (255.9 °F)
Critical pressure	105.4 lbf in^{-2} 71.7 atm	107.2 lbf in^{-2} 72.9 atm	73.7 lbf in^{-2} 50.14 atm	79.8 lbf in^{-2} 54.2 atm
Critical density	7.26 MN m^{-2} 457 g/l	7.38 MN m^{-2} 468 g/l	5.08 MN m^{-2} 410 g/l	5.49 MN m^{-2} −

(29.9 oz). Thus each ounce of nitrous oxide is equivalent to 15.2 litres of gas and each gram is equivalent to 0.537 litres. The average weight of an empty 100-gallon N_2O cylinder is 9.5 lb (4.32 kg).

Consider the weight of an empty '2 lb' (0.908 kg) CO_2 cylinder. This holds 106.6 gallons of CO_2 when allowed to expand to the conditions of 15 °C and 760 mmHg. This is equivalent to 485 litres and has a mass of 33 oz (0.934 kg). Thus each ounce of CO_2 is equivalent to 14.7 litres. The weight of an empty 80-gallon (364 litres) cyclopropane cylinder is 9.5 lb (4.32 kg) and this contains 364 litres when allowed to expand to the conditions of 15 °C and 760 mmHg. The mass of cyclopropane is 22.85 oz (0.648 kg), each ounce being equivalent to 16 litres and each gram being equivalent to 0.562 litres of gaseous cyclopropane. *Table 6.2* gives the principal physical characteristics of nitrous oxide, carbon dioxide, oxygen and cyclopropane.

The production of pre-mixed nitrous oxide and oxygen

When the pressure inside a nitrous oxide cylinder is raised above 51 atmospheres (749 lbf in^{-2}, 5.165 MN m^{-2}), liquid nitrous oxide condenses. If the cylinder is first filled with gaseous nitrous oxide to a pressure of 750 lbf in^{-2}, and then filled with oxygen to a total pressure of 2000 lbf in^{-2} (13.790 MN m^{-2}) the percentage of nitrous oxide by volume in the mixture will be 38 per cent assuming that Dalton's law of partial pressures is obeyed. On this basis it would appear that 38 per cent v/v is the maximum concentration of nitrous oxide that could be prepared in a cylinder filled to 2000 lbf in^{-2} (13.790 MN m^{-2}) at 20 °C. There is an obvious need for a more concentrated mixture (50% N_2O, 50% O_2) for use as an analgesic in obstetrical practice, and for the relief of post-operative pain (Tunstall, 1961) and in ambulances.

Experimentally, it has been found possible to prepare mixtures of concentrations up to 70% N_2O, 30% O_2 by using the proper technique. Attention has been concentrated by the British Oxygen Company on the manufacture of a 50% N_2O, 50% O_2 analgesic mixture (Entonox) in lightweight cylinders. Initially, this was intended for domiciliary midwifery practice (Tunstall, 1961), but the market is expanding into dentistry (Bracken, Brookes and Goldman, 1968) and the relief of pain generally (Baskett and Bennett, 1971). For example, Snook (1969) and Baskett (1972) describe its use in ambulances and Baskett *et al.* (1969) describe its use with phenoperidine and droperidol as an anaesthetic during the removal of burns dressings in children. A good account of the method for producing such mixtures is that of Gale, Tunstall and Wilton-Davies (1964). Basically, the correct amount of liquid nitrous oxide is first introduced into an empty cylinder. The cylinder is then inverted, and oxygen bubbled up through the liquid nitrous oxide. Some of the oxygen dissolves in the nitrous oxide, and the remainder in passing through the liquid carries up droplets into the gas above. As a consequence, the amount of liquid gradually diminishes until none remains. By this means, a cylinder filled to 2000 lbf in^{-2} (13 790 kN m^{-2}) is filled with a purely gaseous mixture containing 50 per cent N_2O.

If it is maintained at room temperature, a cylinder containing a mixture of 75% N_2O, 25% O_2 may be used without any change occurring in the composition of the issuing mixture. At no time during the withdrawal of gas will a liquid phase form in the cylinder. Because of this need to keep anaesthetic concentrations of nitrous oxide at normal room temperature, they have not come into widespread use in pipeline systems.

In the case of 50/50 analgesic mixture, separation of the components may take place if the cylinder is cooled below −6 °C. Crawford *et al.* (1966) found that separation occurred in a cylinder which had been cooled to −7 °C. The separation of the mixture into its two components could be dangerous, since if the nitrous oxide became liquefied, gaseous oxygen would be drawn off first, the last part of the cylinder contents becoming progressively more anoxic until in the finish pure nitrous oxide is drawn off.

The probability of a cylinder of pre-mixed gas being exposed to a sufficiently low temperature to produce separation is slight in the United Kingdom, but it cannot be ignored. Crawford *et al.* (1966) mention that during the months of December, January and February temperatures of −7 °C or lower are experienced on average two or three days each year in several cities. A possibility exists that cylinders could be exposed to such temperatures during transit to a hospital, or whilst stored in the boot of a car or in a hospital yard. If any doubt exists concerning the state of a cylinder containing a 50 per cent mixture, Gale *et al.* (1964) suggest two simple precautions which should be taken. The cylinder should be warmed until any frost or ice disappears and then inverted three times after warming. This procedure may not be feasible with large cylinders. Bracken, Broughton and Hill (1968) showed that it is equally satisfactory to store cylinders for a minimum of 24 hours in a horizontal position in a room whose temperature does not fall below 5 °C. Macgregor, Bracken and Fair (1972) showed that in a properly designed hospital pipeline for Entonox, the delivered mixture will never contain less than 20 per cent oxygen. The maximum volume flow rate is set at 300 litres per minute.

The changes in composition which occur in a cylinder containing nitrous oxide and oxygen at 0 °C when the pressure is varied are shown in the 0 °C isotherm of *Figure 6.7.* The curve obtained by joining all

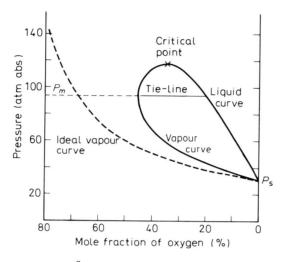

Figure 6.7. 0 °C isotherm for mixture of nitrous oxide and oxygen. Reproduced from Bracken, Broughton and Hill (1970), by courtesy of the Journal of Physics

the points giving the vapour compositions is known as the 'vapour curve' or 'dew-point curve', since if it is approached from a point outside the loop e.g. during compression at a constant mole composition, it gives the point where the first droplet of liquid occurs. Similarly, the points giving the compositions of the condensed liquid phase produce the 'liquid curve' or 'bubble-point curve', since, if it is approached from a point outside the loop, it gives the point where the first bubble appears. For example, if the pressure is reduced in a cylinder containing a liquid phase at a constant temperature, then at a certain pressure, evaporation will commence and a bubble will form. When the mole-fraction of oxygen is zero in the mixture, the bubble-point and dew-point curves meet at the vapour pressure for pure nitrous oxide at the temperature of the isotherm. In this case, 30.87 atmospheres at 0 °C. The broken line adjacent to the vapour curve represents the composition which would be found with an ideal vapour phase composition based on the assumption that the gas and vapour obeyed Dalton's law of partial pressures. That is, the vapour pressure of the nitrous oxide remains constant and independent of the total pressure of the mixture, i.e. $N_2O=(P_s/P)\times 100$ where P is the total pressure and P_s is the saturated vapour pressure at the temperature of the isotherm. At the critical point, the liquid and vapour phase compositions become equal. At $0\,^\circ C$ and a 50/50 mixture, the points for all pressures lie to the left of the closed loop so that no condensation can occur. Following the vapour curve round the diagram, above a certain pressure P_m (approximately 94 atmospheres) in *Figure 6.7* the percentage of nitrous oxide in the vapour increases rather than decreases with an increase in pressure. In *Figure 6.8* pressure–temperature curves for

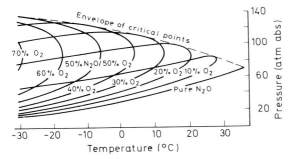

Figure 6.8. Pressure-temperature curves for a nitrous oxide-oxygen mixture of constant composition. Reproduced from Bracken, Broughton and Hill (1970), by courtesy of the Journal of Physics

nitrous oxide–oxygen mixtures of constant composition are shown. It can be seen that the effect of adding oxygen to nitrous oxide is to lower the critical temperature of the mixture. The critical temperature of the 50/50 mixture is $-5.5\,^\circ C$ and for a 75/25 nitrous oxide-oxygen mixture it is $+20\,^\circ C$. It will be recalled that above the critical temperature it is not possible to liquefy the mixture.

The maximum temperature at which a liquid phase can form inside a cylinder of Entonox mixture is $-5.5\,^\circ C$, and the isotherm for this temperature is shown in *Figure 6.9*. The line corresponding to the 50/50 composition just touches the dew-point curve. Hence, if a cylinder of this mixture is maintained above $-5.5\,^\circ C$, no condensation can occur whatever the pressure. It should be pointed out that at $-5.5\,^\circ C$, condensation will only occur when the filling pressure of the cylinder is approximately 115 atmospheres (1700 lbf in^{-2}g or 11.723 MN m^{-2}g). For pressures above or below this value, condensation will take place at a lower temperature. This fact accounts for the range of temperatures reported in practice with Entonox cylinders.

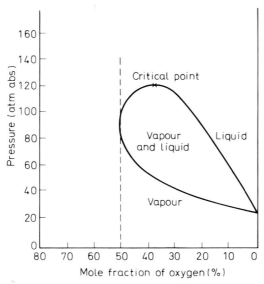

Figure 6.9. −5.5 °C isotherm for mixtures of nitrous oxide and oxygen. (After Broughton, 1969)

As a result of the evaporation process, the issuing gas mixture becomes very cold (−60 °C), and the Entonox demand valve becomes covered in frost. Crawford *et al.* (1966) report that this did not affect the functioning of the valve, nor gave rise to any separation of the gas mixture.

The variation of atmospheric pressure with height

In considering the problems involved in administering anaesthetic agents at high altitudes, it is necessary to take into account the fact that the atmospheric pressure decreases with height above the earth's surface. It is an interesting exercise in the development of a simple exponential equation to determine the law governing this process. Let P be the atmospheric pressure in N m^{-2} at a height of H m in an atmosphere at a constant temperature of T K. At a slightly greater height $(H+h)$ m, the pressure will be less than P by an amount equal to the weight of a layer of air h m thick and 1 m^2 in cross-section. If d is the density of air in kg l^{-1}, then $p = -dgh$ N m^{-2} where g is the acceleration due to gravity = 9.81 m s^{-2}. If it is assumed that air obeys the Ideal Gas law at this pressure, then PV/T = a constant = R (R is the gas constant for a gram-molecule of gas and has a value of 8.313 J per gram-molecule per deg C). Dividing both sides of the equation by M, the effective molecular weight of air, $P/d = RT/M$ so $d = PM/RT$, giving $p = -(PM/RT)\, gh$. Re-arranging, $p/P = -(Mg/RT)h$. Integrating both sides yields the simple exponential equation $\ln (P) = -(Mg/RT)H$ + a constant. At $H = 0$, let p = the barometric pressure B. Then $\ln (P/B) = -(Mg/RT)H$. That is $P = B \exp [-(Mg/RT)H]$. This means that the pressure should fall off exponentially with height. When an altitude of (Mg/RT) m is reached, the pressure should be $1/e$ of atmospheric. If the simple theory held, this would occur at a height of 7137 metres (23 400 feet), but in practice, the pressure is found to be 280 mmHg at 7625 metres (25 000 feet).

References

BASKETT, P.J.F. (1972). The use of Entonox in the ambulance service. *Proc. R. Soc. Med. Lond.* **65**, 7

BASKETT, P.J.F. and BENNETT, J.A. (1971). Pain relief in hospital : the more widespread use of nitrous oxide. *Br. Med. J.* **2**, 509

BASKETT, P.J.F., HYLAND, J., DEANE, M. and WRAY, G. (1969). Analgesia for burns dressings in children. *Br. J. Anaesth.* **41**, 684

BRACKEN, A.B., BROOKES, R.C. and GOLDMAN, V. (1968). New equipment for dental anaesthesia using pre-mixed gases and halothane. *Br. J. Anaesth.* **40**, 903

BRACKEN, A.B., BROUGHTON, G.B. and HILL, D.W.(1968). Safety precautions to be observed with cooled pre-mixed gases. *Br. med. J.* **3**, 715

BRACKEN, A.B., BROUGHTON, G.B. and HILL, D.W. (1970). Equilibria for mixtures of oxygen with nitrous oxide and carbon dioxide and their relevances to the storage of N_2O/O_2 cylinders for use in analgesia. *J. Phys. D.* **3**, 1747

BROUGHTON, G.B. (1969). An investigation into the stability of mixtures of gases and vapours at high pressures. M. Phil. Thesis, London University

COUCH, E.J. and KOBE, K.A. (1961). Volumetric behaviour of nitrous oxide. *J. chem. engng. Data* **6**, 229

CRAWFORD, J.S., ELLIS, D.B., HILL, D.W. and PAYNE, J.P. (1966). Effects of cooling on the safety of premixed gases. *Br. med. J.* 2, 138

DITTMER, D.S. and GREBE, R.M. (Eds.) (1958). *Handbook of Respiration.* Philadelphia; Saunders

GALE, C.W., TUNSTALL, M.E. and WILTON-DAVIES, C.C. (1964). Premixed gas and oxygen for midwives. *Br. med. J.* 1, 732

HILL, D.W. (1961). The production of accurate gas and vapour mixtures. *Br. J. appl. Phys.* 12, 410

JONES, P.L. (1974). Some observations on nitrous oxide cylinders during emptying. *Br. J. Anaesth.* 46, 534

MACGREGOR, W.G., BRACKEN, A. and FAIR, J.A. (1972). Piped premixed 50% nitrous oxide and 50% oxygen mixture (Entonox). *Anaesthesia* 27, 14

SAFAR, P. and TENICELA, R. (1964). High altitude physiology in relation to anesthesia and inhalational therapy. *Anesthesiology* 25, 515

SNOOK, R. (1969). Resuscitation at road accidents. *Br. med. J.* 4, 348

TUNSTALL, M.E. (1961). Use of a fixed nitrous oxide and oxygen mixture from one cylinder. *Lancet* 2, 964

WULF, R.J. and FEATHERSTONE, R.M. (1957). A correlation of Van der Waals constants with anesthetic potency. *Anesthesiology* 18, 97

7 Heat

Heat is simply another form of energy, and is interchangeable with energy existing in other forms, such as electrical and mechanical energy. The addition of heat to a system will, in general, increase the total energy of the system and its temperature. Thus, if a closed volume of gas is heated, the energy of motion of its atoms or molecules is increased, and this is indicated by a rise in temperature as they make more energetic impacts with the walls of the container. The heating or cooling of a body is expressed in terms of its temperature. This is an expression of the average kinetic energy of the constituent molecules.

Temperature scales

One of the SI system base units is that of thermodynamic temperature and the kelvin (K) is the unit. It is the fraction $1/273.16$ of the thermodynamic temperature of the triple point of water. The quantity thermodynamic temperature (T) is expressed in kelvins. Celsius temperature (T) is defined by the equation $t = T - T_0$ where T_0 is equal to 273.15 K by definition.

The thermodynamic temperature scale and its unit employ the triple point of water, a thermometric point obtainable with higher accuracy than is the melting point of ice.

The zero for Celsius temperature is now defined as being 0.01 K below the triple point of water, hence the value of 273.15 in the equation $t = T - T_0$, in contrast to the value of 273.16 encountered in the definition of the kelvin.

For many problems, the common approximation $T_0 = 273$ K will still be sufficiently accurate. The term degree Centigrade is no longer used, the correct symbol is °C (a composite symbol) for degree Celsius. Temperature differences may be expressed in degrees Celsius and for this purpose 1 °C = 1 K.

In dealing with Gas Law calculations, it is necessary to use the thermodynamic scale of temperature. The zero point (0 K) on this scale is the absolute zero, which is the lowest temperature it is possible to obtain. It is the temperature at which the volume and temperature of ideal gases become zero, and has a value of -273.16 K which for most practical purposes can be taken as -273 K. Thus degrees Celsius (°C) can simply be converted to thermodynamic temperatures in kelvins by adding 273. Thus the melting point of ice which was taken as 0 °C would be equal to 273 K and the temperature of the boiling point of water at a pressure of 760 mmHg (101.06 kPa) which used to be taken as 100 °C equals 373 K.

Modern low temperature techniques of adiabatic demagnetization enable temperatures of within a fraction of a degree of the absolute zero to be realized. Many hospitals now employ a cryogenic method to supply oxygen to a central pipeline system (Wilke, 1964). Liquid oxygen is supplied in bulk to a thermally insulated container, and by controlled evaporation of the liquid gaseous oxygen is supplied to the pipeline. The liquid oxygen boils at -183 °C (90 K), and is stored in double-walled vessels having a vacuum between the walls. Cryogenic systems are also employed to pressurize with air hyperbaric operating and treatment rooms (Heringman *et al.,* 1964). Liquid oxygen and nitrogen are evaporated separately to yield the gases which are then mixed in the right proportion and supplied at the desired pressure by means of a special proportioning valve. Liquid nitrogen which boils at -196 °C (77 K), has made possible the development of compact cryogenic probes for use in the welding of detached retinas and in neurosurgery (Harper, 1966). The cold of the liquid nitrogen supplied to the probe head can be counterbalanced by heat supplied from a built-in electrical heater. In this way it is possible to set the temperature of the probe tip anywhere between room temperature and -196 °C.

Units of heat

A unit of heat was defined as the calorie in terms of the amount of heat required to raise the temperature of 1 g of water by 1 °C. However, heat is simply one form of energy and on the SI system the calorie is no longer allowable and is replaced by the joule as the SI unit of energy. One calorie $= 4.1868$ joules.

The most convenient way of expressing energy production and utilization in the living organism has been in terms of the kilocalorie (Calorie spelled with a capital C). The kilocalorie has been the unit normally used in considering the energy of metabolism. In the SI system the Calorie is replaced by the kilojoule where 1 Calorie $= 4.186$ kilojoules. If 1 g of each of the three basic foods is ignited in a bomb calorimeter, the following values are obtained: protein 22.19 kJ, carbohydrate 18.00 kJ and fat 39.77 kJ. When 1 g each of the same substance is oxidized in the body the values become 17.16 kJ for protein, 17.16 kJ for carbohydrate and 38.93 kJ for fat. The discrepancy in the protein values suggests that protein is not completely oxidized in the body. The basal metabolism (or basic metabolic rate, B.M.R.) is the minimal heat output produced by the fasting individual, physically and mentally at rest, at room temperature (approx. 20 °C). The basal metabolism is primarily dependent on the surface area of the body, and therefore it depends on the individual's age and sex. The average surface area of women is about 1.6 square metres and for men it is about 1.8 square metres. In the age group 30—40 years, an average metabolic rate for men is 165.3 kJ and for women 152.8 kJ per hour per square metre of body surface area.

The cooling capacity of refrigeration units used to provide hypothermia, or the output of air-conditioning plants associated with operating rooms and intensive care units is expressed in terms of kilojoules or megajoules per hour. Forrester (1958) describes a refrigeration unit for hypothermia capable of extracting 5.064 MJ per hour at −5 °C.

The use of a hypothermic technique is now commonplace, particularly during cardiac surgery, and anaesthetists are often responsible for the functioning of the equipment which may be considerable. In the profound hypothermia technique of Drew (1961), two artificial circulations are established. On the left side, blood from the left atrium passes into a reservoir and is then pumped through a heat exchanger where it is cooled and then returned to a femoral artery. A similar circulation, but without a heat exchanger, takes blood from the right atrium and returns it to the pulmonary artery. The patient's lungs still function as oxygenators. Each combination of a reservoir and pump takes the place of an atrium and ventricle, so that even if the natural cardiac output is diminished or stopped, the circulation is maintained. At a body temperature of 15 °C, the heart can be stopped for periods of up to an hour. A comprehensive review of hypothermia and associated anaesthesia is that of Hunter (1964).

Specific heat

The quantity of heat required to raise 1 kg of each of various substances through 1 K (the units of kelvin and Celsius temperature interval are identical) will not be the same as that required in the case of 1 kg of water. The *specific heat* of a substance is defined as the quantity of heat energy required to raise 1 kg of that substance through 1 kelvin. In the SI system it is expressed in joules per kilogram per kelvin ($J kg^{-1} K^{-1}$). On the CGS system specific heats are expressed in terms of calories per gram, and these units are still in use in some North American textbooks (Epstein and Kuzava, 1976). The specific heat of water is 1 calorie per gram. Assuming that 1 calorie is equivalent to 4.186 joules and since 1 cubic metre will contain 10^6 cubic centimetres, the specific heat of water on the SI system is 4.186 kJ kg^{-1} K^{-1}. The specific heat of copper is 0.4186 kJ kg^{-1} K^{-1}, of ether 2.093 kJ kg^{-1} K^{-1} and that of whole blood 3.642 kJ kg^{-1} K^{-1}.

Any substance of specific heat s and mass m can be expressed in terms of its water equivalent mass W in kg in respect of the amount of heat required to raise its temperature by t kelvins. Equating the amounts of heat required for the substance concerned and water respectively $m.s.t. = W.w.t.$ where m and W are the mass of the substance and the equivalent mass of water in kg, s and w are the specific heats of the substance and water in kJ kg^{-1} K^{-1}. Thus $W = m(s/w)$. In the case of a composite body, e.g. a soda-lime cannister of interest to anaesthetists, the various component parts made of different materials can be readily expressed in terms of their equivalent masses of water and these are then summed to give the total equivalent mass. This approach was adopted by Ainley-Walker (1959) to determine the temperature rise occurring in a soda-lime cannister during the absorption of carbon dioxide.

The heat required to raise a body of mass m kg and specific heat s kJ kg^{-1} K^{-1} through 1 kelvin represents the amount of heat energy put into that body i.e. its thermal capacity, assuming no heat losses.

The specific heats of gases

The specific heats of gases, and hence their thermal capacity, are much smaller than those of solids or liquids. This fact is illustrated in striking fashion by the fact it is possible to smoke a cigarette in relative comfort when the end is glowing red hot. Unless careful precautions are taken, gases quickly attain ambient temperature when passing along a tube. For example, a mixture of nitrous oxide and oxygen when issuing from a pre-mixed cylinder may attain a temperature of −60 °C. Yet, after passing through three feet of metal and rubber tubing the temperature of the gas may be +20 °C.

The specific heat of a gas reflects the amount of work that has to be done on it in order to raise the temperature of the gas by 1 kelvin (1 °C). A gas really has an infinite number of specific heats, their values depending on whether the volume of the gas is held constant during the heating, or if not, as to how it is allowed to expand. In practice, there are two main specific heats for gases, these are the specific heat at *constant pressure* C_p and the specific heat at *constant volume* C_v. C_p is the number of joules required to raise the temperature by 1 kelvin

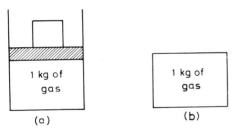

Figure 7.1. The volume of 1 kilogram of gas contained under (a) constant pressure conditions and (b) constant volume conditions

of the gas contained in a cylinder fitted with a frictionless piston loaded with a constant force (*Figure 7.1(a)*) and C_v is the number of joules required to raise the temperature of 1 kg of the gas contained in a fixed volume by 1 kelvin (*Figure 7.1(b)*). In the SI system both C_p and C_v are expressed in terms of J kg^{-1} K^{-1}.

Isothermal and adiabatic changes
When work is performed on a mass of gas in order to compress it, the temperature of the gas would generally be expected to rise. If the compression is performed sufficiently slowly, the heat generated can be conducted away through the walls of the containing vessel and the temperature of the gas remains constant. Such a compression is said to be isothermal in nature. Similar considerations apply to the cooling

which would be expected on an expansion. Under these conditions Boyle's law applies and $PV = $ constant.

If the compression or expansion is sudden, a change in temperature of the gas will occur, and the compression or expansion is said to be adiabatic in nature. Under these conditions the equation $PV^\gamma = $ a constant applies, where $\gamma = C_p/C_v$. For air at $20\,^{\circ}$C, $C_p = 1.009$ kJ kg^{-1} K^{-1} and $C_v = 0.7158$ kJ kg^{-1} K^{-1} giving $\gamma = 1.41$.

When testing automatic ventilators and breathing systems in the laboratory, it is often convenient to make use of an 'artificial thorax'. Such a device consists of a rigid vessel of a suitable volume chosen to simulate the compliance of the chest wall plus lungs. Elastic forces are not involved, but a definite increment of pressure applied to the vessel will force into it a definite increment of gas volume. The slope of the graph of volume increment plotted against pressure increment gives the effective 'compliance' of the vessel. This is proportional to the volume of the vessel, and can be chosen to simulate the compliance of adults, children or neonates.

The theory of such an artificial thorax has been discussed by Hill and Moore (1965). Consider a given mass of gas contained in a volume V at a pressure P. If the temperature remains constant (isothermal conditions), Boyle's law is obeyed and PV is a constant, i.e., $PV = C$. Differentiating both sides of this equation gives $PdV + VdP = 0$. Hence the compliance of the vessel is $(dV/dP) = -(V/P)$. With a barometric pressure of 76 cmHg, a vessel of 51.7 litres capacity would give a compliance of 0.05 litres per cm of water pressure.

If adiabatic conditions are assumed then $PV^\gamma = K$, where K is a constant. Differentiation yields $V\gamma dP + P\gamma V^{\gamma-1}dV = 0$. So that the compliance

$$\frac{dV}{dP} = \frac{-V}{\gamma P}$$

For an atmospheric pressure of 76 cmHg = 1033.6 cmH$_2$O, $V = 50$ litres and $\gamma = 1.41$, the compliance becomes 0.03 litres per cm of water pressure.

Figure 7.2 taken from Hill and Moore (1965) shows the relationship between the pressure rise in a glass bottle of 6.7 litres capacity when a fixed 63 ml tidal volume was delivered at various respiratory rates, and the values to be expected under fully isothermal or adiabatic conditions. At rates greater than four per minute the pressure swings are within 5 per cent of the adiabatic value. Glass is to be preferred for

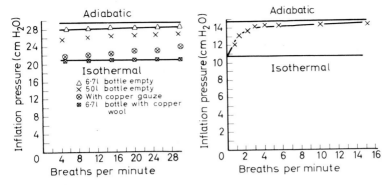

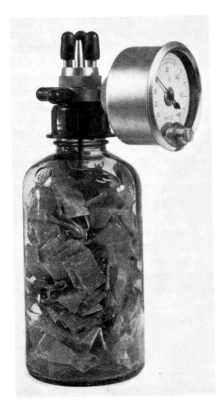

Figure 7.2. The relations between experimental results and the theoretical isothermal **and** adiabatic conditions for an empty 6.7 litre glass bottle

Figure 7.3. A small artificial thorax designed for use in testing an infant's ventilator

the container because of its rigidity, and isothermal conditions can be maintained by filling the vessel with copper wool. *Figure 7.3* illustrates a small artificial thorax designed for use in testing an infant's ventilator.

Latent heat and change of state

Matter can normally exist in one or more of three states; solid, liquid, and gas or vapour. Work must be done on the system in order to bring about a change of state, and heat is often the form of energy used. Normally the addition or subtraction of heat is accompanied by a change in temperature. However, whilst a change of state is being brought about, the temperature remains constant in the case of a pure substance. The heat used to bring about the change of state is known as *latent heat*. This is because the action of the heat is apparently hidden since the temperature stays constant. Consider a pure substance such as naphthalene placed in a test tube containing a thermocouple and gently heated in a water bath. The form of the graph of naphthalene temperature plotted against time is illustrated in *Figure 7.4*. At first the temperature of the solid naphthalene rises steadily, assuming a uniform rate of heating. When the naphthalene starts to melt, the temperature

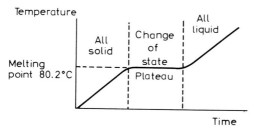

Figure 7.4. The temperature 'plateau' occurring at the melting point of pure naphthalene

of the mixture of solid and liquid naphthalene remains constant whilst the change of state is taking place. This gives rise to the characteristic temperature 'plateau' at the melting point. Once all the naphthalene is melted, the temperature rises uniformly again. If the substance is impure, a series of steps would be obtained, rather than a single well-defined plateau. The lower fixed point (0 °C) occurs at the change of state from ice to water, and the upper fixed point (100 °C) at the change of state from water to water vapour. The latent heat of fusion of ice is approximately 334 kJ kg^{-1} (80 calories per gram) at 10 °C. The melting point of ice is little affected by changes in the atmospheric pressure, and an increase of one atmosphere reduces the melting point by only 0.0075 degrees. (Note that this behaviour is anomalous; increasing the pressure will normally raise the melting point.) This is in marked contrast to the boiling point of water which is raised by an increase in the atmospheric pressure. At 100 °C, the latent heat of vaporization of water is 2.257 MJ kg^{-1} (540 calories per gram).

Another example of a change of state from solid to liquid occurs in the case of calcium chloride crystals which if heated to 30 °C will change to liquid. On cooling through 30 °C, the latent heat of crystallization is given out. This fact was used in the Oxford ether vaporizer to hold the temperature of the evaporating liquid ether constant at 30 °C. A similar principle has been employed during mountain warfare in order to maintain the temperature of intravenous fluids during exposure to cold weather.

Evaporation

The change of state occurring from liquid to gas or vapour is of particular interest to anaesthetists, the process being known as evaporation. As a result of their thermal energy, the molecules of a liquid are continually in a state of random motion. A molecule present in the bulk of the liquid will be surrounded by adjacent molecules on all sides, and attractive forces existing between the chosen molecule and the others will tend to cancel. For a molecule at the surface, however, there will be many more molecules surrounding it in the liquid phase than there will be in the vapour phase above the liquid. Thus such a molecule will experience a net attractive force inwards towards the bulk of the liquid. In order for a molecule to be able to evaporate and escape from the liquid it must, by means of a series of fortunate collisions with other molecules, be able to overcome this attractive force. Thus only the most energetic molecules can escape. When this happens the mean energy of the remaining molecules falls, and this is reflected in a fall in the temperature of the liquid.

A marked cooling can occur when liquefied gases such as nitrous oxide are evaporated, and a layer of frost or condensation forms on the cylinder and reducing valve (this latter effect is due to expansion of the gas through the valve). In neurosurgery, it is sometimes convenient to produce a state of hypothermia by the simple means of swabbing down the patient with iced water, and then evaporating this water with a stream of air produced by electric fans. The evaporation of the water aids cooling, as in sweating. The rate of perspiration varies with the temperature but even at low temperatures there is still some perspiration. This is known as *insensible water loss* and averages about 1000 ml per day. Marked local cooling giving rise to local analgesia can be produced by the evaporation of a ethyl chloride as a jet of vapour directed at the skin (Furnas, 1965).

The effects of the cooling resulting from the evaporation of anaesthetic agents such as ether and halothane have a pronounced effect on the design of anaesthetic vaporizers, and these will be discussed in detail in the next chapter.

The transfer of heat

The transfer of heat from one body to another can take place by one or more of three main mechanisms: conduction, convection and radiation. In the case of man, the total thermal resistance may be considered as that of the air or other environment such as clothing, outside the skin plus that of the tissues between the skin surface and tissue where the deep body temperature is maintained (Chao *et al.,* 1979). Change in the thermal conductivity of tissue brought about by circulatory change forms the main control of heat loss.

Below a 25 °C ambient temperature, the nude body at rest loses more heat than it produces, and as a natural response to cold there is a rise in heat production which precedes the onset of visible shivering and this is due to the stimulation of peripheral receptors. Other thermogenic processes contributing to the pre-shivering rise in heat production include the liberation of adrenaline, noradrenaline or adrenal cortical activity (Chao *et al.,* 1979). There is also a reduction in peripheral blood flow. Between 25 °C and 29 °C vasomotor regulation prevails. Above 29 °C, comparatively little heat is lost by convection alone and sweating begins, increasing in intensity until the maximum as reached. Above 35 °C the body loses heat almost entirely by evaporation.

Conduction

This involves a direct transfer of heat energy from molecule to molecule. Hence it cannot take place across a vacuum. Consider a block of material of cross-sectional area A, thickness d, and having two opposite faces maintained at temperatures t_1 and t_2 respectively, where t_1 is greater than t_2. Experiment shows that the quantity of heat transferred per unit time between the two opposite faces is proportional to the area A, proportional to the temperature difference $(t_1 - t_2)$, and inversely proportional to the thickness d. If Q is the quantity of heat conducted per second, then Q is proportional to $A(t_1-t_2)/d$. This can be written as $Q = KA(t_1-t_2)/d$. The constant of proportionality K is known as the coefficient of thermal conductivity of the substance. On the CGS system its units are ergs per centimetre per second per degree Celsius, and on the SI system watts per metre per degree Celsius. The thermal conductivity of copper is 0.918 cal s^{-1} cm^{-1} $°C^{-1}$ (0.0384 W m^{-1} $°C^{-1}$). The values for other common materials are: aluminium 0.504 (0.021 W m^{-1} $°C^{-1}$); brass 0.260 (0.011 W m^{-1} $°C^{-1}$); steel 0.108 (0.0045 W m^{-1} $°C^{-1}$) and glass 0.0025 (0.0001 W m^{-1} $°C^{-1}$). These are all at 180 $°C$. The value for copper is 8.5 times that for steel.

The high thermal conductivity of copper was a prime consideration in its choice for the manufacture of the copper kettle type of anaesthetic vaporizer. An additional reason for using copper is that it has a high thermal capacity. Consider a volume of one cubic metre of water whose specific heat is 4.186 kJ kg^{-1}. The mass of the water is 10^3 kg so that the water equivalent is 4186 kJ. The density of copper is 9000 kg m^{-3} and its specific heat 0.1 × 4.186 kJ kg^{-1}. Thus the water equivalent of one cubic metre of copper is 0.9 that of water. In practice, a copper kettle vaporizer is mounted on a wide metal base so that the latent heat required during the evaporation of the anaesthetic agent is supplied from the high thermal capacity of the copper. Additional heat is obtained from the atmosphere of the room via the good thermal conductivity of the copper in order to continue the supply of heat to the evaporating liquid. Thus within the limit of the amount of heat which can be transferred from the copper the evaporation of the liquid continues at a constant rate with its temperature remaining constant.

Heat transfer by conduction occurs when a patient is in contact with a hot or cold object. It is the process by which the ear of an unconscious patient, in contact with the lamp of an earpiece oximeter, may become burnt. In some systems for the production of hypothermia, the patient is cooled by being placed upon a rubber mattress through which circulates cold water. On the other hand, Winder and Vale (1970) have described a heat retaining mattress for temperature control during surgery. Brock (1975) deals with the importance of the environmental temperature in the operating room and intensive care unit. Ross *et al.* (1969) report on the observation of central and peripheral temperatures in the understanding and management of shock while Dyde and Lunn (1970) describe heat loss during thoracotomy.

Thermal balance aspects of burns

In a person with normal skin perfusion, damage leading to a burn will occur if the skin temperature is allowed to exceed about 45 °C for a sufficient period of time.

The amount of heat required to produce damage will be affected by the rate at which it can be removed from the site of application by the local perfusion. A common occurrence is the combination of a low level source of heat and an inadequate local perfusion. Thus to avoid a burn, there must be an adequate balance between the supply and removal of the heat. A very common cause for an inadequate perfusion is a low local blood flow caused by pressure over a bony prominence or by a low systemic blood flow as can arise during cardio-pulmonary bypass or in hypovolaemic shock. Under these circumstances sufficient local heating can arise under the plate electrode for a surgical diathermy unit where the plate makes a poor contact with the patient. Stainless steel or foil electrodes plus a conductive gel will obviate this situation.

Gases are poor conductors of heat; the thermal conductivity of air is some sixteen thousand times less than that of copper. Thus garments such as string vests act as efficient retainers of body heat by trapping a layer of static air above the skin. Hyperthermia is being evaluated in the treatment of cancer (Dickson, 1979). Pettigrew *et al.* (1974) heated a series of patients to 41–42 °C with warmed anaesthetic gases, enclosing the body in an envelope of wax to prevent heat loss; treatments were given weekly for up to 18 months. Eighteen (47 per cent) of the 38 patients showed a short-term objective response to heat, as judged by a measurable regression of lesions or histologically confirmed tumour necrosis.

Convection

This is the process by which a stream of gas or water can bring heat to or from a patient. The fact that warm air is less dense than cold air and therefore rises is an example of natural convection. Since a moving medium such as a gas or liquid is involved, again the process cannot take place in a vacuum.

The action of forced convection due to the action of a fan in an incubator on the temperature of neonates has been studied by a combination of thermography to make the surface temperature distribution visible and Schlieren photography to visualize the convection currents from the baby. Forced air circulation increased the baby's heat loss by about 25–30 per cent. For a baby the surface area of the head is 21 per cent on average of the total surface area compared with only 7 per cent for an adult. In contrast for the trunk the percentages are respectively 32 per cent and 35 per cent. Thus heat loss from a baby's head is important.

During anaesthesia, the process of breathing gives rise to a heat loss, since the inspired gases will be at almost ambient temperature, and the temperature of the expired gases will be some 34–36 °C. Let the minute volume of a patient be 5 litres, the temperature of the inspired gas (oxygen) be 20 °C, and that of the expired gas caused by the warming of the gas be 36 °C. The specific heat of oxygen is $1.256\,J\,l^{-1}$. The heat loss caused by the warming of the gas during respiration is $5 \times 16 \times 1.256 = 100.5\,J\,min^{-1}$. There will also be an additional heat loss introduced by the fact that water is being evaporated from the patient in order to saturate the expired gases with water vapour. The oxygen supplied from a cylinder can be assumed to be dry, whilst the water vapour concentration in the expired gases is approximately 6 per cent. Hence the loss of water vapour per minute amounts to 6 per cent of the minute volume of 5 litres, i.e. 300 ml. At body temperature, 1 ml of liquid water vaporizes into 1400 ml of water vapour, so that a mass of approximately 0.2 g of water is vaporized per minute. The latent heat of vaporization of water is $2.26\,MJ\,kg^{-1}$, so that the heat loss per minute due to this cause is $452.1\,J\,min^{-1}$, giving a total heat loss of $552.6\,J\,min^{-1}$. Holdcroft and Hall (1978) have investigated heat losses in man during anaesthesia and found that the observed temperature changes correlated with both the type of anaesthesia and the percentage of body weight of subcutaneous fat. One per cent of halothane decreased the rate of heat loss during the third hour of anaesthesia.

The problem of maintaining a heat balance in patients is particularly acute in children because of their high surface area to weight ratio compared with adults and their markedly reduced ratio of basal to maximum metabolic output. It is important to be able to control the effects of heat loss during the management of neonates particularly where there is a cardiovascular or metabolic compromise. In this respect the minimizing of evaporative heat losses from the respiratory circuit is important in the stabilization of heat loss. Berry *et al.* (1973) have placed an electric heating tape around the carbon dioxide absorber to allow the inspiratory gases to equilibrate with the temperature and moisture of the absorber and thus minimize the respiratory heat loss in infants during anaesthesia. Chalon *et al.* (1978) described an infant circuit with a water vaporizer warmed by carbon dioxide neutralization.

Smith (1978) reviewed the practice of paediatric anaesthesia and states that the conservation of body heat is more important than the application of external heat. Warm operating rooms and maximal coverage of the body, limbs and head have been found to be most essential. Heating lamps are valuable at the commencement of the operation and water blankets are now regarded as of secondary importance.

Radiation

Radiation consists in the emanation, in the form of electromagnetic radiation, of heat energy from a body. Radiant electric fires immediately give rise to the idea of the emission of heat by radiation. Radiation can traverse a vacuum, that is, it does not need a physical medium to support its passage. Because of this fact the sun's heat can reach the earth through the vacuum of space. The greater the temperature difference between a body and its surroundings, the greater will be the radiant heat loss from the body. Thus radiant heat lamps are employed for drying purposes, and in physical medicine departments for the heat treatment of joints. Heat is lost from the human body principally by radiation from the body surface to objects at lower-than-body temperature. When cutaneous arterioles and capillaries dilate, a large volume of blood is enabled to flow close to the body surface, and the heat loss is increased. Heat losses due to convection and radiation are minimized by keeping the patient covered as much as possible. The mechanisms of body heat loss are important in the design of incubators for neonates. About 45 per cent of the heat loss from the baby occurs by radiation, 35 per cent by convection, 20 per cent due to the evaporation of water, and 1 per cent by conduction through the mattress. Hey (1975) discusses the concept of 'thermal neutrality' in regard to neonatal care. He has plotted the heat produced in watts per square metre against the environmental temperature for six babies of approximately 2.5 kg body weight when 7–11 days old. They were each lying naked in draught-free surroundings of uniform temperature and moderate humidity. The zone of minimum heat production extended from 32.5 °C to about 36.5 °C but thermal balance is maintained by sweat loss above a temperature of 33.5 °C. Hey and Katz (1970) discuss the optimal environment for naked babies.

In addition to incubators, infra-red heaters are employed to maintain the temperature of infants by radiant heating in intensive care units (Agate and Silverman, 1963). In one particular device with an infra-red source temperature of 140 °C with a peak emmission at 6.9 μm the maximum surface temperature produced was 36.5 °C, the irradiance at wavelengths greater than 1.4 μm was 4.25 mW cm^{-2}. A thermistor temperature probe is placed on the skin of the infant and used to control the power supplied to the heaters to maintain the skin temperature at the desired value.

Hardy and Muschenheim (1934) describe the radiation of heat from the human body and Kaletzky, Proctor and Crankshaw (1964) describe the use of panels cooled down to −25 °C to provide surgical hypothermia in man due to heat loss by radiation.

The Dewar vessel or vacuum flask.

Good radiators of radiant heat are also good receivers of radiant heat, and poor emitters make poor absorbers. Thus a polished shiny surface will be both a poor emitter and a poor absorber of radiant heat. Methods of minimizing heat loss from a body to its surroundings are well illustrated in the design of a Dewar or vacuum flask. Small types much used for the storage of blood samples, consist of a double-walled glass container, having the walls silvered on the inside and the space between them evacuated. The vacuum stops heat losses by convection and conduction from the inner container to the outside and the silvering reduces radiation losses. The large Dewar vessels used to hold liquid oxygen employ a metal construction, with activated charcoal to absorb any gases which may be liberated from the metal and which would otherwise spoil the vacuum. A more modern approach is to dispense with the vacuum, and to fill the space between the inner and outer shells with an expanded type of material resembling the mica 'vermiculite' material used for thermally insulating the lofts of houses. This material contains plenty of air and is an efficient thermal insulator.

Pipeline systems for medical gases

When more than 5000 ft^3 (141 600 litres) of oxygen is used by a hospital per week, it is more economical to derive the oxygen from a bulk liquid storage tank rather than from separate cylinders. The storage tank normally holds the equivalent of 30 000 ft^3 of gaseous oxygen, and is fitted with a blow-off valve set at 20 lbf in^{-2} (0.414 MN m^{-2}). A compressor raises the pressure to 60 lbf in^{-2} (1.24 MN m^{-2}) and the gas is stored for use in a bank of reservoir cylinders. Nitrous oxide is supplied from a bank of cylinders, an electric heating element in the vicinity of the manifold pipes preventing the formation of frost due to high rates of evaporation. For smaller pipeline systems the oxygen will also be obtained from a bank of cylinders. When the pipeline pressure drops below a pre-set value, electrically operated valves automatically bring a reserve bank of cylinders into operation.

Heat exchangers for use during blood transfusion

Dybkjaer and Elkjaer (1964) report that it is important to warm blood for massive blood transfusion in order to avoid the complications of local cardiac and generalized hypothermia. Russell (1969a) describes a disposable blood-warming unit. This is a rectangular single-walled plastic bag containing welded plastic strips to form 14 linked channels. The bag is suspended in a water bath thermostatically held at 39–40 °C. With an inflow to the bag of 128 ml per minute at 8 °C, the output temperature was 32.6 °C. Insertion of the unit in the line from the drip bottle resulted in a 21 per cent decrease in flow, but this was almost completely offset by the increase in flow which resulted from the change of viscosity due to the warming of the blood.

Russell (1969b) shows that for this type of heat exchanger it is possible to calculate an overall coefficient of heat transfer h_c such that

$$h_c = (\Delta t_1 sm)/(\Delta t_2 A)$$

where h_c = coefficient of heat transfer in J s^{-1} m^{-2} K^{-1}

Δt_1 = temperature difference between the output and input blood temperatures in °C

Δt_2 = temperature difference between the bath temperature and the mean blood temperature in °C

A = area of heat exchange in m^2

m = mass flow in kg s^{-1}

s = specific heat of blood in J kg^{-1} K^{-1}

For Russell's unit with $A = 0.045$ m^2, $m = 0.002$ kg s^{-1} and $s = 1$, $h_c = 0.444$ J s^{-1} m^{-2} K^{-1} for water, and provides a criterion for comparing the efficiencies of similar designs of heat exchanger. Bjoraker (1978) has pointed that electrically powered blood warmers can be a source of potentially dangerous electrical leakage currents.

Heat exchangers for use with an extracorporeal circulation

Heat exchangers are used as part of an extracorporeal circulation to: maintain normothermia; to induce varying degrees of hypothermia and to restore normothermia. These functions are achieved by a secondary circuit of hot or cold water passing close to the flow of blood through the heat exchanger. An extracorporeal circulation requires a small heat exchanger with a low blood priming volume and small temperature differences. Bethune *et al.* (1975) have recommended that water flow rates of 15–20 l min^{-1} at 140 kPa should be available in cardiothoracic operating rooms. In order to produce a blood stream surrounded by a water stream some heat exchangers use the shell technique with an inner core and an outer jacket water flows surrounding an annula blood flow, all the fluid streams being confined to circular annuli. With such a design, Flower *et al.* (1979) found that over a period of 204 seconds 0.081 kilojoules of heat was extracted with a blood flow rate of 1.27 l min^{-1} and a water flow of 2.37 l min^{-1}. The water temperature was 12 °C and the initial blood temperature was 41 °C.

The use of a warm mattress to prevent heat loss during surgery

Lewis, Shaw and Etchells (1973) have described a contact mattress fed with warm air from a thermostatically controlled blower unit and used to prevent heat loss in neonatal and paediatric surgery.

References

AGATE, F.J. and SILVERMAN, W.A. (1963). The control of body temperature in the small newborn infant by low energy infra-red radiation. *Pediatrics* **31**, 725

AINLEY-WALKER, J.C. (1959). The heat mechanics of the Waters canister. *Br. J. Anaesth.* **31**, 2

BERRY, F.A. Jr., HUGHES-DAVIES, D.I. and DIFAZIO, C.A. (1973). A system for minimizing respiratory heat loss in infants during operation. *Curr. Res. Anesth. Analg.* **52**, 170

BETHUNE, D.W., GILL, R.D. and WHEELDON, D.R. (1975). Peformance of a heat exchanger used in whole body perfusion circuits. *Thorax* **30**, 569–573

BJORAKER, D.G. (1978). Blood warmers as a source of significant leakage currents. *Anesthesiology* **49**, 286–288

BROCK, R.C. (1975). The importance of environmental conditions especially temperature in the operating room and intensive care unit. *Br. J. Surg.* **62**, 253–258

CHALON, J., SIMON, R., PATEL, C., RAMANATHAN, S., SESSER, S. and TURNDORF, H. (1978). An infant circuit with a water vaporizer warmed by carbon dioxide neutralization *Anesth. Analg.* **57**, 307–312

CHAO, K.N., EISLEY, J.G. and YANG, W.-J. (1979). Heat and water migration through normal skin: Part 1 – Steady state. *Med. Biol. Engng. & Comput.* **17**

DICKSON, J.A. (1979). Hyperthermia in the treatment of cancer. *Lancet* **1**, 202–205

DREW, C.E. (1961). Profound hypothermia in cardiac surgery. *Br. med. Bull.* **17**, 37

DYBKJAER, E. and ELKJAER, P. (1964). The use of heated blood in massive blood replacement. *Acta anaesth. scand.* **8**, 271

DYDE, J.A. and LUNN, H.F. (1970). Heat loss during thoracotomy. *Thorax* **25**, 355–358

EPSTEIN, L.I. and KUZAVA, B.A. (1976). *Basic Physics in Anesthesiology.* Chicago; Year Book Medical Publishers

FLOWER, K.A., SHAW, E.A. and MORRIS, P. (1979). Performance of a shell-type heat exchanger in extracorporeal circulation. *Br. J. Anaesth.* **51**, 199–204

FORRESTER, A.C. (1958). Hypothermia using air cooling. *Anaesthesia* **13**, 289

FURNAS, D.W. (1965). Topical refrigeration and frost anaesthesia. *Anesthesiology* **26**, 344

HARDY, J.D. and MUSCHENHEIM, C. (1934). The radiation of heat from the human body. *J. Clin. Invest.* **13**, 817

HARPER, P.J. (1966). 'A new cryo-surgical instrument.' *Bio-med. Engng* **1**, 164

HERINGMAN, E.C., MASSEL, T.B., GREENSOME, S.M. and GARON, R.J. (1964). A new approach to the design, construction and operation of a hyperbaric chamber. In *Clinical Application of Hyperbaric Oxygen,* p. 235. Ed. by I. Boerema, W.H. Brummelkamp and N.G. Meijne. Amsterdam; Elsevier

HEY, E.N. (1975). Thermal Neutrality. *Br. med. Bull.* **31**, 69–73

HEY, E.N. and KATZ, G. (1970). The optimal thermal environment for naked babies. *Arch. Dis. in Child.* **45**, 328–334

HILL, D.W. and MOORE, VIRGINIA (1965). The action of adiabatic effects on the compliance of an artificial thorax. *Br. J. Anaesth.* **37**, 19

HOLDCRAFT, A. and HALL, G.M. (1978). Heat loss during anaesthesia. *Br. J. Anaesth.* **50**, 157–164

HUNTER, A.R. (Ed.) (1964). *Intravenous Anaesthesia, Hypothermia,* Vol. 2. Boston; Little, Brown

KALETZKY, E., PROCTOR, C.R. and CRANKSHAW, T.P. (1964). Some observations on surgical hypothermia by means of extensive radiant cooling. *Lancet* **1**, 1365

LEWIS, R.B., SHAW, A. and ETCHELLS, A.H. (1973). Contact mattress to prevent heat loss in neonatal and paediatric surgery. *Br. J. Anaesth.* **45**, 919

PETTIGREW, R.T., GALT, J.M., LUDGATE, C.M. and SMITH, A.N. (1974). Clinical effects of whole-body hyperthermia in advanced malignancy. *Br. med. J.* **4**, 679–682

ROSS, B.A., BROCK, R.C. and AYNESLEY-GREEN, A. (1969). Observations on central and peripheral temperatures in the understanding and management of shock. *Br. J. Surg.* **56**, 876–882

RUSSELL, W.J. (1969a). A new approach in heat exchangers for massive transfusion. *Br. J. Anaesth.* **41**, 338

RUSSELL, W.J. (1969b). A discussion of the problems of heat exchange blood warming devices. *Br. J. Anaesth.* **41**, 345

SMITH, R.M. (1978). Pediatric anesthesia in perspective. *Anesth. Analg.* **57**, 634–646

WILKE, H.J. (1964). Central gas supply systems. *Wld med. Electron. Instrum. Lond.* **2**, 217

WINDER, A.F. and VALE, R.J. (1970). Heat retaining mattress for temperature control in surgery. *Br. med. J.* **1**, 161

8 Anaesthetic vaporizers

The saturated vapour pressure of most volatile anaesthetic agents is sufficiently high that the saturation concentration is substantially above the range of concentrations required for the maintenance of clinical anaesthesia. Thus some means has to be provided for diluting the vapour generated by the evaporation of the liquid agent to the required concentration. In one type of system, the correct amount of liquid agent can be supplied to a known minute volume of gas by the anaesthetist dripping-in the liquid, or supplying it from a syringe. More commonly use is made of an anaesthetic vaporizer to automatically supply the desired concentration of vapour. If accuracy is required, provision must then be made to make good the heat loss from the liquid agent arising from the process of evaporation.

Simple plenum vaporizers

The term *plenum* vaporizer is derived from the plenum system of air-conditioning in which air is forced into a plenum chamber in which it is warmed and cleaned.

The saturation concentrations of ether and halothane at room temperature and normal atmospheric pressure are respectively approximately 50 and 33 per cent by volume corresponding to saturated vapour pressures of one half and one third of an atmosphere. In order to dilute this vapour to clinical concentrations a minor portion of the gas flow perfusing the vaporizer is passed through a vaporizing chamber (*Figure 8.1*) and then rejoins the major portion which has bypassed the

Bypass

Gas
in →

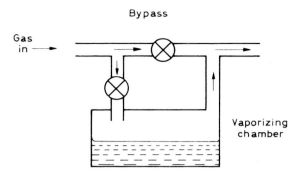

Vaporizing
chamber

Figure 8.1. Schematic diagram of simple plenum vaporizer

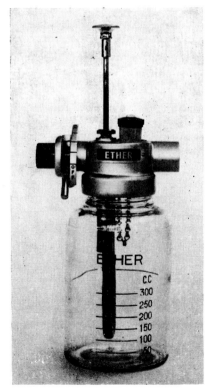

Figure 8.2. Boyle bottle vaporizer for ether.
(By courtesy of British Oxygen Co. Ltd)

chamber. This is the principle used in the well known Boyle's bottle (*Figure 8.2*). This is a simple, inexpensive type of vaporizer, but it does suffer from some disadvantages. The controls of a vaporizer should permit reproducible settings, when the vapour concentration is both increased and decreased, and these should be as far as possible independent of the duration of use and of the perfusing minute volume. Early designs of the Boyle bottle suffered from an almost 'all-or-none' action of the control lever. A fine control of the issuing vapour concentration is possible by raising or lowering the rod protruding from the top of the vaporizer. This varies the distance above the surface of the liquid of the port through which gas enters the chamber. The variation of the output from a Boyle ether bottle with the setting of the lever and plunger has been discussed by Macintosh *et al.* (1958). Stability of the output with time really means stability in relation to the falling temperature of the evaporating liquid. Since glass is a poor conductor of heat, the temperature of the ether falls markedly as evaporation proceeds, and the output concentration of the vapour decreases significantly with the passage of time. Halothane is not so volatile as ether, and because the anaesthetic concentrations required are less, cooling problems are less severe in halothane vaporizers. Since lower concentrations are required for halothane than ether, the Boyle halothane bottle uses only the control tap and has no moving plunger, the gas entering the vaporizing bottle from fixed holes cut in the inlet pipe. A glass bottle holding the liquid agent does not always provide fully saturated vapour, and this makes the provision of a repeatable calibration difficult for this simple type of arrangement. When the vaporizer has been switched off for some time, a considerable volume of vapour builds up above the liquid. This leads to a significant surge of vapour when the vaporizer is first switched on (Jennings and Hersant, 1965). Seed (1967) describes the fitting of a baffle device to a halothane Boyle bottle in order to prevent agitation of the halothane when the vaporizer is moved.

Improved plenum vaporizers

Loosco vaporizer

An improvement on the simple type of plenum vaporizer for halothane has been described by Pearce (1962), and is manufactured by the Loosco Company of Amsterdam (*Figure 8.3*). It has a single rotary

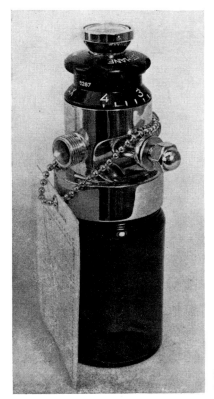

Figure 8.3. Loosco halothane vaporizer.
(By courtesy of Loosco)

control tap, and is fitted with a bimetallic strip thermometer to indicate the temperature of the liquid halothane. The output concentration is read from a calibration chart which relates to the dial setting, the concentration delivered, the fresh gas flow rate into the vaporizer and the halothane temperature. Bronze plungers with nylon liners are fitted to minimize the need for maintenance.

Vapor vaporizer

The principle of the single concentration control knob is used in the German Dräger range of 'Vapor' vaporizers for ether, halothane and methoxyflurane. Provision is made for manual compensation for the falling temperature of the agent, obviating the need for a calibration chart. A schematic diagram of a Vapor is shown in *Figure 8.4*. The body of the vaporizer is made from a heavy block of copper having a high thermal capacity to produce a thermal stability. The actual temperature of the liquid halothane can be read on a built-in mercury-in-glass thermometer. The dial for setting the output concentration of halothane carries several scales each corresponding to a specific temperature concentration. In use, the dial is rotated until the line corresponding to the desired concentration intersects the temperature scale at the value indicated by the thermometer. A mechanical interlock ensures that the vaporizer cannot be turned off until the concentration dial is set at zero.

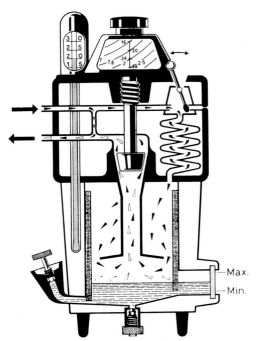

Figure 8.4. Schematic diagram of 'Vapor' vaporizer.
(By courtesy of Drägerwerk, Lübeck)

The Vapor vaporizers are probably the most accurate yet made. They are extremely useful as substandards for the calibration of halothane or ether analysers. Another exceptional property lies in the fact that the calibration of the Vapor is accurate down to flow rates of 100 ml per minute. This performance is achieved by the use of a pair of specially designed needle valves for controlling the vaporizing chamber and bypass gas flows. The opening of the bypass valve is pre-set by the manufacturers, the chamber valve acting as the variable concentration control. The pressure drop across each valve is linearly related to the volume flow of gas in both the forward and reverse directions. This fact enables the flow-splitting ratio set by the two valves to be little affected by the value of the gas flow into the vaporizer over the range 100 ml to 10 litres per minute. Each valve consists of a male and a female cone, the ratio of the length of a cone to the gap being of the order of 100 to 1. Filters are provided to prevent any particles of grit from damaging the cone surfaces. The vaporizing chamber is provided with wicks to ensure that the vapour it contains is fully saturated. This fact also prevents the vaporizer from giving a high output if it is shaken (Hill, 1963). A similar consideration arises in the case of the Fluotec which also uses wicks. Munson (1965) reports on a case of cardiac arrest due to an overdose of halothane arising from the accidental tipping of a Fluotec vaporizer, while Jennings and Hersant (1965) discuss the increased output concentrations found after refilling some vaporizers.

Fluotec Mark 2 vaporizer

The need for a manual adjustment of the temperature setting can be eliminated by the use of an automatic temperature compensation device, but at the expense, in some cases, of making the output concentration dependent on the value of the gas flow rate at the lower flows. An example of this technique occurs in the well known Fluotec Mark 2 vaporizer (*Figure 8.5*) shown in section in *Figure 8.6*. Descriptions of the original Fluotec Mark I vaporizer are those of Mackay (1957) and Brennan (1957). The concentration control adjusts the value of the splitting ratio between the vaporizing chamber and bypass flows. The gas passing into the chamber flows over a series of wicks to ensure that it is fully saturated. The outlet port from the chamber is controlled by a bimetallic strip valve. As evaporation proceeds and the temperature of the liquid halothane falls, so the valve opens allowing more vapour to emerge and this keeps the output concentration reasonably constant. The vaporizing chamber should be drained at regular intervals to remove any accumulation of thymol from the halothane. The output concentration is independent of the value of the volume flow of gas at 4 l min^{-1} and above. Below this the concentration rises to a peak at around 1 l min^{-1} (*Figure 8.7*) due to

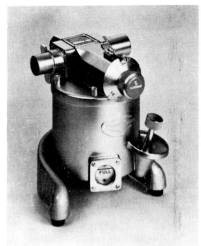

Figure 8.5. Fluotec Mark 2 vaporizer for halothane. (By courtesy of Cyprane Ltd)

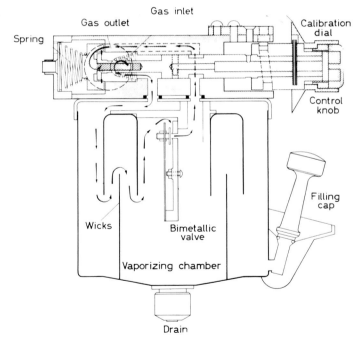

Figure 8.6. Schematic diagram of Fluotec Mark 2 vaporizer. (By courtesy of Cyprane Ltd)

non-linearities occurring in the flow-splitting ratio, and falls to zero as the flow diminishes below 500 ml min^{-1}. There is then insufficient pressure drop developed across the resistance of the bypass to force enough gas through the vaporizing chamber to push out the necessary amount of the relatively heavy anaesthetic vapour. The calibration

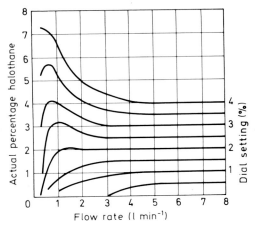

Figure 8.7. Calibration curves for a Mark 2 Fluotec vaporizer. (By courtesy of Cyprane Ltd)

control is provided with a positive lock in the OFF position and a calibration card for use at the lower flow rates is provided with each instrument.

M & IE halothane 4 vaporizer

A vaporizer employing similar principles is the M & IE 'Halothane 4' (*Figure 8.8*). The calibration curve is reasonably accurate down to 1 l min^{-1} and does not exhibit a peak like that of the Fluotec Mark 2. A mercury expansion type of thermal compensation device is employed.

The need for the regular servicing of anaesthetic vaporizers employing automatic temperature compensators is stressed by Adner and Hallen (1965).

Fluotec Mark 3 vaporizer

The design of the Fluotec Mark 3 vaporizer is aimed at producing a vaporizer whose calibration is almost independent of temperature over

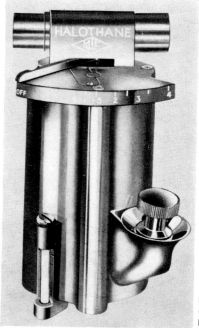

Figure 8.8. M & IE Halothane 4 vaporizer.
(By courtesy of Medical & Industrial
Equipment Ltd)

the range 18 to 36 °C and of flow from 250 ml min^{-1} up to 10 l min^{-1}.
Figure 8.9 shows a cutaway drawing of the Fluotec Mark 3 in the ON
position. The fresh gas inflow is split into two streams by the rotary
valve C. One stream passes through port H and enters the vaporizing
chamber. It then passes through a helical channel formed by two
cylindrical wicks and a nickel plated copper spiral. The gas, fully
saturated with halothane vapour leaves the chamber at J, passes into the
control channel F and rejoins the second gas stream in the sump cover
D. The mixed gas and vapour stream leaves at G. The output concentration of halothane vapour is set by the relative resistances to flow of
the two gas streams, that is, the relative restrictions of the temperature-
sensitive valve E and the control channel F. The resistance of F is
adjusted by turning the control knob K. F is a long, wide but very
shallow groove which gradually deepens from 0.05 mm to 0.275 mm
in order to add more vapour to the bypass at the high percentage
settings. The bimetallic strip valve opens as the temperature of the
halothane rises. This is in contrast to the action of the bimetallic strip
valve in the Fluotec Mark 2. The control channel F is machined into the

face of the rotary valve C, and the opposite face of the valve is coated with a PTFE layer in order to provide a non-stick surface. Paterson, Hulands and Nunn (1969) quote test figures they obtained using a Fluotec Mark 3. Its flow resistance was found to be high (approximately 50 cmH$_2$O at 10 l min^{-1}) and the vaporizer is heavy. In these respects it resembles the Dräger Vapor. The design of the control valve in the Fluotec Mark 3 is such as to virtually eliminate the possibility of it sticking due to an accumulation of thymol arising from the liquid halothane.

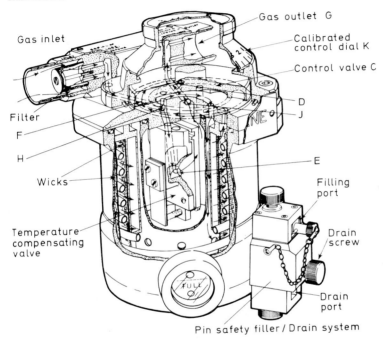

Figure 8.9. Schematic diagram of Fluotec Mark 3 halothane vaporizer. (By courtesy of Cyprane Ltd)

Since the Fluotec Mark 3 vaporizer was introduced, the following modifications have been made. The control valve C is now surfaced with a dry bearing material and the PTFE coating is no longer used; a low resistance bypass circuit has been incorporated which at the OFF setting reduces the pressure drop through the vaporizer to approximately 5 cmH$_2$O at a gas flow rate of 5 l min^{-1}. The resistance to gas flow when the dial is turned ON is unaltered; a positive lock has been introduced which operates at the OFF setting of the control valve. This is in the form of a catch which automatically engages when the dial is turned to the OFF position. The catch must be released to turn the dial to an operating position; versions of the Fluotec Mark 3 are now available for use with the most commonly used volatile anaesthetic agents.

Latto (1973) has investigated the performance of both the Mark 2 and Mark 3 Fluotec vaporizers in regard to the concentration produced in the region of the concentration dial between 0 per cent and the first calibration mark at 0.5 per cent halothane. More variation was possible with the Mark 3, but the output concentration was influenced by the fresh gas flow rate.

Foregger Fluomatic vaporizer

The requirement to compensate for temperature variations while providing a vaporizer calibration which is reasonably independent of the gas flow rate has been tackled in an ingenious fashion in the Foregger 'Fluomatic' vaporizer. A sectional diagram of this is shown in *Figure 8.10*. The fresh gas stream entering the vaporizer at (1) is divided, the bypass stream passing through the fixed restriction (2)

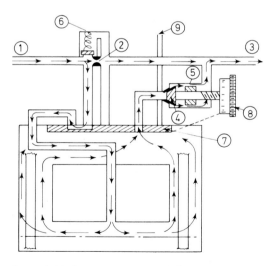

Figure 8.10. Schematic diagram of Fluomatic halothane vaporizer. (By courtesy of Foregger Ltd)

to the outlet (3). The vaporizing chamber stream flows through the wicks and chamber which has a small gas volume and emerges through the variable control valve (4) which is in series with a fixed restriction (5) to merge with the bypass flow. The relief valve (6) limits the pressure of the inlet gas if high flows are applied to the vaporizer. The control needle valve (4) has a relatively large needle fabricated from PTFE which has a high coefficient of thermal expansion relative to the valve seating. As the temperature of the emerging gas and vapour stream

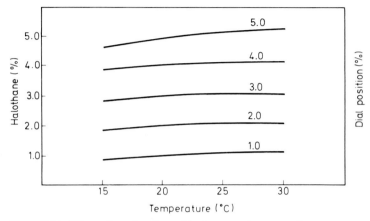

Figure 8.11. Effect of varying the ambient temperature upon the output of a Fluomatic vaporizer. (By courtesy of Foregger Ltd)

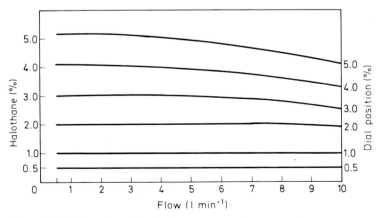

Figure 8.12. Effect of varying the flow rate upon the output of a Fluomatic vaporizer. (By courtesy of Foregger Ltd)

from the chamber alters, so the valve opens or closes to adjust the flow through it in such a way as to hold the output concentration sensibly constant. A similar arrangement operates with the fixed restriction (5) in series with the control valve. The elegance of this arrangement is that no additional moving parts are needed. *Figures 8.11* and *8.12* illustrate the performance of the Fluomatic vaporizer under conditions of varying temperature and gas flow rate.

Foregger Pentomatic vaporizer

The much lower saturated vapour pressure of methoxyflurane means that a vaporizer developed for this substance must pass more of the fresh gas through the vaporizing chamber than would occur for vaporizers designed to operate with other, more volatile, agents. *Figure 8.13* shows a cross-section through a Foregger 'Pentomatic' vaporizer.

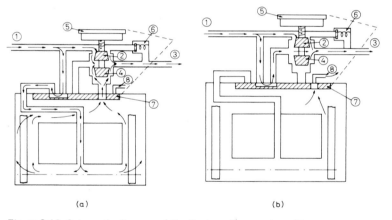

(a)   (b)

Figure 8.13. Schematic diagram of the Pentomatic vaporizer. (By courtesy of Foregger Ltd)

The upper section (2) of the control valve controls the bypass flow, while the lower section (4) controls the outlet from the vaporizing chamber. The two sections move up or down as a unit when the concentration control dial (5) is adjusted. The valves provide automatic temperature compensation as described for the Fluomatic vaporizer. The isolation valve (7) is moved through a linkage to the control knob (5) to close both the inlet and outlet of the vaporizing chamber (*Figure 8.13*). A low-resistance channel completely bypasses the vaporizing

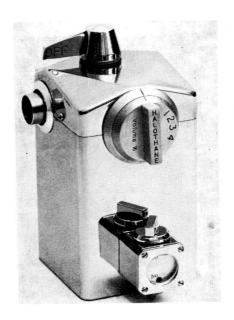

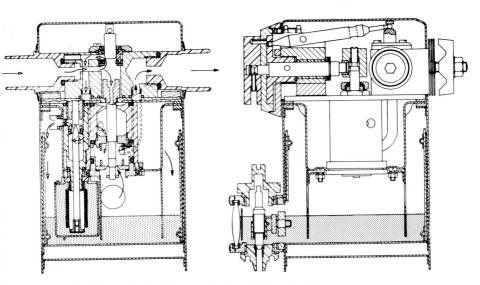

Figure 8.14. (Top) Abingdon halothane vaporizer; (Bottom) section
of Abingdon vaporizer. (By courtesy of Penlon Ltd)

chamber, and the chamber is vented to the atmosphere at (8). The pressure applied to the vaporizer is limited by the relief valve (6).

Abingdon vaporizer

The Abingdon range of plenum vaporizers by Penlon has models for ether, halothane and methoxyflurane. As in the Fluotec Mark 3, the volume of the vaporizing chamber is made small and the resistance of its inlet and outlet channels made relatively high in order to minimize pumping effects from the action of intermittent positive pressure ventilation. A positive ON-OFF control is provided together with a single calibration control (*Figure 8.14*). It is possible to detach the vaporizing chamber for cleaning with ether. A bellows type of thermal compensation valve is fitted. In previous models of the Abingdon vaporizer the bellows was filled with a Freon vapour. However, it was found that changes in atmospheric pressure affected the bellows and could cause a change in the vaporizer's calibration. For example, a vaporizer which was correctly calibrated in England was found to read 1.5 per cent halothane low over the whole scale in Johannesburg. This effect has now been eliminated by filling the bellows with liquid ether. When the vaporizer is turned on a valve automatically vents the vaporizing chamber to atmosphere in order to dissipate any surge of vapour which might have accumulated on standing, for example, in the sun. The maximum available output concentrations are 4.5 per cent v/v halothane, 2.4 per cent methoxyflurane and 20 per cent ether.

Copper kettle vaporizer

In the temperature compensated vaporizers so far described, it has not been necessary to measure individually the vaporizing chamber and bypass gas flows. If these, and the vapour pressure and temperature of the agent are all known, then the output concentration can be calculated from first principles. This is the basis of copper kettle type vaporizers (Morris, 1952). In this arrangement the vaporizing chamber is made from copper and is fixed to the copper table top of the anaesthetic machine. This provides a reservoir of heat when ether is used. A cross-section of a copper kettle vaporizer is shown in *Figure 8.15*. The inflow of oxygen enters at tube (1) and surge chamber (2). It leaves the chamber via the concentric tube (3) leading to the annular chamber (4) of the sintered bronze disc diffuser (5). The multitude of

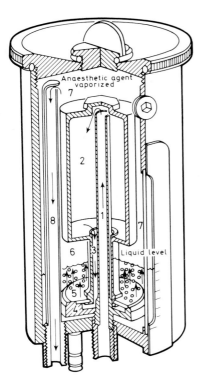

Figure 8.15. Copper kettle vaporizer.
(By courtesy of Foregger Company)

fine bubbles generated produces a fully saturated vapour. The bubbles rise through the liquid agent (6) and pass into the chamber (7) above the liquid, the saturated vapour leaving via the exit tube (8) to join the bypass gas stream coming from the flowmeters of the anaesthetic machine. The inlet (1) to the kettle is supplied from its own flowmeter. A copper kettle of 400 ml capacity is normally used for the vaporization of ether and methoxyflurane, a 160 ml capacity kettle being used for halothane (Feldman and Morris, 1958). Gartner and Stoelting (1974) have compared the performance of the copper kettle vaporizer with that of the Fluotec Mark 2 and Pentec vaporizers. They found that the copper kettle has the advantage of being able to deliver predictable concentrations of potent inhalational agents over a wide range, especially low concentrations, uninfluenced by the carrier gas density. The main disadvantage of the copper kettle lay in its incomplete temperature compensation with continuous gas flows. It is interesting that Stoelting (1971) found that with a Fluotec Mark 2 vaporizer, the halothane output for settings below 1 per cent was increased by the use of a mixture of 60 per cent nitrous oxide—40 per cent oxygen in comparison with the use of 100 per cent oxygen. Dobkin *et al.* (1963) have compared the performance for enflurane of a number of vaporizers including the copper kettle.

Halox vaporizer

The temperature problems are easier in the case of halothane, and a glass container can be used as in the British Oxygen Halox vaporizer (*Figure 8.16*) (Young, 1966). A schematic diagram of the arrangement

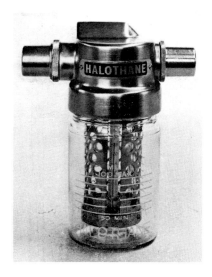

Figure 8.16. Halox vaporizer. (By courtesy of British Oxygen Co. Ltd)

for using the Halox with a Boyle anaesthetic machine appears in *Figure 8.17*. The saturated vapour pressure of halothane is 243 mmHg at 20 °C. This corresponds to a saturation concentration of 31.2 per cent v/v if the barometric pressure is 760 mmHg. Let the flow of gas plus vapour out of the kettle be 250 ml min^{-1}. This corresponds to a flow of 172 ml min^{-1} of gas into the kettle. Then in order to dilute this by a factor of ten to give an output concentration of 3.1 per cent v/v the total of bypass plus kettle flow must equal 2.5 l min^{-1}, i.e. the bypass flow must equal 2250 l min^{-1}. In order to aid the anaesthetist, slide rule type calculators are available so that for a given temperature and desired concentration, the kettle and bypass flows can be quickly determined.

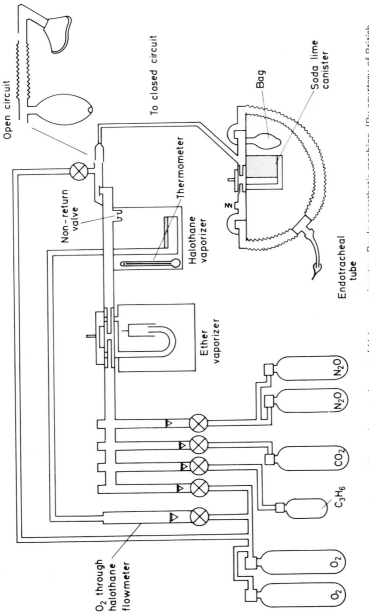

Figure 8.17. Schematic diagram illustrating attachment of Halox vaporizer to a Boyle anaesthetic machine. (By courtesy of British Oxygen Co. Ltd)

From a knowledge of the kettle flow and the saturation concentration and density of the agent, it is straightforward to calculate the mass of halothane delivered to the circuit per minute. Collis (1966) and Jennings, Taylor and Young (1967) describe calibration graphs and the use of a calculator for the Halox vaporizer.

Vaporizers for use with intermittent flows (draw-over vaporizers or inhalers)

The plenum vaporizers so far described are intended for use with unidirectional gas flows obtained from an anaesthetic machine or gas cylinders. Their resistance to gas flow is sufficiently high to render them unsuitable for use as draw-over vaporizers where the minute volume of gas is pulled through the vaporizer as a result of the patient's respiratory efforts. The design of the latest plenum vaporizers such as the Fluotec Mark 3 and the Penlon Abingdon series deliberately increases the resistance of the vaporizer in order to minimize the 'pumping effect' of intermittent positive-pressure respiration. The high resistance of most plenum vaporizers makes it difficult for the patient to draw enough gas through the vaporizing chamber. In addition to possessing a low resistance, the draw-over vaporizer must be able to provide a reproducible calibration when perfused with the fluctuating gas flow pattern of respiration.

EMO vaporizer

A popular type of calibrated draw-over vaporizer for either ether or halothane is the EMO (Epstein and Macintosh, 1956; Leatherdale, 1966) (*Figure 8.18*). The unit contains an outer jacket filled with water to act as a reservoir of heat. The water jacket also serves, by local convection, to even out cold spots appearing on the surface of the wick from which it is separated by a thin wall of copper. The vaporizing chamber outlet is fitted with a thermal compensating valve. This consists of a metallic bellows filled with ether vapour. As the temperature of the evaporating agent falls, the bellows contract and open up the valve port allowing more gas and vapour to emerge from the chamber. The calibration of the EMO is accurate only for intermittent gas flows. The fact that the calibration holds over a wide range of respiratory rates and volumes is stated by the makers to depend upon

the carefully determined relationship between the volumes of the
various chambers and the flows directed between them by bell-mouthed
and sharp-edged orifices. The outlet communicates with a small
chamber in the centre of the control rotor which lies below the concentration pointer. This passageway is always fully open irrespective
of the position of the pointer. The chamber has two inlet ports both of

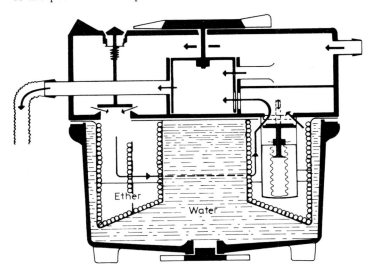

Figure 8.18. Cross-sectional diagram of the EMO vaporizer for ether.
(By courtesy of Penlon Ltd)

which vary in their size of opening, depending upon the position of the
pointer. One of these ports leads from the large chamber of the main
top casting which is full of fresh air drawn in through the inlet to the
vaporizer. This port is fully open when the control pointer is at the
'Close for transit' position so that in this position there is no
obstruction between the inlet and outlet of the EMO. The other port
leads via the temperature compensator valve from the vaporizing
chamber. In the 'Close for transit' position this port is completely
closed. As the control pointer is turned towards 20 per cent the first
(fresh air) port steadily closes while the second (ether vapour) port
steadily opens. The EMO is fitted with a pressure relief valve. Normally
this is closed by a light spring, but should the main inlet of the EMO
be blocked, the relief valve will open. The internal resistance is quoted
as being less than 1.25 cmH_2O at 40 $l\,min^{-1}$. The ether EMO is

calibrated from 2 to 20 per cent by volume with an accuracy of ±0.75 per cent v/v at the 8 per cent setting between 13 and 32 °C and 4 to 12 1 min^{-1}. In conjunction with the Oxford Inflating Bellows (Macintosh, 1953), the EMO ether vaporizer is widely used for the administration of anaesthesia under emergency conditions. Stetson (1968) describes a modification to the EMO vaporizer in order to prevent sticking of the concentration control. This involves the replacement of a rotor inside the vaporizer with one made from PTFE. Bryce-Smith (1964) has described a limited dosage unit using either halothane or trichloroethylene in conjunction with the EMO ether vaporizer. The use of the induction unit is said to greatly reduce the resistance of the patient to ether and enables surgical levels of ether anaesthesia to be attained much more rapidly. The Bryce-Smith induction unit has no controls and its wicks will soak up only approximately 3 ml of the agent. Its performance depends upon both the rate and depth of respiration, but typically about 2 per cent of halothane vapour will be delivered for approximately 4 minutes.

Oxford miniature vaporizer (OMV)

The Oxford Miniature Vaporizer (OMV) is a compact vaporizer designed primarily for use with halothane and it can deliver concentrations up to 3.5 per cent v/v. The vaporizer can also be used with trichloroethylene or chloroform provided that the corresponding scales are substituted. Although not temperature compensated, the OMV incorporates in its base a small, sealed, water-filled compartment which

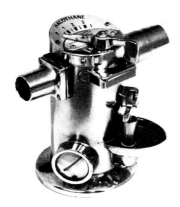

Figure 8.19. Oxford Miniature Vaporizer OMV. (By courtesy of Penlon Ltd)

acts as a reservoir of heat. The body of the OMV is made from stainless steel (*Figure 8.19*) and contains stainless steel wicks. While the OMV can hold 30 ml of halothane, it can work while containing as little as 5 ml. The OMV can be attached to an EMO ether vaporizer in order to precede the ether-air anaesthesia with a halothane-air induction. The clinical performance of the OMV with halothane has been discussed by Parkhouse (1966) and by Jensen (1967).

The Oxford Miniature Vaporizer was originally conceived as an accessory for the EMO ether vaporizer but has subsequently proved of considerable use in other applications, for example, in compact anaesthesia machines for hospital casualty departments. This fact has led to the development of the OMV 50 vaporizer (*Figure 8.20*). For some years

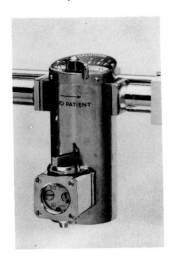

Figure 8.20. Oxford Miniature Vaporizer OMV 50. (By courtesy of Penlon Ltd)

the OMV vaporizer has been available in two versions — one right-to-left flow for attachment to an EMO; the other a left-to-right flow for use with anaesthesia machines. In the latter application the OMV has been limited by the fact that it only held 30 ml of halothane and had no means of mounting it on the back bar of an anaesthetic machine. In the OMV 50, the body has been deepened to hold 50 ml of agent which is sufficient for a 3-hour anaesthetic with halothane, a combined sight glass and filler has been fitted as has a clamp for back bar mounting. There has also been a change in the internal gas passage to improve the vaporizer's performance when used on fairly low constant flows. The OMV can be used to feed a circle system at 4 litres per minute and yet is still quite suitable for use as an inhaler. The original OMV vaporizer gave only very low output concentrations below about 6 litres per minute continuous flow. The cost of these alterations in terms of performance is a reduction of the maximum obtainable output concentration from approximately 4 per cent to approximately 3 per cent. Each OMV 50 vaporizer is supplied with a plastic card showing the output concentration at various ambient temperatures and continuous flow rates. The OMV and OMV 50 vaporizers will only deliver their maximum output for a short period after which they will return to a safer maintenance level even if the anaesthetist forgets to reset the concentration pointer.

Univap vaporizer

A compact draw-over vaporizer for halothane is incorporated in the Haloxair apparatus designed for emergency anaesthesia (Stephens, 1965). This vaporizer does not need a water jacket and may be used with either spontaneous or controlled respiration. Hedstrand (1966) describes the AGA 'Anestor Militar' emergency anaesthetic apparatus which used the Socsil draw-over vaporizer for ether, halothane or chloroform (Hallen and Norlander, 1966, Martinez, Norlander and

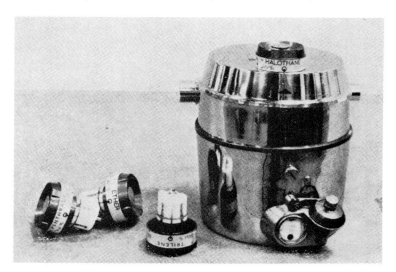

Figure 8.21. Blease Univap Universal Vaporizer. (By courtesy of Blease Medical Equipment Ltd)

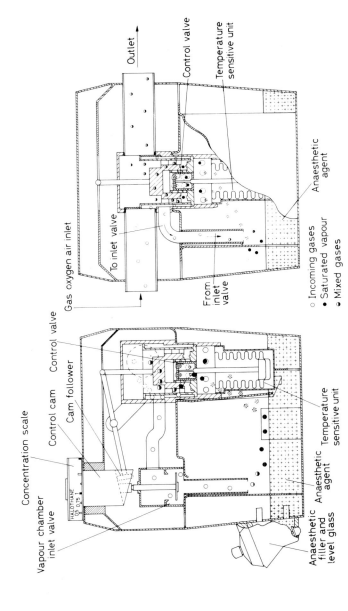

Figure 8.22. Schematic diagram of the Blease Univap universal vaporizer. (By courtesy of Blease Medical Equipment Ltd)

Santos, 1966). The Blease Univap universal vaporizer can be used as a plenum or draw-over vaporizer, and it can be provided with a series of interchangeable control cams so that it can be used with almost any volatile anaesthetic agent. The Blease Univap is shown in *Figures 8.21* and *8.22*. The pressure drop across it is 10 mmH$_2$O at a gas flow rate of 30 l min^{-1}. It offers the advantage that it can be used with an anaesthetic machine in order to familiarize anaesthetists with its characteristics during normal lists. As in the EMO, the vaporizing chamber contains wicks, and a bellows-type of thermal compensation valve is employed. The cam controlling the output concentration can be changed for one cut to suit any volatile agent if the saturated vapour pressure versus temperature characteristic is known. In order to change cams, a special tool must be used. This minimizes the risk of an incorrect cam being placed on the vaporizer body, but the chance of the wrong agent being poured into the vaporizing chamber still remains. When it is desired to change agent, any liquid left is drained off, and that remaining in the wicks can be quickly cleared by using bellows to pump air through the vaporizer. It is described by the makers as being 'Universal'. Although its resistance is sufficiently low, Merrifield, Hill and Smith (1967) found that it was not possible to use it inside a circle anaesthetic system. The output fell markedly with the passage of time, possibly due to the uptake of water by the wicks. Merrifield, Hill and Smith (1967) have extensively studied the characteristics of the Blease Univap and Haloxair vaporizers. Chatrath (1973) has studied the effect of intermittent positive pressure respiration on the halothane output from the Blease Univap vaporizer. He found a considerable effect at low flow rates and recommends that I.P.P.R. should only be used with the Univap for flow rates of not less than 6 litres per minute. The Blease universal vaporizer is an improved version of the former Gardner universal vaporizer (Dobkin *et al.,* 1963). Schreiber and Weiss (1965) report inaccuracies present in the calibration of a Gardner universal vaporizer.

Inhalers for midwifery

Suitable trichloroethylene inhalers for use by midwives to administer analgesia during childbirth have been available for a number of years (Epstein and Macintosh, 1949). Each inhaler made in the United Kingdom is checked to give selectable outputs of 0.35 or 0.5 per cent v/v in the minute volume range of 7–10 litres with tidal volumes from

250 to 1000 ml and respiratory rates from 12 to 30 per minute. The inhalers must be capable of working over the tempeature range 12.5 to 35 °C and the resistance to breathing must not exceed 1.25 cmH$_2$O at 30 litres per minute. Inhalers are now available for methoxyflurane, and an account of inhalers for methoxyflurane and trichloroethylene is given by Cole (1968).

The action of trichloroethylene on soda lime

Trichloroethylene undergoes chemical changes when it comes into contact with warm alkali. Some oxidation to phosgene occurs, but the more dangerous product formed is dichloracetylene which is both neurotoxic and explosive. The concentration of this substance builds up slowly, so that it is not usually the first, but subsequent, patients who are at risk (Adriani, 1962). In order to prevent the accidental use of a trichloroethylene vaporizer with the soda lime carbon dioxide absorber in a closed circle system, some anaesthetic machines are provided with an interlock unit which prevents the vaporizer being turned on with the circle in use.

The use of vaporizers in series

In some techniques, two vaporizers are used in series, for example, Scott (1968) describes the use of a halothane vaporizer in series with a trichloroethylene vaporizer. The possibility exists with this arrangement of one agent contaminating the other. This could lead to an explosion if inflammable agents are used, apart from any undesirable clinical aspects. In order to facilitate the induction of ether anaesthesia, the Oxford Miniature Vaporizer or the Bryce-Smith Induction Unit (Bryce-Smith, 1964) both using halothane can be placed in series with an EMO ether vaporizer.

Dorsch and Dorsch (1973) have investigated the cross-contamination which can arise when two vaporizers are used in series. They suggest that the vaporizers should be connected with that containing the lowest boiling point agent nearest to the patient. Thus a penthrane vaporizer would be proximal and a halothane vaporizer distal to the patient.

The use of vaporizers with circle anaesthetic systems

When using a circle system, it is possible to place the vaporizer in one of two positions. In *Figure 8.23,* the vaporizer is placed in the fresh gas

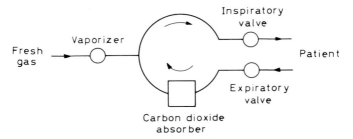

Figure 8.23. Vaporizer placed outside a circle system (V.O.C.)

supply line to the circle. This is the V.O.C. (vaporizer outside circle) position. In a fully closed circle, it is only necessary to supply the basal oxygen requirement, about 250 ml min⁻¹. In practice with circle systems which are in regular use, the presence of leaks makes it difficult to work with fresh gas flows of less than 500 ml min⁻¹. Such low flow rates are encountered on the Continent and in America. In the United Kingdom, fresh gas flow rates into a semi-closed circle system are more likely to be of the order of 4–8 l min⁻¹. When low fresh gas flow rates are employed, an efficient vaporizer must be used, capable of supplying the required output of vapour at these flow rates. For example, Hill and Lowe (1962) used a fresh gas flow rate of 500 ml min⁻¹ of oxygen into a circle system. The ventilation around the circle was 7.2 l min⁻¹ produced by a ventilator. With the output from the vaporizer measured as 4.25 per cent v/v, the inspired concentration presented to the patient rose from 1 to 2 per cent v/v over a period of one hour from the start of induction (*Figure 8.24*). The output of the Fluotec vaporizer was reduced to 1 per cent v/v at 87 minutes, and then maintained at 0.5 per cent v/v for the final twenty minutes of anaesthesia. Approximately 9 ml of liquid halothane was used during two hours of anaesthesia. The patient, a 72 year old woman undergoing surgery on an ovarian tumour, was absorbing 17 ml and 14 ml of halothane vapour per minute at 80 and 100 minutes respectively.

Mushin and Galloon (1960) in a detailed treatment of the use of vaporizers with circle systems, conclude that—

'if the anaesthetist is less experienced with potent anaesthetics such as halothane, he is better advised to use a calibrated and preferably thermostatically controlled vaporizer outside the breathing circuit, especially if he intends to control the ventilation. By this means the somewhat unpredicatable effects with the vaporizer inside the circle

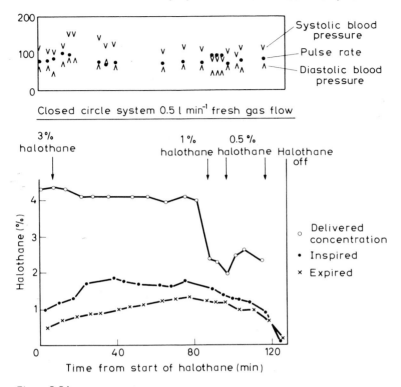

Figure 8.24

of alterations in the patient's ventilation on the inspired concentration of anaesthetic are avoided, particularly if controlled respiration is performed.'

With the vaporizer outside the circle, a change in the ventilation around the circle has no effect on the vaporization of the anaesthetic. As the ventilation is increased, the inspired concentration falls, and there is some rise in the alveolar concentration (Mapleson, 1960). Mushin and Galloon (1960) mention that with fresh gas flow rates of less than 2 l min^{-1}, and ventilations greater than 4 l min^{-1} changes in ventilation produce very little effect on the alveolar concentration and hence on the level of anaesthesia.

Referring to *Figure 8.24*, the fact that the output concentration produced by the Fluotec Mk 2 was 4.1 per cent v/v when the dial

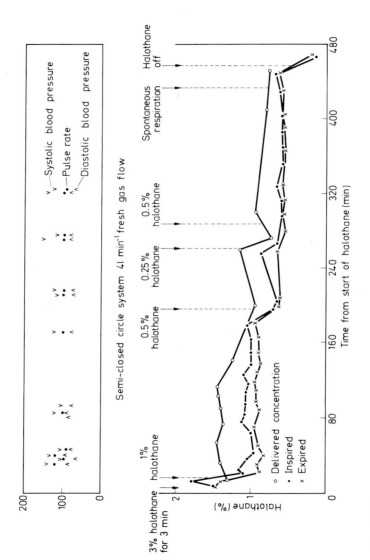

Figure 8.25

setting was only 3 per cent v/v is a result of the action of the pressure fluctuations produced by the ventilator on the vaporizer. This so-called 'pumping effect' will be discussed in detail later in this chapter.

With the vaporizer situated outside the circle, as the fresh gas flow rate is increased, so the vaporizer output concentration must be decreased in order that the inspired concentration does not rise excessively. This is shown clearly in *Figure 8.25*, where the fresh gas flow into the circle is 4 l min⁻¹. The inspired concentration is about 1 per cent v/v, and the vaporizer output concentration is little higher than this. With a high fresh gas flow, the inspired concentration is much more quickly responsive to changes in the vaporizer setting than with a low value of fresh gas flow. The patient of *Figure 8.25* was a 53 year old man with carcinoma of the left cheek and undergoing a left radical neck dissection, superficial parotidectomy and resection of the left temporal and preauricular areas. It was particularly interesting to have a duration of anaesthesia of nearly 8 hours. Approximately 86 ml of liquid halothane was used during this time. The patient absorbed about 10 ml of halothane vapour per minute during the first four hours of anaesthesia, and less than 4 ml min⁻¹ during the remaining period of anaesthesia.

It is important to check that the gas flow is in the correct direction through the vaporizer. In some vaporizers such as the Blease Universal and the Oxford Miniature Vaporizer, it is possible to arrange for the gas to enter from either the left or the right hand side. Adams (1969) states a Fluotec Mark 2 will deliver twice the concentration indicated on the dial if the correct gas direction is not observed.

Neff *et al.* (1968) describe a twin jet venturi circulator. This is driven by the fresh gas flow into a circle system, typically 3 litres per minute. The suction action produced is used to circulate the gas around the circle. This gives a better mixing of the gas and the vapour from the vaporizer located outside the circle and it also reduces the pumping effect of I.P.P.R. on the vaporizer as the jets of the venturi are interposed between the circle and the vaporizer.

The inspired vapour concentration in a circle system fed from a vaporizer outside the circle

With reference to the circle arrangement shown in *Figure 8.26,* the following symbols will be used:

v_d = volume of vapour delivered to the circuit per minute

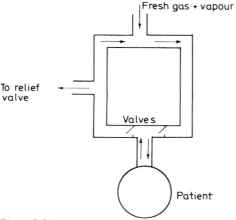

Figure 8.26

v_i = volume of vapour inspired by the patient per minute
v_e = volume of vapour expired by the patient per minute
V_d = volume of fresh gas delivered to the circuit per minute
V_i = volume of gas inspired by the patient per minute
V_e = volume of gas expired by the patient per minute
V_r = volume of gas vented through the relief valve per minute
C_d = concentration of vapour in the fresh gas
C_i = concentration of vapour inspired by the patient per minute
C_e = concentration of vapour expired by the patient per minute

Neglecting the amount of vapour absorbed by the rubber components of the circle, the volume of vapour supplied to the circle per minute is equal to the volume taken up by the patient plus the volume lost through the relief valve in that time, i.e.

$$v_d = (v_i - v_e) + V_r$$

giving

$$v_i = v_d + v_e - V_r$$

The fractional uptake by the patient is

$$U_p = v_e/v_i$$

so that

$$v_e = U_p \times v_i$$

and

$$v_i = v_d + v_i \times U_p - V_r$$

Taking a respiratory quotient of unity

$$V_i = V_e$$

and letting

$$K = V_d/V_i = V_r/V_e$$

i.e. assuming no leaks; so that

$$v_i = v_d + v_i \times U_p - V_e \times K$$

since

$$K = V_r/V_e = v_r/v_e$$
$$v_i = v_d + v_i \times U_p - v_i \times U_p \times K$$
$$v_i(1 - U_p + U_p \times K) = v_d$$

In terms of concentrations of anaesthetic vapours

$$C_d = v_d/V_d$$

so that

$$v_i = C_i \times V_i$$
$$V_d \times C_d = C_i \times V_i (1 - U_p + U_p \times K) =$$
$$= C_i \times V_i (1 - U_p + U_p \times V_d/V_i)$$

giving

$$C_i = \frac{V_d \times C_d}{V_i (1 - U_p) + U_p \times V_d}$$

It can be seen that an increase in the inspired concentration presented to the patient will follow from: an increase in the fresh gas concentration of vapour, an increase in the fresh gas flow rate, a decrease in the minute volume round the circle, a decrease in the uptake of vapour by the patient (the circuit uptake could also be included in this figure).

Consider the semi-closed circuit conditions previously described with $V_d = 0.5$ litres per minute, $C_d = 4.25$ per cent v/v, $V_i = 7.2$ litres per minute and U_p approximately 0.8. Then

$$C_i = \frac{0.5 \times 4.25}{7.2\,(1 - 0.8) + 0.8 \times 0.5}$$

$$= 1.15 \text{ per cent v/v}$$

Vaporizers for use within circle systems

When a vaporizer is placed inside a circle system (V.I.C.) (*Figure 8.27*), the whole of the patient's ventilation passes through the vaporizer. For this reason, the resistance of the vaporizer must be low.

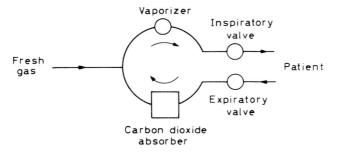

Figure 8.27. Vaporizer placed inside a circle system (V.I.C.)

The vaporizer must be designed to be inefficient, since it will receive not only a substantial minute volume, but also this gas (since it comes from the patient) will already contain anaesthetic vapour. It will also be fully saturated with water vapour. Current practice is to make use of small, glass dental-type vaporizers such as the Rowbotham or Goldman (Burton, 1958; Gusterson, 1959; Hall *et al.,* 1966). The Goldman vaporizer (*Figure 8.28*) (Goldman, 1962) is so constructed that even at high minute volumes it cannot produce more than 3 per cent v/v of halothane vapour. Bodman *et al.* (1967) measured the inspired concentration in a circle system using a Goldman vaporizer and an ultraviolet halothane meter. With this simple vaporizer the cooling effect is not negligible, and there is also a surge of vapour when it is first switched on. However, it was designed basically as a dental vaporizer and not as a precision vaporizer (Goldman, 1966). After a period of time in use, water vapour from the patient's expirate condenses on top of the liquid halothane, and should be removed when it reaches substantial proportions. The only moving parts of the

Goldman vaporizer are those involved in rotating the gas pipe in such a way that none, some or all of the gas flow passes through the vaporizing chamber.

It is usual to allow the patient to breath spontaneously when the vaporizer is placed inside the circle. In this way, a compensatory action is achieved. If the patient lightens, his increased minute volume

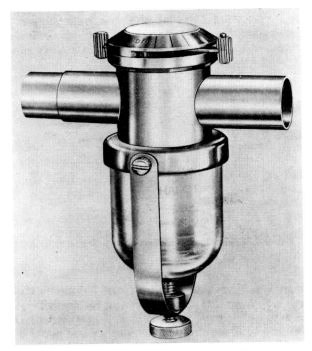

Figure 8.28. Goldman vaporizer. (By courtesy of British Oxygen Co. Ltd)

vaporizes more anaesthetic which gives rise to a deeper level of anaesthesia, and hence reduces the ventilation. There is a risk with intermittent positive pressure respiration (I.P.P.R.) of vaporizing an excessive amount of anaesthetic (Marrett, 1959; Mushin and Galloon, 1960). Intermittent positive pressure respiration is feasible with a vaporizer such as the Goldman placed inside a circle if a halothane analyser is available to monitor the inspired halothane concentration.

Salamonsen (1978) has described a vaporizer using a liquid feed mechanism designed for closed circuit 'programmed' anaesthesia.

Despite its location within the circuit, the vaporizer is designed to directly control the input of volatile anaesthetic agents irrespective of fluctuations in the ventilation of the anaesthetized patient. The digital syringe pump is driven from a digital controller and the vaporizer has an accuracy approaching one per cent under laboratory conditions. During experimental anaesthesia it maintained stable end-tidal concentrations of halothane at 1.2 MAC.

A comparison of the V.I.C. and V.O.C. configurations

When the vaporizer is located outside the circle, the concentration delivered by the vaporizer is normally greater than that inspired by the patient, whereas when a vaporizer is located inside the circle the concentration added to the gas perfusing the vaporizer is normally less than the inspired concentration. A reduction in the patient's minute volume will produce a rise in the inspired concentration with the vaporizer outside the circle and a fall in the inspired concentration when the vaporizer is inside the circle. In both situations, increasing the fresh gas flow rate will cause the concentration of vapour added by the vaporizer and the inspired concentration to tend to become equal, assuming that in the V.I.C. case the fresh gas does pass through the vaporizer before reaching the patient. Jennings and Styles (1968) have produced a nomogram for the prediction of the inspired levels of halothane with circle systems.

The effect of I.P.P.R. on a vaporizer situated outside a circle

When the fresh gas flow passed through a vaporizer situated outside a circle anaesthetic system is $1 \ 1 \ min^{-1}$ or less, consideration must be given to the action of intermittent positive pressure respiration on the concentration of anaesthetic vapour delivered by the vaporizer. It should be emphasized that this 'pumping effect' is negligible at fresh gas flows of more than $1 \ 1 \ min^{-1}$. The pumping effect has been investigated by Hill and Lowe (1962) and by Gordh *et al.* (1964). In the case of *Figure 8.24*, Hill and Lowe used an inflation pressure of $25 \ cmH_2O$, the tidal volume being 800 ml, the ventilation rate 12 breaths per minute. A manometer connected to the drainage outlet of the vaporizer showed that the pressure inside the vaporizer attained a value equal to the circle pressure, as measured on an aneroid manometer connected to the carbon dioxide absorber. The effect is pronounced at a pressure of $20 \ cmH_2O$, but increasing the inflation

TABLE 8.1. Effect of circle pressure on Fluotec Mark 2 calibration

Steady flow (makers') calibration

Fluotec dial setting (% v/v)	*Halothane concentration* (% v/v)	
	500 ml min^{-1}	4 l min^{-1}
0.5 v/v	0.2	0.49
1.0	0.5	0.99
2.0	1.1	2.03
3.0	3.3	2.98
4.0	5.7	3.96

Inflation pressure	*Inspiratory time*	*Respiratory rate*	*Fluotec dial setting*	*Halothane concentration*
10 cmH_2O	1 second	10/minute	0.5% v/v	0.9% v/v
			1.0	1.7
			2.0	2.4
			3.0	3.4
			4.0	5.7
20 cmH_2O	1 second	10/minute	0.5	2.7
			1.0	2.5
			2.0	3.1
			3.0	4.1
			4.0	5.8
30 cmH_2O	1 second	10/minute	0.5	3.2
			1.0	2.6
			2.0	3.1
			3.0	4.1
			4.0	6.0
30 cmH_2O	2 seconds	10/minute	0.5	2.9
			1.0	2.9
			2.0	3.7
			3.0	4.4
			4.0	5.2

Mean oxygen flow through vaporizer 500 ml min^{-1}.

pressure further to 30 cmH_2O produces little further change (*Table 8.1*). Similar effects were found with a copper kettle type of vaporizer.

During the course of the development of the 'Vapor' range of vaporizers, the effect on them of intermittent positive pressure respiration was studied extensively by the development laboratory of the Dräger company. The I.P.P.R. can be produced either by an automatic ventilator or by manual bag-squeezing. During the expiratory phase of ventilation, fresh gas flows steadily through the vaporizers (*Figure 8.29a*). Gauges A and B read the pressure required to keep the gas flowing steadily through the vaporizer. During inflation, the inflation pressure is transmitted up the tube connecting the circle to the vaporizer and raises the pressure on gauge C. Except at fresh gas flow rates of less than 300 ml min^{-1}, fresh gas continues to flow from the anaesthetic machine to the circle, so that gauge A reads higher than gauge C (*Figure 8.29b*). The contents of the vaporizer bypass and vaporizing chamber are now at an elevated pressure. At the commencement of expiration, this elevated pressure is released. The saturated vapour contained in the vaporizing chamber emerges not only through

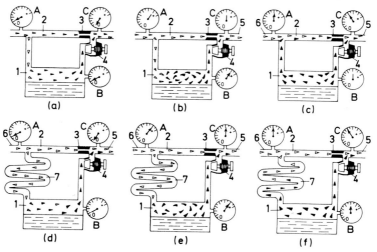

Figure 8.29. Effect of intermittent positive pressure respiration on a Dräger Vapor vaporizer

the normal outlet of the chamber but also through the pipe which normally acts as the chamber inlet (*Figure 8.29c*). This vapour emerging from the normal inlet channel joins the bypass gas stream and is responsible for the enhanced concentration generated by the vaporizer under I.P.P.R. conditions unless precautions against this are taken in the design.

In the 'Vapor' range of vaporizers, the pumping effect is eliminated by the incorporation of a long inlet tube to the vaporizing chamber. When the pressure inside the chamber is released, the volume of saturated vapour entering the lengthened inlet pipe is insufficient to emerge into the bypass (*Figure 8.29d–f*). By this means the vaporizer is rendered insensitive to the action of I.P.P.R. This action can be demonstrated by means of a rigorous experiment. The outlet from a

'Vapor' is taken to a solenoid-operated valve which is caused to open and close at normal ventilation frequencies. When the valve is closed, the pressure inside the vaporizer is arranged to be raised to 30 cm of water. This is suddenly released when the valve is opened. In spite of the resulting severe pressure fluctuations at the outlet, the concentration of halothane delivered by the vaporizer agrees well with its dial setting.

A full discussion of the precautions taken in the Fluotec Mark 3 to avoid a pumping effect is given by Paterson, Hulands and Nunn (1969). The additional volume of gas which is forced into the vaporizing chamber can be calculated by applying Boyle's law. Thus (additional volume of gas) = (volume of gas in vaporizing chamber) × [airway pressure/(barometric + airway pressure)]. For a barometric pressure of 760 mmHg, an airway pressure of 27 cmH$_2$O (2 cmHg) and a volume of 150 ml of gas in the vaporizing chamber, the additional volume of gas forced into the vaporizing chamber is approximately 4 ml. Assuming a saturation concentration of 33 per cent each millilitre of gas leaving the chamber will carry with it 2 ml of halothane vapour. At a respiratory rate of 15 per minute this amounts to 30 ml of vapour per minute. If this is added to a fresh gas minute volume of 500 ml this amounts to an additional 6 per cent by volume of halothane. At a minute volume of 1 litre the added concentration is 3 per cent. The value will also increase as the volume of liquid halothane in the vaporizing chamber falls thus increasing the available gas volume.

In the Fluotec Mark 3 the maximum gas volume of the vaporizing chamber has been reduced to about 150 ml compared with about 630 ml for the Mark 2. In addition the resistance to gas flow of the chamber outlet in the Mark 3 has been made higher than the resistance of the chamber inlet. As a result, during inflation, most of the gas tends to pass into the bypass and enters the chamber via the normal inlet. The inlet is provided with a small, annular, expansion chamber and does not pass near any wicks. This arrangement prevents the gas forced back into the vaporizer from picking up any substantial amount of halothane vapour.

Earlier approaches to this problem aimed at raising the pressure inside the vaporizer to a value above that of the peak inflation pressure, so that the I.P.P.R. would be unable to affect the vaporizer. In practice, a needle valve can be placed distal to a Fluotec vaporizer so that the internal pressure is maintained at 30–40 cmH$_2$O above the circle inflation pressure (Hill and Lowe, 1962) or by the incorporation in the vaporizer of a pressurizing valve which is a miniature pressure regulator (Edmondson and Hill, 1962; Kapfhammer and Atabas, 1965). Other approaches to the action of I.P.P.R. on vaporizers are those of Keenan (1963), Keet, Valentine and Riccio (1963) and Lowe *et al.* (1962).

The Foregger 'Fluomatic' also has a small-volume vaporizing chamber, and operates with a significant pressure drop of 8 cmH$_2$O per litre per minute into it. This discourages any flow of vapour out of the normal chamber inlet when the pressure is released.

Dental vaporizers

The original Goldman vaporizer (Goldman, 1962) was designed for dental practice and was made as simple as possible. Because it uses only a glass vaporizing chamber it will produce a higher output on shaking, and also the output will tend to fall significantly with time due to the cooling of the halothane. Young (1969) reported that the addition of a blotting paper wick to a Goldman or McKesson dental vaporizer increased the halothane output concentration by about 1 per cent v/v and increased the clinical efficiency. The pressure 'pot' vaporizer of Bracken, Brookes and Goldman (1968) is also intended for use in dental anaesthesia with halothane and pre-mixed nitrous oxide and oxygen.

Vaporization from a drip feed or direct injection of a volatile anaesthetic

It is possible to maintain a given concentration of anaesthetic vapour by vaporizing the required mass of the agent into a known volume of gas. In the case of halothane, the molecular weight is 197.4. It can be assumed, for the volatile anaesthetics (Hill, 1961), that the gram-molecular weight volatilizes into a volume of 22.4 litres at STP. This is equivalent to 24.04 litres at 20 °C. Thus 1 g of liquid halothane is equivalent to 122 ml of halothane vapour at 20 °C. Suppose that in a non-rebreathing circuit it is required to produce a concentration of 1 per cent v/v of halothane vapour, when the minute volume is 5 l min^{-1}. To do this, 50 ml of halothane vapour must be generated per minute, i.e. a mass of 0.41 g of liquid halothane must be vaporized per minute. In practice it is more convenient to work in terms of the volume of liquid halothane. The density of halothane is 1.87 g ml^{-1} at 20 °C, so that a volume of 0.22 ml min^{-1} of liquid halothane is needed. For a concentration of 2 per cent v/v it will have to be doubled, and so on. A simple halothane drip feed is described by Hart (1958a, b), and for divinyl ether by Hedstrand (1966). One possible disadvantage of a drip feed lies in the fact that should the gas flow become interrupted and the drip feed inadvertently allowed to continue, then when the gas flow is resumed, the pool of liquid can give rise to a surge of vapour.

This situation is unlikely to arise if the liquid halothane has to be injected at regular intervals from a syringe. Such an arrangement has been described by Wolfson (1962) for a closed circle system.

The calculations associated with the production of a known concentration of a volatile anaesthetic agent are illustrated by the following example. It is required to produce a concentration of 1 per cent v/v of halothane in a minute volume (gas plus vapour) of 6 litres. The following data is provided; molecular weight of halothane 197.4, density of halothane 1.86 g ml^{-1} at 22 °C, ambient temperature 22 °C, saturated vapour pressure of halothane 270 mmHg at 22 °C, barometric pressure 760 mmHg.

Method A. Drip feed or direct injection of liquid halothane

Assume that the gram-molecular weight of halothane vaporizes into a volume of 22.4 litres at STP (0 °C, 760 mmHg). By Charles' law, this volume becomes 24.2 litres at 22 °C. The specific volume of halothane vapour is then $24\,200/197.4 = 123$ ml g^{-1}. In order to produce a 1 per cent v/v concentration of halothane vapour in a total volume of 6 litres, 60 ml of halothane vapour must be produced each minute. This is equivalent to vaporizing a mass of $60/123 = 0.49$ g of liquid halothane per minute. Since the density of liquid halothane is 1.86 g ml^{-1}, 0.49 g is equivalent to 0.26 ml of liquid halothane. Thus approximately 0.25 ml of liquid halothane must be added to a gas flow of 5940 ml min^{-1}.

Method B. The use of a plenum vaporizer

Since the saturated vapour pressure of halothane is 270 mmHg, at 22 °C, the saturation concentration at 22 °C is 35.5 per cent v/v. In order to produce a 1 per cent v/v vapour concentration, 1 part of this vapour must be added to 34.5 parts of fresh gas. This means that of the total 6000 ml, 170 ml must emerge from the vaporizing chamber and 5830 ml pass through the bypass per minute. Of the 170 ml, 35.5 per cent is halothane vapour, i.e. 60 ml of halothane vapour as before, requiring the vaporization of 0.26 ml of liquid halothane per minute. The gas flow into the chamber is $(170-60) = 110$ ml min^{-1}.

Fuel injector vaporizer

A logical extension of the drip feed approach is to utilize a fuel injector to inject increments of a liquid anaesthetic agent into a gas stream under microcomputer control. This arrangement was adopted by Cooper *et al.* (1978) as part of a microcomputer controlled anaesthesia machine.

Gas flows from two digitally controlled valves are joined to produce a known mixture of oxygen and nitrous oxide. Approximately 5 microlitres of liquid agent are injected as a pulse via a modified automatic fuel injector which functions as a solenoid-operated on-off valve. The pulse time, width and liquid driving pressure are all kept at constant values. The frequency of the pulses is set by the microcomputer and is a multiplicative function of the selected gas flow rate, the desired anaesthetic concentration, the calibration constant, the known ratio of the liquid volume to the vapour volume at standard temperature for the particular anaesthetic. Complete vaporization of the liquid is achieved in a copper vaporizing coil so that no temperature compensation is necessary.

The liquid agent is supplied in pre-filled plastic containers which are made of transluscent material to show the liquid level. Each is labelled to show its contents and can be loaded into a socket on the top of the anaesthesia machine and pressurized to 34.5 kPa (5 lbf in^{-2}). A magnetically coded key on the cannister base protects against incorrect mounting. A magnetic sensing device checks for the microprocessor that a cannister is in place and indicates the nature of the liquid.

The performance of anaesthetic vaporizers under hyperbaric and hypobaric conditions

The effect of a low ambient pressure on the working of an anaesthetic vaporizer is important when anaesthesia has to be produced in cities lying at a high altitude, and in the design of portable anaesthetic equipment for use with high altitude expeditions. On the other hand, the use in recent years of an increasing number of hyperbaric operating rooms has made it necessary to have available anaesthetic vaporizers which can be used at ambient pressures several times greater than normal.

The saturated vapour pressure of a volatile anaesthetic agent is, for practical purposes, a function of its temperature only. In the case of halothane it is 243 mmHg at 20 °C. If the barometric pressure is normal (760 mmHg) then the saturation concentration will be 32 per cent v/v. When the ambient pressure is increased by an additional one atmosphere to 2 ata, the saturated vapour pressure remains at 243 mmHg assuming that the temperature is still 20 °C, but the saturation concentration is halved to 16 per cent v/v. However, from the viewpoint of the depth of anaesthesia produced, it is not the volume concentration which is of importance, but the mass of the agent delivered per unit time. Although the concentration has been halved, the mass of vapour delivered remains almost constant. This follows because the increase in pressure has doubled the density of the mixture. The constancy is not exact because the increased density will have an effect on the splitting ratio between the bypass and vaporizing chamber flows. In practice it has proved possible to operate a calibrated vaporizer such as the Fluotec Mark 2 at normal settings in a hyperbaric chamber (McDowall, 1964; Vermeulen-Cranch, 1964). Vermeulen-Cranch used a Fluotec placed outside a circle. The dial setting was 0.5–1.5 per cent v/v with a 4 l min^{-1} fresh gas flow. The chamber pressure was 3 ata. The rate of induction of anaesthesia should be approximately the same as under normal pressure conditions.

Safar and Tenicela (1964) deal with high-altitude physiology in relation to anaesthesia and inhalational therapy. They mention that standard gas flowmeters can be safely used at high altitudes, the calculated error of a Foregger rotameter being only 1 per cent high per 1000 feet (305 metres) of altitude. Although the concentration of vapour delivered by the vaporizer at low atmospheric pressure will be increased, the mass of vapour delivered will be approximately constant.

Pressurized vaporizers

The majority of anaesthetic vaporizers use a dynamic dilution with a bypass gas stream to dilute the fully saturated vapour produced in the vaporizing chamber. However, it is possible to use a static dilution as described by Bracken, Brookes and Goldman (1968). Oxygen or Entonox (50/50 N_2O/O_2) at 60 lbf in^{-2} g (412.8 kN m^{-2}) from a pipeline is applied to a stout metal 'pot' of 0.5 litres capacity. The pressure is equivalent to 5 ata, i.e. four atmospheres above atmospheric. Assuming that the saturation concentration of halothane at normal atmospheric pressure is approximately 33 per cent by volume, then at 5 ata this becomes 6.7 per cent. If the minute volume supplied to the pot at 5 ata is 500 ml, this expands on exit at atmospheric pressure to become 2.5 litres. In order to produce a 2 per cent concentration the output from the pot must be diluted with an additonal bypass gas flow of 5.9 litres per minute, so that a total minute volume of 8.4 litres is available.

Another form of pressurized vaporizer is that of Titel *et al.* (1968). The pressure inside the vaporizer is maintained at twenty times the saturated vapour pressure of halothane. Compensation is provided for changes in the ambient temperature and the output is calibrated directly in terms of millilitres of halothane vapour delivered per minute.

The calibration of anaesthetic vaporizers

The refractive index method

The method employed by all manufacturers of calibrated vaporizers in the United Kingdom is an optical one, based upon the measurement of the refractive index of the gas and anaesthetic vapour mixture. It is also used for the calibration of on-demand anaesthetic machines. Measurements are performed with an instrument known as a refracto-meter, often of the Rayleigh type (Edmondson, 1957; Luder, 1964). The refractometer measures accurately the refractive index of the gas and vapour mixture and it can be calibrated directly in terms of the percentage of vapour if either the refractive index of the vapour is known or the refractometer has been calibrated against known mixtures. The great advantage of the refractometer method lies in the stability of its calibration, and this makes it particularly useful for factory purposes. It is also the method employed by the Test House of the British Standards Institution to test the accuracy of trichloro-ethylene inhalers intended for analgesic use in obstetric practice. The calibration of the refractometer is affected by the composition of the diluent gas mixture, so that the method requires care when other than simple binary mixtures are used. It cannot be directly applied to the measurement of anaesthetic concentrations in a circuit where the water vapour and gas concentrations will be changing. Hulands and Nunn (1970) have given a detailed account of the use of a portable refracto-meter for measurements during anaesthesia. Details of the operating principle of the Rayleigh refractometer are given in the chapter on optical instruments.

Ultraviolet and infra-red analysers

The fact that halothane vapour will absorb the ultraviolet radiation at 254 nm emitted by a low pressure mercury discharge lamp makes possible the construction of a simple halothane analyser (Robinson, Denson and Summers, 1962; Wolfson, 1968). Two ultraviolet photo-cells are used, each feeding one side of a balanced cathode follower. One photocell monitors the output of the lamp, the other receives light which has passed through a stainless steel sample cell fitted with quartz windows. With no halothane vapour in the cell, the intensities of the two beams are first made equal by introducing a wire gauze screen into the reference beam. A pump draws a sample of gas from the anaesthetic circuit through the cell and the difference in the photo-cell outputs is proportional to the percentage of halothane present. The calibration range is 0–5 per cent. The system is insensitive to water vapour, nitrous oxide and carbon dioxide so that it is attractive for use with circle systems. The specific absorption by many gases and vapours of anaesthetic interest makes possible the application of a range of infra-red gas analysers. Both ultraviolet and infra-red instruments are described in Chapter 10. They all need to be calibrated against known vapour concentrations during manufacture and then at regular intervals. A convenient method for routine checks is to employ an accurately calibrated, stable vaporizer such as one of the Dräger Vapor models. For more fundamental work, known vapour mixtures can be prepared in cylinders under pressure (Hill, 1961).

Even though an accurately calibrated analyser is available, faulty sampling techniques can often lead to erroneous results being obtained when measuring anaesthetic vapour concentrations. Halothane vapour is notoriously difficult to mix with gas, and hence it is desirable to follow the vaporizer under test with a metal mixing baffle. Metal, glass or PTFE tubing and connections are essential in order to minimize any uptake of vapour by plastic or rubber. Care must be taken to ensure that the sampling pump of the analyser does not entrain room air along with the vapour mixture, thus diluting the true concentration.

The Dräger Narkotest

This instrument operates on the principle that strips of silicone rubber will expand when exposed to halothane vapour. In order to minimize the condensation of water vapour the Narkotest is connected in the inspiratory limb of a circle system, so that the minute volume passes through four strips of silicone rubber connected in parallel. The expansion of the strips is magnified by a mechanical linkage to cause a pointer to move over a scale calibrated 0–3 per cent halothane. The meter responds slightly to nitrous oxide, so that if this is to be used, the meter zero is first set using the appropriate oxygen–nitrous oxide mixture. The Narkotest is a simple non-electrical device; it will however respond to vapours other than halothane. Lowe and Hagler (1971) found that the deflection of the Narkotest was the same for the MAC of each agent and were able to scale the instrument in MAC's. This greatly facilitated the giving of an equipotent anaesthetic concentration with a range of volatile agents or mixtures of them. However, White and Wardley-Smith (1972) although satisfied with the clinical performance of the Narkotest as a halothane analyser found that their tests did not support the accuracy of the Narkotest in terms of an MAC meter. Velazquez and Feingold (1978) have calibrated a Narkotest apparatus in terms of the concentration of the new volatile anaesthetic agent isoflurane.

Gas chromatography

Gas chromatography is a physical method capable of separating multi-component gas and vapour mixtures. It is thus a versatile technique and can be adapted to the measurement of blood–gas contents (Hill, 1966; Davies, 1970). The heart of a gas chromatograph is the column (*Figure 8.30*). This is a glass or metal tube of $\frac{1}{8}$ in (3 mm) internal diameter and commonly about 6 feet (2 m) long, although columns up to 20 feet (6 m) in length are encountered. Through the column is swept a steady stream of a carrier gas such as helium, hydrogen or nitrogen, at a flow rate of the order of 20–60 ml min^{-1}. The column is mounted in a thermostatically controlled hot-air oven, the temperature lying between 40 and 100 °C for anaesthetic analyses. The column is filled with an inert support material such as crushed firebrick which is impregnated with 10–20 per cent by weight of a stationary phase such as dinonyl phthalate or silicone fluid. A sample of the gas or vapour mixture to be analysed is injected into the front end of the column, either from a gas-tight syringe through a rubber septum, or by means of a gas sampling valve (Hill and Hook, 1960). Suppose that the mixture consists of oxygen plus halothane vapour. As the sample is swept along the column, the halothane vapour has a higher affinity for the stationary phase and emerges after the oxygen. Thus oxygen might emerge from the column after one minute and halothane after four minutes. The presence of an emerging component is sensed by passing the effluent from the column into a detector. When both gases and

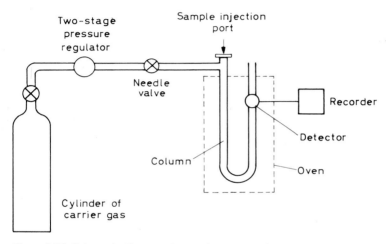

Figure 8.30. Schematic diagram of a gas chromatograph

vapours have to be detected with only a modest sensitivity, the detector might be a katharometer (thermal conductivity cell) which measures the difference between the thermal conductivity of the carrier gas plus sample component and that of the carrier gas alone. The electrical output voltage from the bridge circuit of which the katharometer forms a part is fed to a potentiometric recorder. As each sample component passes through the detector the bridge is unbalanced and the recorder pen traces out a peak on the chart. The peak height, or more accurately, the peak area is proportional to the concentration present in the sample mixture of that component. Application of this type of chromatograph to anaesthetic research is described by Hill (1960). The individual components of a mixture are identified by the time each takes to emerge from the column. When it is required to separate a combination of several gases such as oxygen, nitrogen, carbon dioxide and nitrous oxide during a blood–gas content analysis, or oxygen and carbon dioxide from ether, halothane or cyclopropane, it is necessary to run two columns in parallel. One is a partition column as previously described, which will separate the vapours but not the gases. The separation of carbon dioxide and nitrous oxide is best accomplished using a column packed with cross-linked polymer beads, for example, Porapak. In blood gas analyses this is run in parallel with a column packed with an artificial zeolite (molecular sieve). This will separate oxygen from nitrogen.

When detecting oxygen, nitrogen, nitrous oxide or carbon dioxide, a thermal conductivity detector must be used. However, for organic substances a far greater sensitivity is obtained by passing the column effluent into a small flame fed with a hydrogen—air mixture. The presence of an organic component in the flame increases the number of ions in the flame by a factor of hundreds or thousands. The resulting change in electrical current between a pair of electrodes placed on either side of the flame and polarized with about 200V is amplified with an electrometer amplifier and produces the usual peaks on the chart recorder as a sample component enters the flame. Sensitivities below one part per million are obtainable. Ether or halothane is first extracted from the blood sample, typically 1 ml in volume, by shaking it with normal heptane (Butler and Hill, 1961; Butler and Freeman, 1962; Wortley *et al.*, 1968), or, in the case of methoxyflurane, by shaking it with carbon tetrachloride (Wolfson *et al.*, 1966). Allott *et al.* (1971) have carefully analysed the accuracy obtainable for the determination of halothane in gas, blood and tissues by chemical extraction and gas chromatography. They used carbon tetrachloride as the extraction agent with a trace impurity of chloroform acting as an internal standard. The mixture is placed on the chromatograph column (1—5 microlitres) and the peak heights or areas calibrated in terms of mg/100 ml for each agent using standard concentrations made up in blood. The method can also be applied to chloroform, trichloroethylene and methoxyflurane. Volatile anaesthetics can be estimated in solid tissues by placing a sample of the tissue in a heated sampling port at the column inlet. The port is removable for cleaning (Lowe, 1964; Douglas, Hill and Wood, 1970). Halothane readings are available in about 2—3 minutes which is invaluable when the results are required during the course of an anaesthetic.

The standing current of the flame is about 10^{-9} A and this increases to more than 10^{-8} A as a peak emerges. The linear dynamic range of concentrations for a flame detector is about 1000 : 1.

Halogenated anaesthetic agents such as halothane and chloroform are capable of being detected both in the atmosphere and in blood at extremely low levels by means of a gas chromatograph fitted with an electron capture detector (Douglas, Hill and Wood, 1970; Atallah and Geddes, 1972). In the gas phase the method is very useful in wash-out studies using a short chromatographic column and also for the measurement of environmental pollution with halothane. Hill, Hook and Mable (1962) describe a high-speed gas chromatograph for anaesthetic vapours utilizing small-bore capillary columns and a cathode-ray tube display.

References

ADAMS, A.P. (1969). Anaesthetic machines. *Br. J. Hosp. Med.* April Equipt Suppl. 35

ADNER, M. and HALLEN, B. (1965). Reliability of halothane vaporizers. *Acta anaesth. scand.* **9**, 233

ADRIANI, J. (1962). *The Chemistry and Physics of Anaesthesia*, p. 184. 2nd edn. Springfield; Thomas

ALLOTT, P.R., STEWARD, A. and MAPLESON, W.W. (1971). Determination of halothane in gas, blood and tissues by chemical extraction and gas chromatography. *Br. J. Anaesth.* **43**, 913–918

ATALLAH, M.M. and GEDDES, I.C. (1972). Gas chromatographic estimation of halothane in blood using electron capture detector unit. *Br. J. Anaesth.* **44**, 1035–1039

BODMAN, R.I., GERSON, G. and SMITH, K. (1967). A simple closed circuit for halothane anaesthesia. *Anaesthesia* **22**, 476

BRACKEN, A.B., BROOKES, R.C. and GOLDMAN, V. (1968). New equipment for dental anaesthesia using pre-mixed gases and halothane. *Br. J. Anaesth.* **40**, 903

BRENNAN, H.J. (1957). A vaporizer for fluothane. *Br. J. Anaesth.* **29**, 332

BRYCE-SMITH, R. (1964). Halothane induction unit. *Anaesthesia* **19**, 393

BURTON, P.J.C. (1958). Halothane concentrations from a Rowbotham's bottle in a circle absorption system. *Br. J. Anaesth.* **30**, 312

BUTLER, R.A. and FREEMAN, J. (1962). Gas chromatography as a method for estimating concentrations of volatile anaesthetics in blood. *Br. J. Anaesth.* **34**, 440

BUTLER, R.A. and HILL, D.W. (1961). Estimation of volatile anaesthetics in tissues by gas chromatography. *Nature, Lond.* **189**, 488

CHATRATH, R.R. (1973). The effect of intermittent positive pressure on the output of halothane from a Blease Univap universal vaporizer. *Br. J. Anaesth.* **45**, 915–918

COLE, P.V. (1968). Apparatus for the relief of pain in labour. *Br. J. Anaesth.* **40**, 660

COLLIS, J.M. (1966). Concentration graphs for the Halox vaporizer. *Anaesthesia* **21**, 558

COOPER, J.B., NEWBOWER, R.S., MOORE, J.W. and TRAUTMAN, E.D. (1970). A new anesthesia delivery system. *Anesthesiology* **49**, 310–318

DAVIES, D.D. (1970). A method of gas chromatography for quantitative analysis of blood-gases. *Br. J. Anaesth.* **42**, 19

DOBKIN, A.B., ISTAEL, J.S., SAMONTE, A.L. and BYLES, P.H. (1963). Universal anaesthesia vaporizer in disasters. *N.Y. State J. Med.*, 1815

DORSCH, S.E. and DORSCH, J.A. (1973). Chemical cross-contamination between vaporizers in service series. *Anaesth. Analg.* **52**, 178–180

DOUGLAS, R., HILL, D.W. and WOOD, D.G.L. (1970). Methods for the estimation of blood halothane concentrations by gas chromatography. *Br. J. Anaesth.* **42**, 119

EDMONDSON, W. (1957). Gas analysis by refractive index measurement. *Br. J. Anaesth.* **29**, 570

EDMONDSON, W. and HILL, D.W. (1962). A pressurizing valve for the Fluotec vaporizer. *Br. J. Anaesth.* **34**, 741

EPSTEIN, H.G. and MACINTOSH, R.R. (1949). Analgesia inhaler for trichloroethylene. *Br. med. J.* **2**, 1092

EPSTEIN, H.G. and MACINTOSH, R.R. (1956). An anaesthetic inhaler with automatic thermocompensation. *Anaesthesia* **11**, 83

FELDMAN, S.A. and MORRIS, L.E. (1958). Vaporization of ether and halothane in the copper kettle. *Anesthesiology* **19**, 650

GARTNER, J. and STOELTING, R.K. (1974). A laboratory comparison of Copper Kettle, Fluotec Mark 2 and Pentec vaporizers. *Curr. Res. Anesth. Analg.* **53**, 187

GOLDMAN, V. (1962). The Goldman halothane vaporizer Mark 2. *Anaesthesia* **17**, 537

GOLDMAN, V. (1966). Correspondence. *Br. J. Anaesth.* **38**, 980

GORDH, T., HALLEN, B., OKMIAN, L., WÅLILIN, Å. and STERN B. (1964). The concentration of halothane by the combined use of Fluotec vaporizer and Engstrom respirator. *Acta anaesth. scand.* **8**, 97

GUSTERSON, F.R. (1959). Halothane in the closed circuit, with special reference to prostatectomy. *Anaesthesia* **14**, 35

HALL, J.M., HELLEWELL, J., FISCHER, E.L., BURNS, T.H.S. and FUZZY, G.J.J. (1966). A test of two types of halothane vaporizer. *Br. J. Anaesth.* **38**, 484

HALLEN, B. and NORLANDER, O.P. (1966). Performance of the AGA-SOCSIL vaporizer for volatile anaesthetics studied by gas chromatography. *Acta anaesth. scand., Suppl.* **26**, 43

HART, W.S. (1958a). Halothane anaesthesia. Drip-feed administration in neuro-surgical and other cases. *Anaesthesia* 13, 385

HART, W.S. (1958b). A simple halothane drip feed. *Anaesthesia* 13, 458

HEDSTRAND, U. (1966). AGA ANESTOR MILITAR in clinical use. *Acta anaesth. scand., Suppl.* 26, 53

HILL, D.W. (1960). The application of gas chromatography to anaesthetic research. In *Gas Chromatography 1960,* p. 334. (Ed. by R.P.W. Scott), London; Butterworths

HILL, D.W. (1961). Production of accurate gas and vapour mixtures. *Br. J. Appl. Phys.* 12, 410

HILL, D.W. (1963). Halothane concentrations obtained from a Dräger Vapor Vaporizer. *Br. J. Anaesth.* 35, 285

HILL, D.W. (1966). Methods of measuring oxygen content of blood. In *Oxygen Measurements in Blood and Tissues,* p. 63. (Ed. by J.P. Payne and D.W. Hill.) London; Churchill

HILL, D.W. and HOOK, J.R. (1960). Automatic gas sampling device for gas chromatography. *J. scient. Instrum.* 37, 253

HILL, D.W. and LOWE, H.J. (1962). Comparison of concentrations of halothane in closed and semi-closed circuits during controlled ventilation. *Anesthesiology* 23, 291

HILL, D.W., HOOK, J.R. and MABLE, S.E.R. (1962). A compact cathode-ray tube gas chromatograph. *J. scient Instrum.* 39, 214

HULANDS, G.H. and NUNN, J.F. (1970). Portable interference refractometers in anaesthesia. *Br. J. Anaesth.* 42, 1051

JENNINGS, A.M.C. and HERSANT, M.E. (1965). Increase of halothane concentration following refilling of certain vaporizers. *Br. J. Anaesth.* 37, 137

JENNINGS, A.M.C. and STYLES, M. (1968). 'A predictor for halothane concentrations during closed-circuit anaesthesia.' *Br. J. Anaesth.* 40, 543

JENNINGS, A.M.C., TAYLOR, T.H. and YOUNG, J.V.I. (1967). Nomograms for the Halox vaporizer. *Br. J. Anaesth.* 39, 598

JENSEN, J.K. (1967). Halothankonzentration erreight durch den 'Oxford Miniature Inhaler.' *Anaesthetist* 16, 54

KAPFHAMMER, V. and ATABAS, A. (1965). Der Fluotec Mark 2 mit angebrauten druckausgleich Venti. *Anaesthetist* 14, 18A

KEENAN, R.L. (1963). Prevention of increased pressures in anaesthetic vaporizers with a uni-directional valve. *Anesthesiology* 24, 732

KEET, J.E., VALENTINE, G.W. and RICCIO, J.S.(1963). An arrangement to prevent pressure effect on the Vernitrol vaporizer. *Anesthesiology* 24, 734

LATTO, I.P. (1973). Administration of halothane in the 0–0.5% concentration range with the Fluotec Mark 2 and Mark 3 vaporizers. *Br. J. Anaesth.* 45, 563

LEATHERDALE, R.A.L. (1966). The EMO ether inhaler (clinical experience in a series of over 1000 anaesthetics). *Anaesthesia* **21**, 504

LOWE, H.J.(1964). Flame ionization detection of volatile organic anaesthetics in blood gases and tissues. *Anesthesiology* **25**, 808

LOWE, H.J., BECKHAM, L.M., HAN, Y.H. and EVERS, J.L. (1962). Vaporizer performance – closed circuit Fluothane anesthesia. *Anesth. Analg.* **41**, 742

LOWE, H.J. and HAGLER, K.J. (1971). Clinical and laboratory evaluation of an expired anesthetic gas monitor (Narkotest). *Anesthesiology* **34**, 378

LUDER, M. (1964). Bestimungen von Halothandampkonzentrationen mit dem Laboratoriumsinterfermometer I, Mitseilung, Methodik. *Anaesthetist* **13**, 360

McDOWALL, R.G. (1964). Anaesthsia in a pressure chamber. *Anaesthesia* **19**, 321

MACINTOSH, SIR R.R. (1953). Oxford inflating bellows. Preparations and Appliances. *Br. med. J.* **2**, 202

MACINTOSH, R., MUSHIN, W.W. and EPSTEIN, H.G. (1958). *Physics for the Anaesthetist.* 2nd edn. Oxford; Blackwell

MACKAY, J.M. (1957). Clinical evaluation of Fluothane with special reference to a controlled percentage vaporizer. *Can. Anaesth. Soc. J.* **4**, 235

MAPLESON, W.W. (1960). The concentration of anaesthetics in closed circuits, with special reference to halothane. (1). Theoretical study. *Br. J. Anaesth.* **32**, 298

MARRETT, H.R. (1959). Halothane, its use in the closed circuit. *Anaesthesia* **14**, 28

MARTINEZ, L.R., NORLANDER, O.P and SANTOS, A. (1966). Laboratory evaluation of a SOCSIL vaporizer. *Acta anaesth. scand., Suppl.* **26**, 75

MERRIFIELD, A.J., HILL, D.W. and SMITH, K. (1967). Performance of the Portoblease and the Fluoxair portable anaesthetic equipment, with reference to use under adverse conditions. *Br. J. Anaesth.* **39**, 50

MORRIS, L.E. (1952). A new vaporizer for liquid anaesthetic agents. *Anesthesiology* **13**, 587

MUNSON, W.M. (1965). Cardiac arrest. Hazard of tipping a vaporizer. *Anesthesiology* **26**, 235

MUSHIN, W.W. and GALLOON, S. (1960). The concentration of anaesthetics in closed circuits with special reference to halothane. (3). Clinical aspects. *Br. J. Anaesth.* **32**, 324

NEFF, W.B., SIMPSON, F.B., and THOMPSON, R. (1968). A venturi circulator for anesthetic systems. *Anesthesiology* **29**, 838

PARKHOUSE, J. (1966). Clinical performance of the O.M.V. vaporizer. *Anaesthesia* **21**, 504

PATERSON, G.M., HULANDS, G.H. and NUNN, J.F. (1969). Evaluation of a new halothane vaporizer: the Fluotec Mark 3. *Br. J. Anaesth.* **41**, 109

PEARCE, C. (1962). A versatile halothane vaporizer. *Anaesthesia* **17**, 540

ROBINSON, A., DENSON, J.S. and SUMMERS, F.W. (1962). Halothane analyser. *Anesthesiology* **23**, 391

SAFAR, P. and TENICELA, R. (1964). High altitude physiology in relation to anesthesia and inhalational therapy. *Anesthesiology* **25**, 515

SALAMONSEN, R.F. (1978). A vaporizing system for programmed anaesthesia. *Br. J. Anaesth.* **50**, 425–433

SCHREIBER, P. and WEIS, K.H. (1965). Konzentrationsmessungen mit dem Gardner-Universal-Verdunster. *Anaesthetist* **14**, 289

SCOTT, L. (1968). Clinical experiences with combined halothane-tri-chloroethylene anaesthesia. *Br. J. Anaesth.* **40**, 632

SEED, R.F. (1967). Vaporization of halothane during movement. *Anaesthesia* **22**, 659

STEPHENS, K.F. (1965). Transportable apparatus for halothane anaesthesia. *Br. J. Anaesth.* **37**, 67

STETSON, J.B. (1968). A simple improvement in the EMO vaporizer. *Br. J. Anaesth.* **40**, 65

STOELTING, R.K. (1971). The effect of nitrous oxide on halothane output of Fluotec Mark Two vaporizer. *Anesthesiology* **35**, 215

TITEL, J.H., LOWE, H.J., ELAM, J.O. and GROSHOLZ, J.R. (1968). Quantitative closed-circuit halothane anesthesia. *Anesth. Analg.* **47**, 560

VELAZQUEZ, J.L. and FEINGOLD, A. (1978). Calibration of the Narkotest gas monitor for isoflurane. *Anesth. Analg.* **55**, 441–442

VERMEULEN-CRANCH, D.M.E. (1964). Anaesthesia in a high pressure chamber. In *Clinical Application of Hyperbaric Oxygen*, p. 206. Ed. by I. Boerema, W.H. Brummelkamp, and N.G. Meijne. Amsterdam; Elsevier

WHITE, D.C. and WORDLEY-SMITH, B. (1972). 'The Narkotest' anaesthetic gas meter. *Br. J. Anaesth* **44**, 1100

WEINGARTEN, M. and LOWE, H.J. (1973). A new circuit injection technique for syringe-measured administration of methoxyflurane: a new dimension in anesthesia. *Curr. Res. Anesth. Analg.* **52**, 634

WOLFSON, B. (1962). Closed circuit anaesthesia by intermittent injection of halothane. *Br. J. Anaesth.* **34**, 733

WOLFSON, B. (1968). Appraisal of the Hook and Tucker Halothane Meter. *Anesthesiology* **29**, 157

WOLFSON, B., CICCARELLI, H.E. and SIKER, E.S. (1966). Gas chromatography using an internal standard for the estimation of methoxyflurane levels in blood. *Br. J. Anaesth.* **38**, 29

WORTLEY, D.J., HERBERT, P., THORNTON, J.A. and WHELPTON, D. (1968). The use of gas chromatography in the measurement of anaesthetic agents in gas and blood: description of apparatus and method. *Br. J. Anaesth.* **40**, 624

YOUNG, J.V.I. (1966). The practical use of the Halox vaporizer. *Anaesthesia* **21**, 551

YOUNG, T.M. (1969). Vaporizers for dental anaesthesia modified by the addition of a wick: an evaluation of performance. *Br. J. Anaesth.* **41**, 120

9 Electrical, fire and explosion hazards in the operating room

Only rarely do accidents occur in the operating room involving an electric shock or a fire and explosions are now virtually unknown. However, burns arising from the use of surgical diathermy apparatus do occur although they may not always be reported. These facts often lead to a state of false security, and the necessary routine precautions become overlooked. It must be remembered that when a shock or an explosion does occur the results may well be fatal. It is worth stressing this point, because although in most countries the use of explosive anaesthetic agents has greatly diminished, the use of electronic monitoring equipment has greatly increased. Ether is still in regular use, for example for tonsillectomies, and is a potentially explosive agent (Walter, 1964). Reminders of this fact arise in the papers of Smith (1968) who described a serious explosion which occurred in a copper kettle vaporizer normally used with halothane, but which was being cleaned with diethyl ether in order to remove any thymol which might have accumulated in the vaporizer. Walter (1966) reports on the explosion of an ether vaporizer arising from static electricity. Another complication arises from the use of hyperbaric chambers for therapy and surgery. The use of large chambers containing equipment has markedly diminished, but strict precautions are necessary to prevent the possibility of a flash fire. Anaesthetists are expected to be responsible for the safe functioning of their anaesthetic apparatus. Additionally, surgeons and anaesthetists should be aware of the necessary maintenance and routine checks which have to be carried out on electrical apparatus such as patient monitors and the indifferent electrode of a surgical diathermy unit. Negligence in this respect can lead to the possibility of a dangerous electric shock or a radio-frequency burn. At some time, most people will have received an electric shock, but this is not usually serious. Contact is generally made via a hand; and this is normally withdrawn rapidly by a reflex action. The situation is very different in the case of an unconscious, paralysed, patient who is unable to move or to indicate his discomfort.

Sources of ignition

Sparks and static electricity

In order to produce a fire or an explosion, there must be a supply of ignitable material and a source of ignition. Obvious sources of ignition could be a lighted match, a gas burner or a glowing cigarette, but fortunately these are not generally found in operating rooms. In practice, the two main sources of ignition are sparks arising from the build-up of electrostatic charges, or produced at electrical contacts, and sparking or arcing generated by the surgical diathermy unit. Only a minute amount of energy (approximately 1 microjoule) is needed to ignite an explosive anaesthetic mixture.

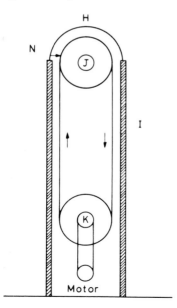

Figure 9.1. The operating principle of a Van de Graaf electrostatic generator

Static electric charges are generated whenever two insulated surfaces are separated, electrons being gained by one surface and lost by the other. The build-up of charge is marked when the surfaces are rubbed together and then rapidly separated. A good example of this occurs in the small Van de Graaf electrostatic generators used in school science demonstrations (*Figure 9.1*). The high voltage terminal is a smooth metal hemisphere H situated at the top of a Perspex tube I about 0.75 m (30 in) long. An endless rubber belt drives continuously over wooden rollers J, K. As a result of the friction between the rubber and the wood, the rubber becomes negatively charged, and a stream of negative charges is carried up until it is opposite a set of pointed conductors N. It then induces a positive charge on N and a negative charge on H. Positive charge streams from the point N to the belt where it neutralizes the negative charge on the belt. As the belt rotates, a high negative potential of the order of 200 000 V is built up on the sphere. Sparks 75 mm (3 in) long can be produced by such a simple arrangement. Van de Graaf generators are used in radiotherapy departments to generate voltages as high as 2 000 000 volts. These are applied to an X-ray tube to produce penetrating X-radiation for the treatment of deep seated tumours.

Prevention of static charge formation

Antistatic flooring

If either of the bodies concerned with the generation of the static charge is connected via a conducting path either to earth or to a conductive floor having a large capacitance to earth then the rate of discharge will exceed the rate of charge and static voltages sufficiently high to produce a spark cannot be produced. An antistatic terrazzo-type floor is often used in operating rooms. It contains a galvanized steel wire netting surrounded by a conducting screed containing carbon black. The netting is not earthed. In the U.K. using electrodes placed 0.6 m (2 ft) apart and each weighing about 1 kg (2 lb) with a tin foil facing 10 cm^2 (4 in^2) in area and having a soft Sorbo rubber between the weight and the foil, the average resistance value should not exceed 2 MΩ between the electrodes with the floor dry (*Hospital Technical Memorandum No. 2*).

It is important that the patient and staff in the operating room should not be connected by a low resistance to earth, as this would increase the risk of a dangerous electric shock should they accidentally come into contact with 'live' metal work. A very low voltage can be very dangerous if it makes contact directly with the heart. It is recommended that the average resistance for antistatic floors with the surface dry should not be more than 2 MΩ and with the surface wet the average resistance to earth should not be less than 50 000 Ω.

Antistatic rubber

The wheels of trolleys and the feet of stools and soles and heels of footwear worn by the staff should be made from antistatic rubber, as should the rubber portions of anaesthetic equipment such as rebreathing bags and anaesthetic tubing. The following limits for the electrical resistance of antistatic rubber items are quoted in British Standard 5724 (1979): Anaesthetic tubing, mattresses and pads 50 kΩ minimum, 1 MΩ maximum; castor tyres — no upper limit: other antistatic items, no lower limit, maximum 1 MΩ. Most antistatic rubber contains carbon black, and hence is black in colour. It must carry the word 'antistatic' in lemon or at least display a yellow mark.

Lichtenthal and Roberts (1973) have investigated the effect of volatile anaesthetic agents upon the electrical conductivity of anaesthetic circuits. They found that ether, halothane and methoxyflurane all decreased the conductivity of six different anaesthetic corrugated hoses. Methoxyflurane caused some types of disposable hoses to become non-conductive as defined by the United States National Fire Protection Association's Code No. 56. They also recommend that certain types of disposable conductive hoses should not be used with flammable anaesthetic agents if they have already been used with methoxyflurane. There is an increasing tendency to use disposable conductive plastic hoses in place of the traditional antistatic rubber hoses in order to minimize problems of cross-infection and to reduce the compliance of the circuit. Attention must be paid to the requirement that the antistatic properties of these hoses remain adequate whilst they are in contact with agents such as ether.

Clothing

Precautions to be taken because of the possible generation of static charges on clothing need some thought because of the human factors involved. Shirts and jumpers made from synthetic fibre materials such as nylon or Terylene are capable of producing a significant charge.

On removing a nylon drip-dry shirt at night, a crackling sound is often heard accompanied by blue sparks. It is desirable that 'scrub suits' and gowns should be made of an inherently antistatic material such as cotton, and boots or overshoes must be antistatic. Underwear is of no consequence, since a charge can only reside on the outer garments. Quinton (1953) has shown that nylon stockings are not a source of hazard, provided antistatic footwear is worn as they are in contact with the body and any charge on the nylon is rapidly transferred to the body and discharged through the footware. Walter (1966) discusses the case of an ether explosion arising from a static spark jumping to an earthed anaesthetist.

Antistatic sprays

The majority of apparatus found in operating rooms is made of metal which is a good conductor of electricity, and antistatic rubber. However, an insulating plastic such as Perspex occurs in the covers of the rotameter banks of anaesthetic machines and the Perspex containers of soda lime canisters used in circle breathing systems. In order to prevent the build up of charge on these sites, it is desirable to spray the Perspex with an antistatic spray such as 'Croxtine' marketed for this purpose by the British Oxygen Company. Tests have shown that before spraying, the surface resistivity of Perspex sheet was 4.4×10^{14} Ω cm^{-2} at 20 °C and 75 per cent relative humidity. After spraying the value was reduced to 3.3×10^9 Ω cm^{-2}. Salt (1964) draws attention to the possible ignition hazard represented by the plastic housing of rotameter banks. Static charges arising from the friction occurring between the bobbin and tube of a rotameter type gas flow meter can cause the bobbin to stick and impair the accuracy (Hargelston and Larsen, 1965). Clutton—Brock (1972) has tested a set of rotameter tubes which had been rendered proof against the effects of static electricity by having a continuous coating of electrically conductive stannic oxide placed on the inside of the tubes. The ends of each tube were coated, inside and out, with gold. Inside the lower end of each tube and making contact with the gold was a coil of soft wire upon which each bobbin rested when no gas was flowing. It was found that the resistance between the gold at the extremity of the tubes through the normal rubber seating at the base of the rotameter block was approximately 2000 MΩ at 1000 V d.c. Clutton-Brock reports that rubbing of the outside of the tubes in a manner which regularly caused sticking of the bobbins in untreated tubes did not do so in the case of the treated tubes. Greenbaum and Hesse (1978) have also discussed the electrical conductivity of flowmeter tubes.

Humidification

The humidification of the atmosphere of an operating room to a relative humidity of some 70 per cent ensures that all the objects in the room are covered with an invisible film of water (Forrest, 1953). The conductivity of this film depends on the presence of substances such as carbonic acid ions in the water, and it takes about ten minutes for the film to form. In modern operating rooms fitted with full air-conditioning, a relative humidity of 70 per cent can be well tolerated by the staff provided that the temperature does not rise above 20 °C. Operating rooms are usually fitted with a hair-type of hygrometer to indicate the relative humidity. When this falls to less than 50 per cent, particular care must be taken to ensure that there are no insulated surfaces present upon which sparking potentials could build up if cyclopropane or ether have to be used.

Sparks from electrical apparatus

When an electrical circuit is opened or closed, a spark often occurs at the switch contacts. This is particularly so when an inductive circuit, such as that of an electric motor, is broken. In extreme cases the spark may continue as an arc. These effects are more pronounced in d.c. than in a.c. circuits because a.c. voltages fall to zero every half cycle. In the past, electrical outlets in United Kingdom operating rooms have commonly used mercury switches. Here the switch contacts are placed inside a sealed tube containing mercury. The switch is closed by tilting the tube to cause the mercury to bridge the gap between the contacts. Any sparking occurs inside the sealed tube and is shielded from the room atmosphere. When the switch is closed, an interlocking lever engages with the earth pin of the plug which has been placed in the socket. This ensures that the plug cannot be withdrawn from the socket whilst the power is on and thus produce a spark. Sparking also occurs regularly at thermostat contacts and at the brushes of d.c. and some universal type electric motors. These types must not be used to power vacuum pumps used in surgical suction apparatus. Explosions have been caused by an accumulation of ether and oxygen in the housing of the surgical suction apparatus.

To render an apparatus such as an automatic lung ventilator completely explosion-proof is a major undertaking. In Germany, electrical apparatus for use in the operating room must comply with the safety regulations devised for use in the coal mines. This means the use in a ventilator of a special electric motor mounted in a stout metal container and the use of spark-proof switches (Hill, 1966). These flame-proof type motors are used, but in the United Kingdom motors of lighter construction and having no sparking source, e.g. capacitor type motors, are frequently used with a special centrifugally operated clutch to overcome the low starting torque associated with this type of motor.

A new British Standard, BS 5724 Part One *Safety of Medical Electrical Equipment – General Requirements* is virtually identical with the International Electrotechnical Commission Document IEC 601–1 having the same title. It specifies Anaesthetics Proof Category G Equipment (APG), a classification applicable to equipment used within an enclosed medical gas system and within 5 cm of places where gas leaks can occur from such a system. At least that part of the equipment specified for use between 5 and 25 cm of an enclosed medical gas system shall be of type AP. In additon to specifying these two types of equipment (APG and AP) BS 5724 covers topics such as: Explosions in medically used rooms; External ventilation with internal over-pressure; Enclosures with restricted breathing; Low energy circuits; Temperature limits.

Sparks from surgical diathermy apparatus

Older type diathermy sets work on the spark-gap principle and these can present a hazard if an explosive mixture finds its way into the diathermy cabinet. All the spark-gap surgical diathermy sets currently manufactured in the United Kingdom are encased in gas-tight enclosures.

In a typical spark-gap diatherm (*Figure 9.2*), the 1500 V r.m.s. secondary winding of the mains power transformer is applied across

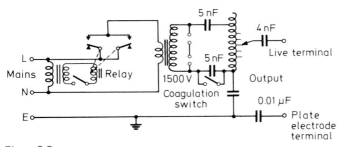

Figure 9.2

two spark-gaps in series. The metal rods forming the gaps are fitted with fins to dissipate the heat. The gaps are in series with two mica capacitors and a tapped inductor. During each half cycle of the mains voltage, the voltage across the secondary winding steadily increases, charging the capacitors. When the voltage is sufficient to break down the air in the gaps, sparking occurs and the capacitors discharge through the coil. As the current decays the back electromotive force produced in the inductor drives current in the reverse direction back into the capacitors. While the gaps are conducting radiofrequency oscillations are generated in the tuned 'tank' circuit. The power available from this circuit can be altered by changing the tapping point on the inductor. The mica coupling capacitor connected to the tapping point prevents d.c. or mains-frequency voltages from reaching the patient. Since the voltage across the gaps peaks twice per mains cycle, the output wave-form consists of trains of damped radiofrequency oscillations produced at 10 millisecond intervals. When the two 5 nF capacitors are in series their effective value is 2.5 nF. This is the condition when the diathermy is set for cutting and the frequency is basically 450 kHz. For coagulation, one capacitor is shorted out and the frequency falls to about 350 kHz. The surgeon's footswitch operates a 6 V relay to apply the mains to the primary winding of the power transformer so that no mains voltage is on the footswitch which can be on a wet floor. The maximum power output is about 150 W into a 150 Ω load.

The latest diathermy sets are compact solid-state electronic systems. *Figure 9.3* shows a typical unit operating at 700 kHz with a maximum output power of 400 W. Separate high frequency outputs are provided for cutting and coagulation. The unmodulated signal is used for smooth cutting of tissues in air or under water without fulguration. Sufficient power is available to cut even heavy layers of fatty or muscle tissue. For 'virtually bloodless' cutting, the output signal is modulated at 26 kHz. Deep coagulation is obtainable with an unmodulated output using a large electrode or with clamps or forceps using a 20 kHz modulation. It is employed for coagulation without cutting and is good for closing up areas of small seeping blood vessels. Dobbie (1969) gives a useful account of the output waveforms from diathermy sets.

The plate electrode can be arranged to be earthed directly, earthed through a capacitor or isolated from earth. An isolated output of up to 12 W at 1.75 MHz is available for microcoagulation in neurosurgical and other procedures.

Explosions have occurred during thoractomy when the diathermy has ignited a mixture of cyclopropane and oxygen in the lungs. Barrkman (1965) reports the case of an intestinal explosion after a colostomy with diathermy. This was due to hydrogen or methane in the gut plus the air let in from the surgical incision. Nagans, Shinya and Wolf (1974) reported on the explosive potential of colonic gas during colonoscopic electrosurgical polypectomy. Explosive mixtures were found in rectal gas in 43 per cent of unprepared patients, but when the

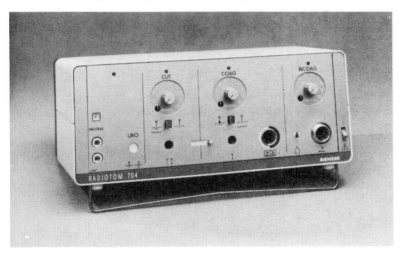

Figure 9.3. Solid-state diathermy unit. (Courtesy of Siemens Ltd)

intestines were cleansed for colonoscopic polypectomy no explosive mixtures were found. Robinson, Thompson and Wood (1975) deal with the explosion hazards arising from the use of nitrous oxide rather than carbon dioxide as the insufflating gas during laparoscopy. A concentration of only 5.5 per cent of hydrogen will explode in mixtures with nitrous oxide at atmospheric pressure. Up to 47 per cent of hydrogen has been found in intestinal gas. The reaction is sensitized by the presence of water vapour, oxygen and traces of organic vapours.

Flammability characteristics of some volatile anaesthetic agents

Modified from Bracken (1965), *Table 9.1* applies under normal atmospheric pressure conditions. With the exception of ethylene, all the agents listed are heavier than air and will tend to gravitate towards the floor. The position in regard to flammability is obviously much worse in oxygen than in air. All the agents require the presence of an atmosphere that can support combustion before a fire or explosion can occur. For a given combination of agent and atmosphere, the proportion of each must lie between certain limits.

TABLE 9.1

Substance	Boiling point (°C)	Relative density (air = 1)	Flammability limits		Limits of concentration used in anaesthesia (% v/v)
			In air (% v/v)	In oxygen (% v/v)	
Diethyl ether	34.6	2.6	1.9−48	2.0−82	3−20
Cyclopropane	−32.8	1.5	2.4−10.4	2.5−60	3−40
Trichloro-ethylene	87	4.5	None	10−65	2−7.5
Divinyl ether	28.4	2.2	1.7−2.7	0.8−45	2−12
Halothane	50.3	6.8	None	None	0.5−10
Halothane ether azeotrope	52.7	5.4	None	Lower limit 8	2−5
Ethyl chloride	12.5	2.3	3.8−15.4	4.0−67	2−6
Ethylene	−103	0.97	3.1−32	3.0−80	60−80
Nitrous oxide	−89	1.5	None	None	35−80
Methoxy-flurane (Penthrane)	104.8	5.7	9.0−28	5.2−28	0.5−3.0
Fluroxene (Fluomar)	42.7	4.4	Lower limit 4.2	Lower limit 4.0	1−5

The most efficient flammable reaction between a fuel and oxygen occurs when the reactants are present in stoichiometric proportions and the reaction goes to completion. Once a fire has been started in such a mixture it will spread rapidly through the mixture since the reaction produces a great deal of heat. Oxidation in one portion of the mixture produces sufficient heat to spread the ignition.

The combustion of cyclopropane in oxygen is given by the equation

$$2C_3H_6 + 9O_2 - 6CO_2 + 6H_2O$$

thus two molecules of cyclopropane will require nine molecules of oxygen for complete combustion. The proportion of cyclopropane in the mixture is 22.2 per cent by volume. However, in practice, percentages of the order of 10–15 per cent cyclopropane in oxygen can produce an explosion.

When air is used as the diluent rather than pure oxygen, it will contain approximately 21 per cent of oxygen and this will react with $(21/9) \times 2$ volumes of cyclopropane, i.e. 4.67 volumes. The volume composition of the mixture is approximately (21 volumes oxygen, 79 volumes nitrogen, 4.7 volumes cyclopropane) giving the percentage of cyclopropane in the stoichiometric mixture as 4.5 per cent.

In a mixture having more than the stoichiometric proportions of the fuel, the excess material together with inert gases such as nitrogen absorb some of the heat of the spreading flame and hinder the ignition process. If pure oxygen is the diluent only the excess fuel acts as a heat absorber and hence the upper limit of flammability is lower in air than in oxygen.

When the mixture contains less fuel than stoichiometric conditions require it makes little difference whether the balance is air or oxygen since both are similar in terms of their heat capacities so that the lower limit for flammability does not differ much between air and oxygen as the diluent.

There is no fundamental difference between the start of a fire (deflagration) and an explosion (detonation). The conditions obtaining in the case of an explosion are favourable to the build-up of a violent reaction leading to the propogation of high pressure shock waves. Here, the heat liberated from the combustion supplies the necessary energy to propogate the shock wave which travels at a velocity greater than the speed of sound. An explosion is more likely to occur than a fire when the mixture is rich in oxygen, but not too close to the lower and upper flammability limits for the concentration of the agent. These conditions promote the rapid combustion and the rise in temperature required to generate the shock wave.

In the United Kingdom, ether and cyclopropane are the flammable agents requiring care, although ethyl chloride sprays must be borne in mind. On the grounds of both economy and safety, cyclopropane – still widely used because of the rapid induction which it produces – is nearly always employed with a closed circuit technique. Ether is often employed in tonsillectomy lists and in developing countries where the cost of non-explosive agents such as halothane is prohibitive. Ether is markedly absorbed by rubber tubing, and at the end of anaesthesia, the breathing tubes which may have been flushed through with pure oxygen can contain a flammable mixture as a result of ether emerging from the rubber. For this reason, an adequate open circuit ventilation should be performed at the cessation of the anaesthetic. Vickers (1965) investigated the duration of the explosion hazard following induction of anaesthesia with ether or cyclopropane. Using a gas chromatograph, he measured the time taken for the concentration of the gases being vented from the anaesthetic circuit to fall to such a level that they would not ignite even if the igniting source was applied directly to them (2 per cent v/v ether or 2.2 per cent v/v cyclopropane). With an adequate ventilation the times were approximately three minutes for ether and one minute for cyclopropane. Even with a closed circuit, an explosion could still arise from the static spark generated inside the circle if the tubing is dry.

Zones of danger and ventilation

The most dangerous region in the operating room itself will be immediately adjacent to the anaesthetic machine, tubing, relief valve, reservoir bag and the patient, particularly his head (Bulgin, 1953). This high risk zone extends out horizontally for about 30 cm (1 ft) and downwards to floor level. There is a further lower risk zone extending out about a further 1 m (3 ft) horizontally and downwards. Beyond this the concentration will generally be below the limit for ignition. These facts should be borne in mind when siting electrical apparatus in the operating room. If there is any doubt about its sparking risk it should be placed more than 1.25 m (4 ft) from the patient and anaesthetic equipment. Because only ethylene is lighter than air, any ether vapour or cyclopropane present in the atmosphere will gravitate towards the floor.

The regulations for the use of electrical equipment in the presence of inflammable anaesthetic agents now differ between the United Kingdom and some other countries such as the U.S.A. and Canada.

In the United Kingdom only spark-proof apparatus may be used in the high risk zone extending outwards 0.3 m (1 ft) from any part of the anaesthetic circuit containing the flammable mixture and downwards to the floor. Outside this zone, electrical apparatus does now not have to be spark-proof and normal mains three-pin electrical outlets can be used. These are normally mounted 0.45 m (18 in) from the floor level so that cleaning of the floor will not affect them. Although interlocking mercury switch outlets are no longer required for U.K. operating and anaesthetic rooms, the floors of these areas must still be of an anti-static construction and conducting rubber must be used for all rubber components. The Association of Anaesthetists of Great Britain and Ireland has published (1971) its recommendations in respect of the precautions to be taken when using flammable anaesthetic agents.

In the U.S.A. and Canada, apparatus which is not spark-proof must be mounted at least 1.5 m (5 ft) above floor level. This applies to permanently installed switches and to switches on portable apparatus if the apparatus is closer than 1.25 m (4 ft) to the anaesthetic circuit. Antistatic flooring and conductive rubber components are also required in all areas where flammable agents may be used. A good ventilation system will greatly reduce the chance of a dangerous concentration of a flammable agent accumulating. From 5 to 10 changes of air per hour is recommended (Report, 1956). The air extraction points should be placed near floor level, and the inlet points as high as possible, certainly not less than 2 m (6 ft). Lidwell (1972) states that the ventilation system should provide an ambient temperature of approximately 18 °C with an air movement of 0.15 m s^{-1} (25 ft min^{-1}). The design of air-conditioning controls for operating rooms has been discussed by Conn (1966).

Halothane as a non-explosive anaesthetic agent

Halothane (2-bromo-2-chloro-1, 1, 1,-trifluorethane) is non-flammable and non-explosive when mixed with oxygen in all proportions (Seiflow, 1957). Mixtures of halothane, nitrous oxide and oxygen are non-flammable at normal atmospheric pressure in the proportions which occur in anaesthetic practice (Lawrence and Bastress, 1959). This is illustrated in *Table 9.2.*

TABLE 9.2

Lowest % v/v of halothane which will ignite	% v/v oxygen	% v/v nitrous oxide
3.8	0	96.2
9.3	30.2	60.5
13.4	43.3	43.3
16.5	50.1	33.4
19.0	54.0	27.0
20.5	56.8	22.7

It is interesting to see that although nitrous oxide on its own is non-flammable and will not support life, it can strongly support a combustion process. Brown and Morris (1966) confirm that even with the most flammable mixtures, there is no ignition risk from a wide variety of ignition sources such as capacitor sparks, coal gas flames and surgical diathermy with nitrous oxide–oxygen–halothane mixtures at ambient pressures provided that the concentrations of halothane recommended for use are not greatly exceeded. Leonard (1975) investigated the lower flammability limits of halothane, enflurane and isoflurane and confirmed that none of these agents were flammable in oxygen under conditions encountered in clinical anaesthesia. However, a high nitrous oxide concentration increased the range of flammability. With a diluent of 80 per cent nitrous oxide, 20 per cent oxygen the flammability limits were: halothane 3.25 per cent; enflurane 4.25 per cent and isoflurane 5.25 per cent.

The use of halothane, methoxyflurane and fluroxene under hyperbaric oxygen conditions

Halothane has been regularly used in a hyperbaric chamber with oxygen as a carrier gas (Vermeulen-Cranch, 1964; McDowall, 1964). Gottlieb, Fegan and Tieslink (1966) found that halothane in the range of 7.6–49 mmHg (1–6.5 per cent of 1 atmosphere) at a total pressure of 1 and 4 atmospheres did not explode, nor did it show any evidence of being flammable when a high voltage spark was generated and held for 5 seconds. Similar results were obtained with methoxyflurane (Penthrane) at 2 per cent of 1 atmosphere. Fluroxene (Fluomar) in the range of 7–35 mmHg did not explode or burn. At 73 mmHg fluroxene exploded and burned. The critical partial pressure for exploding and for burning of fluroxene is in the range of 35–73 mmHg.

For comparison, Miller and Dornette (1961) found that the flammable level of fluroxene in dry oxygen at normal atmospheric pressure was 4 per cent. Patterson, Adams and Johnson (1965) measured the flammability of moist samples of fluroxene in nitrous oxide–oxygen taken from a circle system in clinical use, where the concentrations of fluroxene were 2.27–6.13 per cent. Concentrations of 4.26 per cent or less were found to be non-flammable, whilst concentrations of 4.5 per cent or more were flammable. The ignition risk leading to a 'flash fire' when pure oxygen rather than air is used in hyperbaric chambers is discussed by Denison, Ernsting and Cresswell

(1966), Purser (1966) and Segal (1966). The vogue for cardiac surgery in hyperbaric chambers has passed, but anaesthetists are sometimes involved in the use of chambers for group respiratory therapy or single person chambers for the treatment of gas gangrene or septic abortion. Large chambers are pressurized with air, the patient breathing oxygen or an anaesthetic gas mixture via a tightly-fitting face-mask. The small plastic chambers are pressurized with oxygen and the only electrical equipment inside is a microphone.

Use of nitrous oxide oxygen halothane mixtures in a hyperbaric chamber

Because of a possible ignition risk at elevated pressures the use of nitrous oxide—oxygen mixtures is not recommended in combination with halothane (Brown and Morris, 1966). They also recommended that surgical diathermy and coal gas flames should be excluded from the tank and that pressures should not exceed 3.5 ata.

Duncalf (1978) has reported on a survey of the use of flammable anaesthetic agents in the U.S.A. He found that apart from teaching aspects, there was a considerable scepticism, even by those still using flammable agents, concerning their need. In 1976 of 37 anaesthetists questioned, 29 used diethyl ether and 34 used cyclopropane while in 1978 six of the 37 had stopped using flammable agents.

The misuse of oxygen cylinders and regulators

It can happen that oxygen issuing from an oxygen cylinder becomes ignited (Ito, Horikawa and Ichiyanagi, 1965). In this case the cylinder will not explode, unlike the case of an oxygen cylinder which is closed and becomes heated in a fire. If it is not too hot, the cylinder valve should be promptly closed. Otherwise the cylinder should be left to burn out, care being taken to prevent the ignition of surrounding objects. A more serious problem can arise in the case of calibration mixtures of ether vapour prepared under pressure in cylinders. Here the diluent gas should be nitrogen (Hill, 1961). If oxygen is used there is a risk of combustion being sustained inside the cylinders. Oil and grease should be excluded from oxygen cylinders, regulators, taps and pipelines. Even at pressures near atmospheric, oxygen can form an ignitable mixture with oil or grease, especially when using high flow rates. Some risk has to be accepted, however, since endotracheal tubes and catheters have to be lubricated. Feeley *et al.* (1978) have reviewed the potential hazards of compressed gas cylinders in anaesthesia.

Patient safety with electrical equipment

Anaesthetists are much concerned with the use of electronic patient monitoring apparatus, not only in the operating room, but in the recovery room and intensive care unit. It is important to realize that the equipment should, for use in the United Kingdom, conform to the standards of the *Hospital Technical Memorandum No. 8.*

In the United Kingdom, single-phase a.c. flexible cables have three leads which are colour coded: line (live), brown; neutral, blue; earth, yellow and green striped. There may still be some existing pieces of equipment fed through cables conforming to the previous standard — live, red; neutral, black and earth, green. The line voltage alternates fifty times per second between the positive and negative values of the peak voltage (325 V for a 230 V r.m.s. supply). The neutral connection is within a few volts of earth. Hence if a patient is earthed, and touches an object carrying the line voltage he will be placed across the mains supply with dangerous results. To guard against this possibility it is proposed that the diathermy indifferent electrode strapped to the patient should be connected to earth via a capacitor of suitable value (e.g $\sim 0.01\ \mu F$) and not directly earthed.

The cardinal rule is to remove the possibility of a dangerous current flowing from a point of higher electrical potential to a point of lower electrical potential via the patient. The lower potential is most commonly earth (ground). Two approaches are obviously possible. One is to allow the patient to become earthed, but to ensure that no circuit connected to the patient is capable of passing a dangerous level of current either to or from the patient. The word 'dangerous' will need interpretation. For example, the danger will be less for d.c. than for a.c. and greater for current passing into the heart rather than through the periphery. This approach depends on the concept of electrically isolated patient circuits. The patient need not be connected to earth, but if he is, then no harm can come to him. The alternative is to ensure that all circuits connected to the patient and any conducting objects with which he might come into contact are made to have a potential close to earth so that a dangerous potential difference cannot exist across the patient. The first approach has been adopted in the United Kingdom and the second in the U.S.A. and Canada.

In the U.S.A., the National Electrical Code requires that in electrically susceptible areas of hospitals the maximum 60 Hz a.c. potential difference between any two conducting surfaces within reach of the patient, or of those persons touching the patient, shall not exceed 5 mV measured across 500 Ω under normal operating conditions or in case of any probable failure. All anaesthetizing areas are stated to be electrically susceptible and careful consideration must be given to acute-care beds, angiographic laboratories, cardiac catheterization laboratories, intensive care units, post-operative recovery rooms, coronary care units and dialysis units. The Code requires that the mains outlets in the susceptible areas be fed from isolating transformers such that the possible maximum total hazard leakage current from the system to the patient is 2 mA. This is the maximum current which can flow from one side of the mains supply to an earthed patient. It is not sufficiently small to prevent the possibility of ventricular fibrillation occurring when an electrode is placed in a ventricle, but under most circumstances the patient would otherwise not come to harm. A leakage current warning device is usually provided to indicate if a fault current is flowing to earth of the order of 300 μA or more.

Basically, an 'isolated' mains supply is available from the well insulated secondary winding of a 1 : 1 ratio mains transformer. The only path existing between either end of the winding and earth is via the insulation resistance and capacitance of the winding. It is this high impedance path which limits the amount of current which can flow through the patient if he touches simultaneously either end of the winding and earth. In North American practice an isolating transformer feeds a cluster of mains outlets close to the patient's bed or in the operating room, each cluster having its own circuit breaker. A separate 'star' earth point allows all the connected equipment to work with an equipotential earth arrangement.

Danger levels of electrical current

When a patient becomes connected between two parts of a circuit having a potential difference between them a current, which may be dangerous, will flow through him. At values of currents smaller than the 'hold-on' value it is possible to let go of the 'live' object. At higher currents due to muscular spasm this become impossible, deterioration of the skin occurs at the point of contact and there is a real risk of electrocution arising from the large current now flowing through the body. Dalziel and Lee (1968) quote an average 'hold-on' current of 10.5 mA r.m.s. at 60 Hz for men and 16 mA for women. For 50 or 60 Hz currents applied to a person through the skin via either the upper or the lower limbs the threshold of sensation is approximately 1 mA r.m.s., muscular spasm and paralysis commence between 10–16 mA and ventricular fibrillation occurs in the region of 70–100 mA. It is the current density actually at the heart which is important and this will depend on the total current and the electrode placement. It must be remembered that patients who have been paralysed with a muscle relaxant drug will be unable to separate themselves from a 'live' object even when the current passing is below the usual 'hold-on' value and thus represent a high electrical risk, as do unconscious or enfeebled patients.

Kouwenhoven, Hooker and Langworthy (1932), Hooker, Kouwenhoven and Langworthy (1933) and Kouwenhoven and Milnor (1957) have investigated a.c. electric current pathways in experimental animals. They found that 10 per cent of the current passing through the body along its vertical axis passed through the heart, but only about 3 per cent passed through the heart if the path was from arm to arm. Using the most dangerous pathway, external shocks with currents of less than 50 mA probably did not produce damage although they rapidly gave rise to pain. Currents in the range 100 mA–3 A could produce ventricular fibrillation while currents in excess of 5 A could also cause burns and respiratory arrest.

Ferris *et al.* (1936) found in animals that the susceptibility to the effects of an a.c. current decreased as the frequency was increased. The risk is maximal for frequencies up to 100 Hz and thereafter decreases rapidly. It is negligible for radiofrequency currents of a few milliamperes so that impedance cardiographs and pneumographs are designed to operate in the range 25–100 kHz. Ferris *et al.* (1936) also found that shocks which coincided with the T-wave of the ECG were most likely to produce ventricular fibrillation.

In most cases the studies referred to were performed with external electrodes. Weinberg *et al.* (1962) showed that the current required to induce ventricular fibrillation in man with endocardial or epicardial electrodes was approximately 100 μA r.m.s. at mains frequencies. There is a spread of values amongst individuals Raftery *et al.* (1975) in the range 80–2000 μA. The smallest current to produce a rhythm disturbance from the right ventricle was 80 μA. Hopps and Roy (1963), Starmer, Whalen and McIntosh (1964) and Geddes and Baker (1971) have also provided data on threshold current levels in man for both sensation and ventricular fibrillation.

Currents of such a magnitude as to give rise to ventricular fibrillation are unlikely to arise due to contact with the skin under a single fault condition if the equipment has been properly designed and maintained. The presence of unearthed metal objects which could become connected to the mains under fault conditons could lead to dangerously high currents. Both the U.K. *Hospital Technical Memorandum No. 8* and the International Electrotechnical Commission Document IEC 601-1 set a maximum level of 0.5 mA r.m.s. for the accidental flow of current through skin contacts under a single fault condition, such as the mains connectors normal or reversed and the earth connected or disconnected but either supply conductor disconnected.

The new British Standard BS 5724 (1979) Part One *Safety of Medical Electrical Equipment* is virtually identical with IEC 601-1. It has more than 200 pages and deals with: Terminology, Marking, Documentation, Electrical and Mechanical Safety Requirements, Requirements for equipment used with flammable anaesthetics and Constructional requirements. In the U.K. National Health Service *HTM8* will be phased out over the two years from May 1979 and during that period equipment which satisfies *HTM8,* BS 5724 Part One or IEC 601-1 will be acceptable. From April 1981 equipment will be expected to comply with BS 5724 Part One or IEC 601-1.

It is important to realise that the compliance tests specified in BS 5724 Part One and IEC 601-1 are type tests which need performing with care as they can be potentially damaging to the equipment. Type tests may involve extensive dismantling of the equipment and the removal of components. Skilled staff will be involved and these type tests must not be confused with simpler acceptance tests for new equipment taken into service on assurance from the manufacturers or a Test House that it has passed type tests.

Patient classification

It is convenient to group patients for the purposes of electrical protection into three categories.

(1) *General patients.* These patients are unlikely to come into more

than a casual contact with electrical equipment and will not be connected directly to instrumentation. They would not usually be in an intensive care area, but are likely to be enfeebled and to have an increased chance of ventricular fibrillation because of their medications. For equipment only making skin contact with the patient, *HTM8* limits the maximum leakage current under single fault conditions to the patient to 100 μA. This is known as Type B apparatus.

(2) *Susceptible patients* include all those who are intentionally connected to electrical equipment via a low impedance external contact such as a skin electrode. They are likely to be in intensive care situations, to be enfeebled and to have an increased susceptibility to ventricular fibrillation. Type BF equipment having isolated input circuitry may be specified for these patients.

(3) *Critical patients* include all those having a direct electrically conductive path to the left or right ventricle such as a pressure transducer catheter or a pacing catheter electrode (Noordijk, Oey and Tebra, 1961; Raftery *et al.,* 1975; Whalen, Stalen and McIntosh, 1964). Type CF equipment must be used with these patients and the International Electrotechnical Commission has proposed a 50 μA limit for the leakage current which can flow to the patient under single fault conditions.

A direct injection of mains frequency leakage current into a ventricle would put the critical category of patients at risk from ventricular fibrillation. Lee and Scott (1973) in dogs, found that at 50 Hz there was a minimum threshold of 130 μA when the current pathway was between a right ventricular catheter and the right leg. Green, Raftery and Gregory (1972) found that currents in excess of 3 mA r.m.s. at 50 Hz in dogs were required to flow into either atrium to produce ventricular fibrillation, but that some dogs fibrillated with only 80 μA into the right or left ventricle. They also found that the danger of fibrillation from leakage current flowing via a floating ventricular catheter is less than for a catheter lodged in the apex of a ventricle. In one dog, failure to pump occurred at a mean current of 1.318 mA with the catheter tip floating in the right ventricle, but this was reduced to 228 μA with the catheter anchored in the apex of the ventricle. Roy (1974) quotes a resistance of 600 kΩ for a 1 m long No. 6 to 8 French gauge catheter having a hole area of 1 mm^2 and filled with physiological saline at 37 °C. With a mains voltage applied of 110 V r.m.s. a leakage current of 180 μA could flow via this catheter into the heart.

Isolated amplifiers and pressure transducers

Isolation-type amplifiers are available in all modern patient monitoring systems; for example, in ECG monitors and pressure transducer amplifiers. The basic design principle is that the input stage pre-amplifier which is connected to the patient or transducer is powered from a low voltage battery supply so that no dangerous voltage can accidently be applied to the patient from the circuitry. The output from the pre-amplifier is fed via an isolator to the main amplifier and display. Isolation may be accomplished by means of modulating a beam of light from a light emitting diode with the physiological signal of interest − the light then falling on to a photocell feeding the main amplifier, or by amplitude-modulating an audio frequency carrier signal which is transformer-coupled from the pre-amplifier to the main amplifier. Using this technique, leakage currents of less than 5 μA can be obtained. The use of photo-isolators has been described by Van der Weide (1968) and Bracale and Marsico (1970). Pocock (1972) has discussed in detail the problems which can be encountered when attempting to implement an earth-free patient monitoring system in an intensive care unit.

Body temperature monitors are available with electrically isolated inputs for use with non-isolated input probes. It should be recalled that should a patient go into ventricular fibrillation there may not be time to remove the electrodes and transducers which are connected to him before the d.c. defibrillator is used. Hence the input of each amplifier must be protected by a zener diode network from damage which would arise from the high voltage discharge from the defibrillator.

In order to prevent leakage currents from flowing down a cardiac catheter into a patient, modern blood pressure transducers are fitted with a disposable plastic cuvette (dome) having a slack plastic diaphragm which provides an electrical isolation between the catheter hydraulic system and the body of the transducer. It is usual to provide additional insulation between the transducer's case and diaphragm. A leakage current of less than 2.5 μA from the transducer to the fluid filled catheter at 115 V 60 Hz is quoted for the Hewlett Packard Model 1280C.

It is also necessary to be certain that no significant leakage currents can be produced from equipment connected to a ventricular catheter. Even with the use of an isolated diaphragm transducer, leakage from a mains-powered injector for contrast medium might produce ventricular fibrillation (Mody and Richings, 1962). The use of battery powered equipment such as cardiac pacemakers and monitors is helpful in reducing risks due to leakage currents.

General electrical precautions

The need for continuing vigilance is emphasized by the paper of Said and El-Shiribiny (1962) who described the case of a patient who received no less than eleven electric shocks resulting from the making of an accidental electrical connection during general anaesthesia. Bruner (1967) gives a useful review of the hazards of using electrical apparatus in hospitals and Bruner, Aronow and Rubin (1972) have discussed their experience of electrical accidents based upon 3½ years experience at the Massachusetts General Hospital. This has 1100 beds and in the period there were 55 incidents, three of which involved ventricular fibrillation. Both surgical diathermy and electrically-powered beds accounted for a substantial number of the incidents, but a wide range of apparatus was involved. The faults were rarely subtle, gross faults including mains connectors and cables were common as was failure of equipment earthing. No problems with microshock to the heart were encountered. Bruner, Aronow and Rubin felt that whilst not particularly glamorous, good maintenance of equipment and user education offered the best approach to the solution of common and predictable problems.

Some points which should be observed are:

(1) Before purchasing equipment ensure that it satisfies the relevant national safety regulations (Meyer, 1973).
(2) Apparatus should be serviced on a routine basis with particular attention paid to mains connectors and cables. Earth cables should be checked by a heavy current test (Albisser, Parson and Pask, 1973).
(3) If possible all the instruments connected to a patient should be fed from a common mains supply and the leakage current from this supply reduced to a minimum by the use of an isolating transformer. Individual equipments may use their own isolating transformers, and they will reduce leakage currents to less than 100 μA.
(4) Use as short a mains cable as is conveniently possible.
(5) Use isolation techniques for critical category patients.

A number of portable test-sets have been described for the routine testing of hospital electrical equipment to national safety standards. That due to Brown *et al.* (1973) is designed to test to the requirements of the U.K. *Hospital Technical Memorandum No. 8.* It tests the earth bonding of equipment at a current of 25 A, the insulation at a voltage of 1000 V d.c. and measures the earth leakage current, the patient isolation and the patient circuit a.c. and d.c. currents.

Burns from the surgical diathermy unit

The output of the valve diathermy units is derived from a radiofrequency transformer, the cutting electrode being connected to one end of the secondary winding and the indifferent electrode to the other. When the indifferent electrode was not earthed many patients received burns if they came into contact with an earthed object since the diathermy current flowed through them to earth. The number of burns was greatly reduced by the simple expedient of earthing the indifferent electrode. However, this increased the risk to the patient of electrical shock with the use of more monitoring apparatus during surgery. As a result, it is now recommended that the low potential end of the radiofrequency generator should be bonded to earth inside the case of the diathermy set, and the indifferent electrode should not be bonded directly to earth, but connected to this point via a capacitor whose impedance is small at the diathermy frequency. A high working voltage 0.01 μF ceramic capacitor is suitable: it must be a low loss, high current component. The impedance of this is 0.3 MΩ at 50 Hz and 30 Ω at 400 kHz.

In practice the patient is not maintained uniformly at earth potential owing to the impedance of his body and the contact impedance at the indifferent electrode. Hence, apparatus connected to him should be earth-free so that it does not provide an alternative return path for the diathermy current which would give rise to burns at the point of contact. Radiofrequency choke coils should be fitted into the leads of other apparatus joined to the patient whilst diathermy is in use. If this is not done an appreciable radiofrequency current might travel up the leads and through their capacitance to earth. This could give rise to a burn at the point of contact of the leads with the patient. An interesting paper on this subject is that of Becker, Malhortra and Hedley-Whyte (1973). This discusses the unwanted paths which diathermy current can take, for example, leading to burns under ECG electrodes. The authors recommend the use of r.f. chokes in the electrode leads. A good practice is to use two indifferent electrodes, one on the thigh and one under the back. This will greatly reduce radiofrequency voltage differences around the body.

The indifferent electrode has usually been a lead plate placed inside a cloth bag soaked in a saline solution. Over a period of time, the plate may become buckled and corroded or more usually the bag dries out, resulting in a high value of contact impedance with the patient. The passage of the diathermy current through this high impedance causes heating and a burn. It will also result in a loss of cutting power at the cutting electrode. As a result, the surgeon may try to correct matters by turning up the power but this will only increase the burning at the indifferent electrode. It is obvious that regular maintenance action is essential, the greatest danger to the patient arising from broken plate electrode leads. Another approach is to employ a thin stainless steel plate as the indifferent electrode. This does not buckle, and hence need not be placed in a cloth bag. A new measure is the use of a disposable metal foil electrode fed by two flexible metal strips in parallel on a plastic strip. A transistor circuit passes a small d.c. current down one strip and back up the other. If the circuit becomes broken the loss of current causes an audible alarm to sound. The self-contained alarm unit and the flexible electrode can be connected to a conventional diathermy unit. Disposable pre-gelled indifferent (plate) electrodes are now available in the U.S.A. The foam electrode provides a good contact with the skin.

By far the most common cause of diathermy burns comes from the fact that the patient's body is not connected to the low potential output terminal of the diathermy set via the plate electrode lead. As a result he assumes a radiofrequency potential of 100–150 V r.m.s. when he is touched with the cutting electrode. The radiofrequency current will flow to earth by any convenient path and this may well result in burns appearing at the point where the current leaves the body, e.g. the patient's cheek or a finger. Masuko and Ichiyanagi (1973) have described how a patient received a diathermy burn on his back due to a broken plate lead and the presence of excess amounts of solution used for aseptic and cooling purposes. The burns arose from contact between the patient's back and the sheet on which he was lying. Whilst the use of a plate lead continuity alarm will guard against a lead which is broken or not plugged in, it will not guard against one which is plugged in but with the plate not attached to the patient! Diathermy burns can also arise from the surgeon accidentally stepping on the footswitch when the diathermy needle is lying on the patient or is placed in a conductive quiver which is touching the patient.

Becker, Malhorta and Hedley-Whyte (1973) have given a good review of the possibilities of burns to patients arising when there is a fault associated with the plate electrode. Under these circumstances a burn can occur under a disposable ECG electrode on the chest if the impedance to earth of the ECG amplifier is not sufficiently high. DeRosa and Gadsby (1979) give quantitative data on the heating produced under ECG electrodes by radiofrequency heating from a diathermy. The time duration of current flow to produce a significant heating was in excess of 30 seconds. The average time of an electro-surgical activation was found to be 10 seconds, but since a large number of activations are used during a surgical procedure cooling may not be adequate and the potential for skin heating and burns from the cumulative effects is very real.

Pearce *et al.* (1979) used a high speed thermal scanner to study the temperature distribution of the skin under metal foil diathermy plate electrodes in patients whose weight ranged from 46 to 84 kg. A radio-frequency current of 700 mA r.m.s. was passed for one minute through either an electrolyte-coated aluminium or copper electrode. The maximum temperature rises occurred at the perimeter of both electrodes and were 3.5 °C and 2.5 °C respectively. Neufeld (1978) has described the principles and hazards of electrosurgery and laparoscopy.

Fires due to surgical diathermy or cautery

Diathermy sets often provide a low voltage, high current, outlet from a transformer secondary winding at the mains frequency to heat a wire loop for use as a cautery. Either the cautery loop or sparks from the diathermy cutting electrode can set alight drapes or dressings which have become soaked in surgical spirit. The ignition temperature of an ether—methylated spirit mixture in air and oxygen has been investigated by Briscoe, Hill and Payne (1976). Plumlee (1972) reported after the use of a skin preparation spray with surgical diathermy.

Low voltage burns

Low voltage burns can be caused to the skin beneath an electrode, such as an ECG electrode to which a voltage as low as 3 V is applied

(Leeming, Ray and Howland, 1970). The effect is due to electrolysis. The writer has knowledge of this happening when an ECG electrode placed on an anaesthetized patient was accidentally connected to a socket carrying 12 V d.c. for approximately 45 minutes.

Regulations applicable to equipment for use in the operating room

Report of a Working Party on Anaesthetic Explosions. 1956
H.M.S.O., London.

Code for the Use of Flammable Anaesthetics. No. 56, 1962
National Fire Protection Association, 60 Battery March Street,
Boston, Mass. 02110, U.S.A.

Code for the Use of Flammable Anaesthetics. Canadian Standard Z 32,
1963 Canadian Standard Association, 235 Montreal Road, Ottawa
7, Canada.

Normen-Verzeichnis und de-Vorschriften der Radiologie und Elektro-medizin.
Verband Deutscher Elektrotechniker, 1958
Beuth-Vertreib GmbH, Berlin, W.12.

Safety Code for Electro-medical Apparatus. 1963
Department of Health and Social Security, Hospital Technical
Memorandum No. 8. H.M.S.O., London.

Antistatic Precautions: Rubber, Plastics and Fabrics.
Department of Health and Social Security, Hospital Technical
Memorandum No. 1. H.M.S.O., London.

Antistatic Precautions: Flooring in Anaesthetizing Areas.
Department of Health and Social Security, Hospital Technical
Memorandum No. 2. H.M.S.O., London.

British Standards Institution, London.
B.S. 2099: Part 1: 1960 Amendment p. 3786.
Castors for hospital equipment

B.S. 2050: 1961
Specification for electrical resistance of conductive and anti-static products made from flexible polymeric material

B.S. 3353: 1961
Specifications for anaesthetic breathing bags made of antistatic rubber

B.S. 3398: 1961
Specification for antistatic rubber flooring

B.S. 2506: 1961
Antistatic rubber footwear

B.S. 3806: 1964
Breathing machines for medical use.

References

ALBISSER, A.M., PARSON, I.D. and PASK, B.A. (1973). A survey of the grounding system in several large hospitals. *Med. Instrum.* **7**, 297

ASSOCIATION OF ANAESTHETISTS OF GREAT BRITAIN AND IRELAND. (1971). Explosion hazards. *Anaesthesia* **26**, 155

BARRKMAN, M.F. (1965). Intestinal explosion after opening a caecostomy with diathermy. *Br. med. J.* **1**, 1594

BECKER, C.M., MALHORTRA, I.V. and HEDLEY-WHYTE, J. (1973). The distribution of radiofrequency current and burns. *Anesthesiology* **36**, 106

BRACALE, M. and MARSICO, M. (1970). A photon-coupled amplifier for measuring and recording physiological signals. *Med. Biol. Engng* **8**, 103

BRACKEN, A. (1965). Fires and explosions. In *General Anaesthesia*. 2nd edn. Vol. 1. (Ed. by F.T. Evans and T.C. Gray.) London; Butterworths

BRISCOE, C.E., HILL, D.W. and PAYNE, J.P. (1976). Inflammable antiseptics and theatre fires. *Br. J. Surg.* **63**, 981–983

BROWN, M.C., JOHNSON, F., RUDDY, T. and McDONALD, T. (1973). An instrument for testing electro-medical equipment for safe performance. *Biomed. Engng* **9**, 24–25

BROWN, T.A. and MORRIS, G. (1966). The ignition risk with mixtures of oxygen and nitrous oxide with halothane. *Br. J. Anaesth.* **38**, 164

BRUNER, J.M.R. (1967). Hazards of electrical apparatus. *Anesthesiology* **28**, 396

BRUNER, J.M.R., ARONOW, S. and RUBIN, I.L. (1972). Controlling the electrocution hazard in the hospital. *J. Am. Med. Ass.*, **220**, 1581

BULGIN, D. (1953). Factors in the design of an operating theatre free from electrostatic risks. *Br. J. appl. Phys.* **4**, S87

CLUTTON-BROCK, J. (1972). Static electricity and Rotameters. *Br. J. Anaesth.* **44**, 86–90

CONN, G.D. (1966). Air conditioning controls for the modern hospital. *Wld Med. Electron. Instrum. Lond.* **4**, 224

DALZIEL, C.F. (1956). Effects of electric shock on man. *I.R.E. Trans. Med. Electron.* **PGME-5**, 44

DALZIEL, C.F. and LEE, W.R.(1968). Re-evaluation of lethal electric currents. *I.E.E.E. Trans.* **IGA-4**, 467

DENISON, D.M., ERNSTING, J. and CRESSWELL, A.W. (1966). Fire and hyperbaric oxygen. *Lancet* **2**, 1405

DeROSA, J.F. and GADSBY, P.D. (1979). Radio-frequency heating under ECG electrodes. *Med. Instrumentation* **13**, 273–276

DOBBIE, A.K. (1969). The electrical aspects of surgical diathermy. *Biomed. Engng* **4**, 206

DUNCALF, D. (1978). Survey of the use of flammable anesthetics. *Anesthesiology* **48**, 298–299

FEELEY, T.W., BANCROFT, M.G., BROCKS, REBECCA A., and HEDLEY-WHYTE, J. (1978). Potential hazards of compressed gas cylinders: A review. *Anesthesiology* **48**, 72–74

FERRIS, L.P., KING, B.G., SPENCE, P.W. and WILLIAMS, H.B. (1936). Effect of electric shock on the heart. *Elec. Eng.* **55**, 498

FORREST, J.S. (1953). Methods of increasing the electrical conductivity of surfaces. *Br. J. appl. Phys.* **4**, S37

GEDDES, L.E. and BAKER, L.E. (1971). Response to the passage of electric current through the body. *J. Ass. Adv. Med. Instrum.* **5**, 13

GREEN, H.L., RAFTERY, E.B. and GREGORY, I.C. (1962). Ventricular fibrillation threshold of healthy dogs to 50 Hz current in relation to earth leakage currents of electro-medical equipments. *Bio-med Engng* **7**, 408

GREENBAUM, R. and HESSE, G.E. (1978). Electrical conductivity of flowmeter tubes. *Br. J. Anaesth.* **50**, 408

GOTTLIEB, S.F., FEGAN, F.J. and TIESLINK, J. (1966). Flammability of halothane, methoxyflurane and fluoroxene under hyperbaric oxygen conditions. *Anesthesiology* **27**, 195

HARGELSTON, J.O. and LARSON, O.S. (1965). Inaccuracy of anaesthetic flowmeters caused by static electricity. *Br. J. Anaesth.* **37**, 637

HILL, D.W. (1961). Production of accurate gas and vapour mixtures. *Br. J. appl. Phys.* **12**, 410

HILL, D.W. (1966). Recent developments in the design of electronically controlled ventilators. *Anaesthesist* **15**, 234

HOOKER, D.R., KOUWENHOVEN, W.B. and LANGWORTHY, O.R. (1933).

The effect of alternating electrical currents on the heart. *Am. J. Physiol.* **103**, 444

HOPPS, J.A. and ROY, O.Z. (1963). Electrical hazards in cardiac diagnosis and treatment. *Med. Electron. biol. Engng* **1**, 135

ITO, Y., HORIKAWA, H. and ICHIYANAGI, K. (1965). Fires and explosions with compressed gas. Report of an accident. *Br. J. Anaesth.* **37**, 140

KOUWENHOVEN, W.B., HOOKER, D.R. and LANGWORTHY, O.R. (1932). The current flowing through the heart under conditions of electric shock. *Am. J. Physiol.* **100**, 344

KOUWENHOVEN, W.B., and MILNOR, W.R. (1957). Field treatment of electric shock. *Trans. Am. Inst. Elec. Eng.* **76**, 82

LAWRENCE, J.S. and BASTRESS, E.K. (1959). Combustion characteristics of anaesthetics. *Anesthesiology* **20**, 232

LEE, W.R. and SCOTT, JANET R. (1973). Thresholds of fibrillating leakage currents along intracardiac catheters: an experimental study. *Cardiovasc. Res.* **7**, 495

LEEMING, M.N., RAY, C. Jr. and HOWLAND, W.S. (1970). Low-voltage direct-current burns. *J. Am. Med. Ass.* **214**, 1681

LEONARD, P.F. (1975). The lower limits of flammability of halothane, enflurane and isoflurane. *Anesth. Analg.* **54**, 238–240

LICHTENTHAL, P. and ROBERTS, R.B. (1973). The effect of volatile anaesthetic agents upon the conductivity of anaesthetic circuits. *Curr. Res. Anaesth. Analg.* **52**, 121

LIDWELL, O.M. (1972). *Ventilation in Operating Suites.* London; Medical Research Council

McDOWALL, R.G. (1964). Anaesthesia in a pressure chamber. *Anaesthesia* **19**, 321

MASUKO, K. and ICHIYANAGI, K. (1973). Still another mode of electrosurgical burns: a report of two cases and an experiment. *Curr. Res. Anaesth. Analg.* **52**, 19

MEYER, J.A.(1973). Publications of the National Fire Protection Association of interest in anesthesiology. *Curr. Res. Anaesth. Analg.* **51**, 821

MILLER, G.L., and DORNETTE, W.H.L. (1961). Flammability studies of fluomar-oxygen mixtures used in anesthesia. *Anesth. Analg.* **40**, 232

MODY, S.M. and RICHINGS, M. (1962). Ventricular fibrillation resulting from electrocution during cardiac catheterization. *Lancet* **1**, 21

NAGANS, H., SHINYA, H. and WOLF, W. (1974). The explosive potential of colonic gas during colonoscopic electrosurgical polypectomy. *Surgery Gynec. Obstet.* **138**, 554–556

NEUFELD, G.R. (1978). Principles and hazards of electrosurgery including laparoscopy. *Surgery Gynec. Obstet.* **147**, 705–710

NOORDIJK, J.A., OEY, F.T.I. and TEBRA, W. (1961). Ventricular electrodes and the dangers of ventricular fibrillation. *Lancet* **1**, 21

PATTERSON, J.F., ADAMS, J.G. and JOHNSON, C.G. (1965). Flammability of fluoroxene. *Anesthesiology* **26**, 825

PEARCE, J.A., GEDDES, L.A., BOURLAND, J.D. and SILVA, L.F. (1979). The thermal behaviour of electrolyte-coated metal-foil dispersive electrodes. *Med. Instrumentation* **13**, 298–300

PLUMLEE, J.E. (1972). Operating room flash fire from use of cautery: a case report. *Anaesth. Analg.* **52**, 202–203

POCOCK, S.N. (1972). Earth-free patient monitoring. *Biomed. Engng* **7**, 21

PURSER, P.R. (1966). Sparks in hyperbaric oxygen. *Lancet* **2**, 1405

QUINTON, A. (1953). Safety measures in operating theatres and the use of a radioactive thallium source to dissipate static electricity. *Br. J. appl. Phys.* **4**, S92

RAFTERY, E.B., GREEN, H.F. and YACOUB, M.H. (1975). Disturbances of heart rhythm produced by 50 Hz leakage currents in human subjects. *Cardiovascular Res.* **9**, 263–265

Report of a Working Party on Anaesthesic Explosions. (1956). London; H.M.S.O.

ROBINSON, J.C., THOMPSON, J.M. and WOOD, A.W. (1975). Laparoscopy explosion hazards with nitrous oxide. *Br. med. J.* **3**, 764–765

ROY, O.Z. (1974). Ventricular fibrillation. *Med. Biol. Engng* **12**, 130

SAID, K. and EL-SHIRIBINY, A. (1962). Accidental repeated electrical shocks during anaesthesia. *Acta anaesth. scand. Suppl.* **12**, 111

SALT, R.H. (1964). Anaesthetic explosions – a possible source of ignition. *Anaesthesia* **19**, 598

SEGAL, L. (1966). Fire suppression in hyperbaric chambers. *Fire Journal* **60**, 17

SEIFLOW, G.H.F. (1957). The non-inflammability of fluothane. *Br. J. Anaesth.* **29**, 438

SMITH, T.C. (1968). Serious explosion during cleaning of a copper kettle. *Anesthesiology* **29**, 386

STARMER, C.F., WHALEN, R.E. and McINTOSH, H.D. (1964). Hazards of electric shock in cardiology. *Am. J. Cardiol.* **14**, 537

VAN DER WEIDE, H. and VAN BEMMEL, J.H. (1968). A photon-coupled amplifier for the transmission of physiological signals. *Med. Biol. Engng* **6**, 447

VERMEULEN-CRANCH, D.M.E. (1964). Anaesthesia in a high pressure chamber. In *Clinical Application of Hyperbaric Oxygen,* p. 205. (Ed. by I. Boerema, W.H. Brummelkamp and N.G. Meijne.) Amsterdam; Elsevier

VICKERS, M.D. (1965). The duration of the explosion hazard following induction with ether or cyclopropane. *Anaesthesia* **20**, 314

WALTER, C.W. (1964). Anesthetic explosions: a continuing threat. *Anesthesiology* **25**, 505–514

WALTER, C.W. (1966). Explosion of an ether vaporizer. *Anethesiology* **20**, 192

WEINBERG, D.I., ARTLEY, J.L., WHALEN, R.E. and McINTOSH, H.D. (1962). Electric shock hazards in cardiac catheterization. *Circ. Res.* **11**, 1004

WHALEN, R.E., STARMER, C.F. and McINTOSH, H.D. (1964). Electrical hazards associated with cardiac pacemaking. *Ann. N.Y. Acad. Sci.* **111**, 922

10 Physical optics, photometry and spectrophotometry

Light and electromagnetic radiation

Light is a form of electromagnetic radiation as are radio waves, X-radiation and the gamma-radiation of radioactivity. The distinguishing feature of the radiations is their wavelength, the distance between successive peaks or troughs of the wave. All electromagnetic radiations travel at the speed of light, i.e. 3×10^8 m s^{-1} (186 000 miles per second). For a wave the velocity is equal to the product of frequency and wavelength (Coulson, 1941). The frequency is the number of cycles of the wave occurring in one second. Thus if the frequency of a surgical diathermy set is two million cycles per second (2 MHz), the wavelength generated is $(3 \times 10^8)/(2 \times 10^6)$ m = 150 m. Light wavelengths are very much shorter, the current unit of light wavelength being the nanometre (10^{-9} m) which replaces the earlier, smaller unit, the Ångstrom (sometimes referred to as the tenth metre since it equals 10^{-10} m). Thus 1 nm = 10 Å.

TABLE 10.1. Spectrum of electromagnetic radiation

Name of radiation	Approximate wavelength range
Gamma rays	Less than 0.0001 nm
X-rays	0.0001–5 nm
Ultraviolet radiation	10–380 nm
Visible light	380–680 nm
Infra-red radiation	680 nm – 0.1 mm
Micro waves	A few millimetres to metres
Radio waves	A few metres and up

White light, as is well known, consists of all the colours of the rainbow, i.e. red, orange, yellow, green, blue, indigo and violet. This occupies a narrow band of wavelengths from about 680 nm in the red to about 380 nm in the violet. Beyond the visible region of the spectrum are regions of ultraviolet on the short wave side and the infrared on the long wave side.

Photobiologists generally divide the ultraviolet spectrum into three portions: UV-A, 320–400 nm; UV-B, 290–320 nm and UV-C, 200–290 nm. UV-C is also called germicidal radiation because of its effectiveness in killing one-celled organisms, and it is also very efficient in causing erythema of normal skin. UV-B is very efficient in causing sub-burning of human skin and hence is often called the sunburn spectrum. UV-A is known as longwave ultraviolet radiation and its photobiological properties have been reviewed in detail by Parrish *et al.* (1978). One application is the treatment of skin disorders.

From the viewpoint of anaesthetists, the region of interest in the ultraviolet is 200–380 nm and in the infra-red 680–~6000 nm. The SI unit of infra-red wavelength is the nanometere. The previous non-SI unit was the micrometre (micron) = 1000 nm. *Table 10.1* lists the wavelength ranges occupied by various types of electromagnetic radiation. X-rays are designated as those electromagnetic waves with a wavelength lying between about 10^{-10} mm and 10^{-5} mm (10 nm). This range overlaps on one side with the gamma rays (wavelengths less than 10^{-10} mm) and on the other side with the ultraviolet rays (wavelengths between about 10^{-5} mm (10 nm) and 3.8×10^{-4} mm (380 nm)).

Light is a form of energy and radiant energy is expressed in terms of joules. The rate of delivery of the radiant energy is the radiant flux expressed in watts, milliwatts or microwatts. The irradiance is the radiant flux arriving over a given area and is expressed in watts, milliwatts or microwatts per square metre. The radiant exposure or dose is equal to the product of the irradiance multiplied by the exposure time in seconds. Since one watt is equal to one joule per second the units of radiant exposure are joules per square metre or millijoules per square metre.

These radiometric terms may also be expressed in terms of wavelength by adding the prefix 'spectral'. For example, spectral irradiance – the irradiance at a particular wavelength – is given in terms of milliwatts per square centimetre at the specified wavelength. A graph of spectral irradiance (at a given distance and position relative to the source) is valuable in describing sources of light radiation. Spectral radiant flux is often used by lamp manufacturers to describe the radiant flux emitted by a lamp as a function of the light wavelength. Parrish *et al.* (1978) quote the following figures for the approximate UV-A irradiance in $W\,m^{-2}$ in the band 320–400 nm: Sunlight at 3 p.m. or 9 a.m. at an angle of 45 °, 25–35; Sylanvania fluorescent UV-A source for photochemotherapy of psoriasis, 100.

In the case of the infra-red, a need to know the spectral irradiance characteristic of an infra-red heat source arises in the case of infra-red radiant heat systems used for warming infants in neonatal intensive care units.

Light as waves or a stream of particles

The intensity of a beam of light is given by the amplitude (squared) of the wave at that instant. It is known that if two waves are exactly in step (in phase), then the resultant amplitude is the sum of the two separate amplitudes. If the two waves are exactly out of step (in anti-phase), the resultant amplitude is equal to the difference between the individual amplitudes. If these were equal the resultant would be zero. This effect is known as the interference of two light waves. It is the working principle of the Rayleigh refractometer which is used by all manufacturers of calibrated anaesthetic vaporizers in the United Kingdom to check the calibration (Edmondson, 1957). Thus for many purposes it is convenient to think of light in the form of waves. However, in considering the *photoelectric* effect (the action of light on photocells and photomultiplers in oximeters and spectrophotometers), it is convenient to think of light as a series of discrete particles or *quanta*. In a similar fashion, it is convenient to think of electrons both in terms of particles and of waves, as in the electron microscope.

Polarized light and optical activity

Light waves are transverse waves, that is to say, the vibrations take place in planes perpendicular to the direction of travel of the wave. Ordinary light consists of a large number of such waves, each having its own plane of vibration. If monochromatic light, from a sodium discharge lamp for example, is passed through a crystal of tourmaline, it is found that the vibrations of the emergent light all lie in one plane, and this is parallel to the optical axis of the tourmaline (*Figure 10.1*). The emergent light is said to be polarized. This plane-polarized light will

Tourmaline crystals

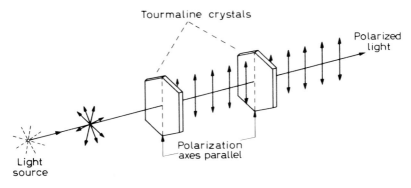

Polarized
light

Polarization
axes parallel

Light
source

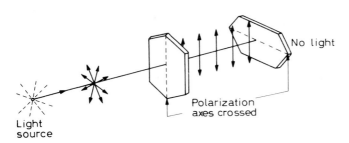

No light

Polarization
axes crossed

Light
source

Figure 10.1. Production of plane polarized light

pass through a second crystal of tourmaline if the optical axis of the
second crystal is made parallel to the first. If the second crystal is now
rotated about the light beam, the intensity of the emergent beam will
be gradually extinguished, until when the optical axes of the two
crystals are mutually at right-angles, the light emerging from the second
crystal will be completely extinguished. When this occurs, the two
crystals are said to be 'crossed'. If a sample of some materials is placed
between the two crossed crystals, the intensity of the light emergent
from the second crystal will be partially restored. These materials are
known as *optically active.* In order to once again extinguish the light
the second (or analyser) crystal will have to be rotated through a
definite angle with respect to the first crystal (or polarizer). Substances
which cause the plane of polarization to be rotated to the right are said
to be dextrorotatory, whilst substances which cause it to be rotated to

384 Physical optics, photometry and spectrophotometry

the left are said to be laevorotatory. The muscle relaxant *d*-tubocurarine is an example of a dextrorotatary compound. Naturally occuring noradrenaline and adrenaline are examples of laevorotatory substances. Sugar solutions exhibit optical activity, and this led to development of the 'saccharimeter' for measuring the amount of rotation of the plane of polarization produced by optically active solutions. The analyser and polarizer are made of Polaroid which is more efficient than tourmaline.

Lighting in the operating room

Photometric units

Luminous intensity
Light is simply another form of energy, but only the luminous energy in the visible region of the spectrum stimulates the sensation of vision. One of the base units of the SI system is the candela. This is defined as the luminous intensity, in the perpendicular direction, of a surface of 1/600 000 square metres of a black body at the temperature of freezing platinum under a pressure of 101 325 newtons per square metre. The symbol for the candela is cd.

Luminous flux
It is next necessary to consider the luminous flux which occurs when the light radiation from the heated platinum sources falls into a particular solid angle. The SI unit of luminous flux is the lumen (lm) and it is equal to 1 cd. sr. The steradian (sr) is the solid angle which, having its vertex in the centre of a sphere, cuts off an area of the surface of the sphere equal to that of a square with sides of length equal to the radius of the sphere. Taking a collecting period of one second for the luminous flux it can be shown that the radiant energy is equivalent to 0.00146 watts. This is a straight energy conversion for the luminous energy once it has been radiated from the source of light. It must not be confused with the actual conversion efficiency of an electric lamp. Thus a fluorescent lamp might have an efficiency of 70 lumens per watt of power fed into the lamp.

Illuminance (intensity of illumination)
The SI unit of illumination is the lux (1 lumen per square metre). Hopkinson (1964) suggests that the illumination level for lighting the operating area should range between 2153 and 32 292 lux. Hopkinson

makes the point that the eye does not have an arithmetic appreciation of light, and that the difference between 538 and 32 292 lux would under operating room conditions appear to be no greater than a magnitude difference of one to three. It must also be borne in mind that the intensity of illumination will fall off inversely as the square of the distance of the source from the area concerned.

Crul (1964) states that a general level of illumination of 800–1000 lux is desirable in operating rooms. The corresponding level on the operating table would be 20 000–40 000 lux.

Brightness of a surface

The brightness of a surface in a given direction is defined as the luminous flux into a steradian coming from the surface in the particular direction. The brightness of a surface must be carefully distinguished from the intensity of illumination of the surface, which is the luminous flux into a steradian incident on the surface. Thus the brightness B and intensity of illumination E are linked by the reflection factor R; $B = R.E$. Hopkinson (1964) suggests that when a cavity is illuminated, visual comfort is best when the brightness of the immediate surroundings to the task have a brightness of about 1/30 of that of the cavity and the general brightness of the environment is about 1/100 that of the cavity. This is achieved by arranging for the illumination to fall away from the cavity plus the use of drapes of low reflectance.

The spectral composition of operating room lighting

In addition to an adequate intensity of illumination, it is most desirable that the lighting chosen should give rise to a skin colour of the patient which can provide a good warning of impending cyanosis. The effects of absorption and reflection must be a maximum for reduced and oxygenated haemoglobin. The incandescent filament lamp is the most versatile source of light at present available. Its colour rendering, although not the same as daylight, is familiar to everyone. When fluorescent lamps are used to obtain high levels of general illumination, the choice of lamp needs care to enable the onset of cyanosis to be distinguished. *Figure 10.2* shows the variation of the molecular extinction coefficients for reduced and oxygenated haemoglobin plotted against the light wavelength. The maximum difference occurs at 650–700 nm. Crul

(1964) found that a lamp with the Philips 34 colour phosphor was the best for this purpose when little or no daylight is present. This choice was confirmed in the *Memorandum No. 43* (H.M.S.O., 1965) of the U.K. Medical Research Council *Special requirements of light sources for clinical purposes.* Currently the choice is the Philips 37 phosphor which satisfies the requirements of the *Memorandum No. 43* but has a greater light output. A Report No. CP29 of the Illuminating Engineering Society of North America* entitled *Lighting for Health Care Facilities* covers all types of rooms encountered in health care

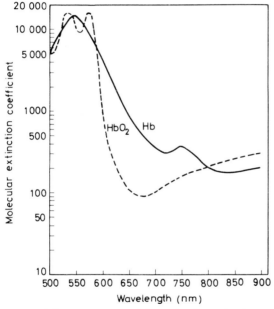

Figure 10.2. The variation of the molecular extinction coefficients for reduced and oxygenated haemoglobin with light wavelength (nm)

facilities and has an extensive table of recommended general and visual-task lighting levels for various purposes and the characteristics of typical light sources are given. The areas discussed in detail include: patient rooms, obstetrics and gynaecology departments, paediatrics, dental suites, and critical care areas.

*Illuminating Engineeering Society of North America, 345 East 47th Street, New York, NY 10017, U.S.A.

Optical instruments of interest to the anaesthetist

Gas analysis by the measurement of refractive index

When a ray of light passes from an optically less dense medium (e.g. air) into an optically more dense medium (e.g. glass) it is refracted so that the angle of refraction *r* is now less than the angle of incidence *i* made with the normal (perpendicular) to the interface separating the media (*Figure 10.3*). The ratio sin *i*/sin *r* is known as the refractive index of the more dense medium with respect to the less dense medium. This is Snell's law. A typical value for the refractive index of glass would be 1.5 with respect to air.

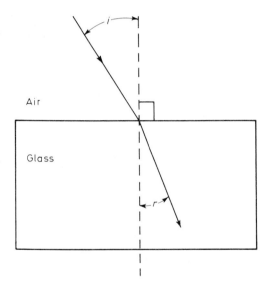

Air

Glass

Figure 10.3

The refractive index of a gas mixture can be measured by means of an optical instrument known as a refractometer and the value depends on the composition of the mixture (Edmondson, 1957; Hill, 1963; Hulands and Nunn, 1970). The refractometer can be calibrated from a knowledge of the refractive index of the gases and vapours concerned and will hold this calibration for years. It is particularly simple to use with binary gas mixtures and is used by makers of anaesthetic vaporizers to calibrate these devices on a mixture of the vapour concerned with air. It is also employed to calibrate dental and analgesic machines with nitrous oxide–oxygen mixtures.

An alternative definition of refractive index which is applicable to a gas mixture is that the refractive index = (velocity of light *in vacuo*)/ velocity of light in the gas mixture). The velocity of light in the mixture depends upon the number of molecules present, i.e. on the density and thus on the temperature and pressure of the gas. The refractive index μ is usually referred to standard conditions of 0 °C and 760 mmHg by assuming that $(\mu-1)\rho$ is a constant where ρ is the density of the gas mixture.

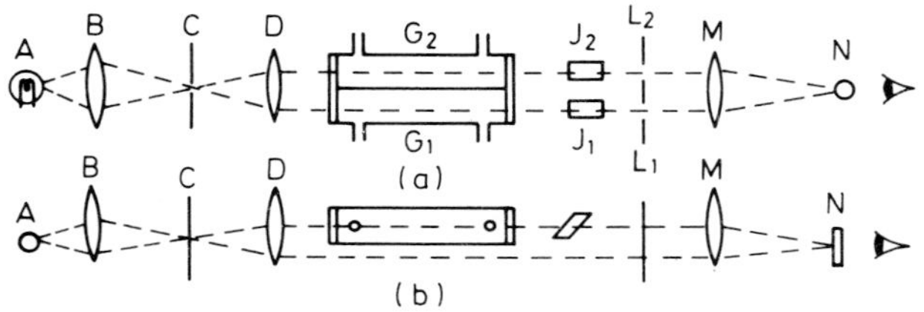

Figure 10.4

The Rayleigh refractometer is often used in laboratories concerned with the calibration of anaesthetic vaporizers (Edmondson, 1957; Luder, 1964). *Figure 10.4* (after Edmondson, 1957) illustrates the principle of the Rayleigh refractometer. White light from the filament lamp A is focussed by lens B on to the vertical slit C which is situated at the focus of lens D. Light emerges from D in a parallel beam and passes through two similar metal tubes fitted with optically flat windows and gas inlet and outlet ports. Each tube can be made gas tight by closing the ports and they do not communicate. Tube G_1 – the sample cell – contains the gas mixture to be analysed, while the reference cell G_2 contains a gas of known refractive index. On emerging from the tubes, the two beams of light pass through a pair of optically flat glass plates J_1 and J_2. The plates are mounted at an angle with J_1 fixed and J_2 capable of being slowly rotated with respect to J_1. On leaving the plates the beams pass through the vertical slits L_1 and L_2 and the lens M which brings them to a focus at N. M is a cylindrical lens eyepiece capable of magnifying only in the horizontal plane. Two other beams of light from lens D pass underneath tubes G_1 and G_2 but not through the plates J_1 and J_2. This light is also seen via lens N by the observer.

If the light from A was monochromatic the observer would perceive a pattern such as *Figure 10.5a*. The horizontal line in the middle is a shadow caused by the bottom wall of tubes G_1 and G_2. The lower vertical lines are produced by optical interference arising between the two beams of light passing beneath G_1 and G_2. The formation of these

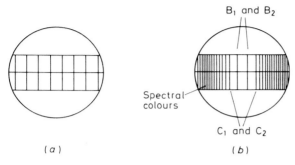

B₁ and B₂

Spectral colours

C₁ and C₂

(a)   (b)

Figure 10.5

fringes is detailed in *Figure 10.6*. Consider a point X located on the axis mid-way between the slits L_1 and L_2, and equidistant from each slit. Light waves passing through the slits are arranged to be exactly in step and since the distances $L_1 X$ and $L_2 X$ are equal the waves will be in step at X where they reinforce each other to produce a band of light. Now consider a point Y such that the distance $L_1 Y$ is one light wavelength less than $L_2 Y$, thus the waves will reinforce again at Y to produce a

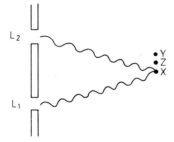

L_2

L_1

Figure 10.6

second bright band of light. Half-way between X and Y at point Z the path length for the two waves will differ by one half a wavelength so the two waves will arrive there exactly out of step. Thus a peak cancels with a trough to produce zero light, i.e. darkness. The view in the eye-piece N consists of a series of alternate vertical bands of light and dark.

When the gas in G_1 is replaced with a gas which has a slightly greater refractive index than that in G_2 the rays passing through G_1 will now be relatively retarded and rays arriving at X will no longer be exactly in step. However, light from L_1 will be in step at some point X with light from L_2 which has taken the longer path $L_2 X$. This effect applies to all the interference bands so that the observer will see the whole of the upper set of fringes move to the left. The lower set of fringes remains stationary since it has not been formed from light which has passed through G_1 and G_2.

With monochromatic light from a laser, all the fringes look much the same and it is difficult to distinguish one from another. It is necessary to be able to do this in order to count the number of fringes moved when the gas mixture in G_1 is changed.

On substituting a white light source the view in the eyepiece changes to that shown in *Figure 10.5b*. At the centre is a fringe of bright light with two sharply defined black fringes B_1 and B_2 on either side. The next pair of dark fringes C_1 and C_2 are less well defined, further fringes being hardly visible. The edges of the field of view show the colours of the rainbow. On changing the composition of the gas in G_1, the upper set of fringes move to the left while the low set of fringes remains stationary. By slowly rotating plate J_2, so that the beam from G_2 now has to pass through a greater thickness of glass, the light from the reference cell G_2 can be retarded by an amount identical to that of the light passing through the sample cell G_1. This has happened when the upper and lower fringe patterns again match. The angle through which J_2 has had to be turned to accomplish this can be calibrated against the refractive index change or against the percentage of one gas or vapour in the sample gas mixture.

Monochromatic light must be used for calibrating the refractometer to read directly in terms of refractive index changes. With the same gas in G_1 and G_2 the black fringes of *Figure 10.5a* are aligned and the reading of the scale attached to J_2 is noted. J_2 is moved to shift the pattern by one fringe and the reading noted. This procedure is repeated for several fringes and the mean dial reading change D_1 found for a shift of one fringe. This is equivalent to a refractive index change of $\Delta\mu$. $D_1 = \Delta\mu = \lambda/L$ where L is the length of the cells G_1 and G_2 and λ is the wavelength of the monochromatic light source.

The source is next changed to white light and the upper and lower fringes of *Figure 10.5b* aligned. The gas or vapour mixture is placed in G_1 and J_2 moved to realign the fringes. If the resulting change in the dial reading is D_2 then the refractive index change arising from the introduction of the mixture is $D_2\Delta\mu$. If the refractive index of the pure vapour concerned at ambient temperature and pressure is μ_1 and that of the pure carrier gas is μ_2 then a 100 per cent vapour in G_1 would produce a refractive index change of $(\mu_1 - \mu_2)$. By simple proportion the percentage of vapour present in the mixture which gave rise to a refractive index change of $D_2\Delta\mu$ can be calculated.

The refractive indices of some gases and vapours at 0 °C and 760 mmHg are given in *Table 10.2.*

TABLE 10.2

Substance	Refractive index
Oxygen	1.000272
Nitrogen	1.000297
Air	1.0002918
Nitrous oxide	1.000515
Carbon dioxide	1.0004498
Chloroform	1.001455
Trichloroethylene	1.001784
Halothane	1.00151 (white light)
Water vapour	1.000257

Rayleigh refractometers are about 1.5 m long as can be seen from the model shown in the Frontispiece of this book. However, portable refractometers which can be hand-held are available and Hulands and Nunn describe their use in anaesthesia. Salamonsen (1978) used a refractometer with a 10 ml cell and monochromatic light obtained from a mercury discharge lamp filtered through a No. 77 Wratten filter to calibrate a vaporizer designed for programmed anaesthesia.

Optical absorption instruments—principles of optical absorption
If I_0 is the intensity of a definite monochromatic wavelength passing into a layer of a substance limited by two parallel planes and of thickness d, and I is the emergent intensity from the layer, then the Lambert–Bouguer law relates I and I_0 by $I=I_0 \exp(-ad)$. These are simple exponential equations where (ad) is called the *optical density* or *absorbance,* and the quantity a is called the Bunsen's extinction coefficient. The layer thickness d is conveniently measured in cm. The optical density is simply the index of a power and must be dimensionless, so that the extinction coefficient is expressed in terms of cm^{-1}.

Thinking back to time constants, the extinction coefficient a can be visualized as the reciprocal of that thickness through which the radiation energy must be passed in order to be reduced to 37 per cent $(1/e)$ of its original value. For $d = 10$ cm, a would be one tenth. Obviously, the larger the thickness d irradiated, the greater the absorption of a body and the larger the extinction coefficient for the wavelength in question. However, the absorption depends on the actual number of molecules irradiated. Hence the extinction coefficient suffices to define the absorption power of a substance provided the number of molecules in the measurement volume remains constant. This will apply to solid and liquid pure substances, but not to mixtures and solutions, or to gases where the molecular density is pressure dependent. A relationship is required between the concentration of a substance and the absorption it produces. Beer's law states that the absorbance is a linear function of the pressure or concentration c. This can be combined with the Lambert–Bouguer law to give the Lambert–Beer law $I=I_0 \exp(-\epsilon c d)$. ϵ is called the extinction coefficient, as was a. Its dimensions depend on the unit selected for the concentration c. If c is in moles/litre, ϵ is called the molar extinction coefficient. It follows that the optical density $D=\epsilon c d$. If the liquid obeys Beer's law a plot of the optical density against concentration for a particular wavelength and absorption cell thickness will yield a straight line. Modern spectrophotometers are usually calibrated directly in terms of both the optical density and the percentage transmission of light by the sample.

Quantitative analysis in spectrophotometry is simplified by the absorption law which states that the optical density varies linearly with concentration, and that the optical densities of the various components in a mixture are additive. When deviations from linearity do occur, then quantitative analysis is only possible by empirical comparison using calibration curves. These deviations are most probably due to interactions between solvent and solute molecules. The following simple theory only applies to solutions whose optical density varies linearly with concentration.

The unknown concentration of one absorbing component in a mixture of non-absorbing components is obtained by a comparison between the pure compound and the sample at one wavelength.

$$\frac{\text{Optical density of compound in mixture}}{\text{Unknown concentration}} = \frac{\text{Optical density of pure compound}}{\text{Concentration of pure compound}}$$

Analysis of two mutually interfering components requires the simultaneous solution of two such equations containing the data at two wavelengths. Additional terms are necessary to correct for the interference of one component at the wavelength position of the other, thus making a total of four optical density terms. The number of terms increases as the square of the number of components. When setting up the spectrophotometer for a two-component analysis, it is necessary to compare the spectra of the pure compounds and to choose for each one a wavelength setting at which its absorption is strongest and the interfering absorption of the other compound is a minimum. In

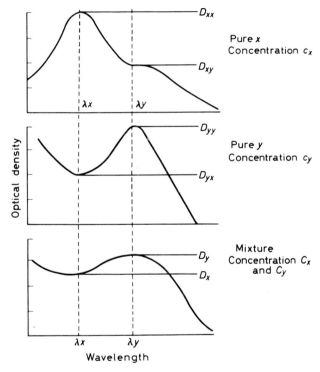

Figure 10.7. The variation of optical density with light wave-length for a binary mixture of absorbing substances

Figure 10.7, if c_x is the concentration of pure x, of optical density D_{xx} at wavelength λ_x, and c_y is the concentration of pure y, of optical density D_{yy} at wavelength λ_y, and C_x and C_y are the concentration of x and y in the mixture, which has an optical density of D_x at λ_x, and D_y at λ_y, then at λ_x,

$$D_x = \frac{D_{xx}C_x}{c_x} + \frac{D_{yx}C_y}{c_y}$$

and at λ_y,

$$D_y = \frac{D_{xy}C_x}{c_x} + \frac{D_{yy}C_y}{c_y}$$

Solution of these two equations enables C_x and C_y to be found. Useful references on spectroscopy are Brügel (1962) and Oster and Pollister (1955).

Ultraviolet spectrophotometric methods are important in the estimation of barbiturates in blood and urine. The methods are based upon the fact that 5,5′-disubstituted barbiturates exist in three forms in solution:

(1) Un-ionized in acid, with no selective absorption at 230–270 nm.
(2) First ionized form, pH 9.8–10.5, with a maximum at 240 nm but no minimum at 230–270 nm.
(3) Second ionized form, pH 13–14 with a maximum at 252–255 nm and a minimum at 234–237 nm.

Barbiturates are characterized by their characteristic absorption spectra between 227 and 260 nm and then estimated from the

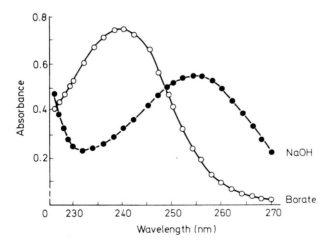

Figure 10.8. The ultraviolet absorption spectra of a barbitone solution. (By courtesy of Pye Unicam)

difference in optical density at pH 13 and pH 10, this difference being proportional to concentration.

Figure 10.8 taken from Broughton (1956) shows the ultraviolet absorption spectra of a barbitone solution (13.5 μg ml^{-1}). The criteria for its presence are seen to be

(1) In borate: maximum at 238–240 nm.
(2) In NaOH: maximum at 252–255 nm and a minimum at 234–237 nm.
(3) Isobestic points (points of equal optical density) at 227–230 nm and 247–250 nm.

For comparison, *Figure 10.9* shows the ultraviolet absorption spectra of a normal blood extract. *Figure 10.10* illustrates the spectra of a barbiturate in urine.

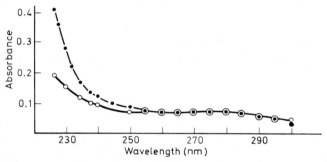

Figure 10.9. The ultraviolet absorption spectra of a normal blood extract. (By courtesy of Pye Unicam)

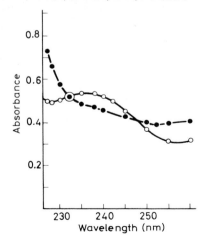

Figure 10.10. The ultraviolet absorption spectra of a barbitone in urine. (By courtesy of Pye Unicam)

If C (μg ml^{-1}) is the concentration of barbiturate in the solution measured and F is a calibration factor, then at 260 nm, $C=F(D_N-D_B)$.

If V_1 = volume (ml) of specimen taken

V_2 = volume (ml) of 0.45N NaOH used for extraction

d = total dilution of extract before measurement

then

$$\text{blood barbiturate} = \frac{dV_2 F(D_N-D_B)}{10\,V_1}\,\text{mg}/100\text{ ml.}$$

The factor F varies with the type of barbiturate, being 43.7 for phenobarbitone, and 48.1 for pentobarbitone.

The identification of barbiturates is also discussed by Curry (1959). Ultraviolet spectrophotometric methods have been employed by Burns *et al.* (1955) for the estimation of pethidine, by Wiser, Knebel and Siefter (1960) for the estimation of promazine and by Crawford (1956) for the estimation of thiopentone.

The absorption spectrum of indocyanine green dye

Indocyanine green dye (Fox *et al.*, 1957, 1960) is now widely accepted for the determination of cardiac output by the dye dilution technique. When the dye is diluted in plasma to a concentration of less than 70 mg l^{-1}, it exhibits a single absorption peak at 805 nm when the spectral range 650–850 nm is considered. An attractive feature of this dye is that its optical absorption occurs at an isobesic point where the absorption of oxygenated and reduced haemoglobin are equal. Thus changes occurring in the oxygenation of the patient's blood will not affect the apparent absorption of the dye in blood. Saunders *et al.* (1970) found that the dye in plasma obeys Beer's law over the range of concentration 0–25 mg l^{-1}. However, these workers also found that in high concentrations of dye the plot of optical density against wavelength is radically altered from that obtaining at concentrations of 70 mg l^{-1} or less (*Figure 10.11*). It can be seen that at high concentrations the absorption is shifted towards regions of lower wavelengths. Thus an optical densitometer centred on 805 nm will read lower than it should under these conditons. Saunders *et al.* found that blood flows calculated from indicator–dilution curves with a bolus injection of indocyanine green overestimated the actual flow in dog right heart-bypass preparations and several models by 20–60 per cent. A low value of the optical density is equivalent to a high flow. The error was similar with blood and plasma and was not due

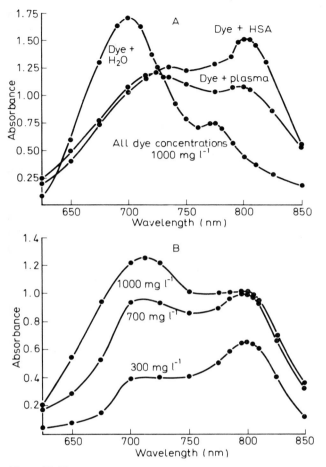

Figure 10.11

to pulsatile flow, negative cuvette pressures (−500 mmHg), instability, hysteresis, or the patterns of alinearity and response to a rising baseline in either Waters XP302 or Gilford 103 IR densitometers. The frequency response of these densitometers was adequate. The error is thought to be due to the delay in changing from the absorption spectrum of concentrated dye (1000 mg l^{-1}) to the different spectrum of dilute dye (1–40 mg l^{-1}). This change is likely to be due to molecular disaggregation since it is known that many organic dyes in aqueous solution form aggregates. The change was found to take about 6–8 seconds to complete at room temperature as verified by delay-loop and stopped-flow experiments. It was faster at 37 °C. The effect could be significant in studies where the dye appearance time is less than 8 seconds, for example in renal flow estimations. Saunders *et al.* found no flow estimations with Evans blue dye (T-1824) which showed a spectral shift on dilution.

Non-dispersive infra-red gas analysers

Infra-red gas analysers are commonly available for the measurement of carbon monoxide, carbon dioxide, nitrous oxide, ether, halothane and any of the other voltaile anaesthetics. They are much used in anaesthetic and respiratory research. The conventional medical infra-red gas analyser works on the Luft principle (Luft, 1943), illustrated in *Figure 10.12*. Two equal strength beams of infra-red radiation from the

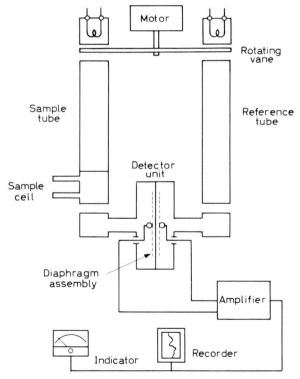

Figure 10.12. Schematic diagram of a Luft-type infra-red gas analyser

hot wire spirals fall one on to each half of the condenser microphone assembly. Each half of the detector is identical, and is filled to a sub-atmospheric pressure with the pure gas or vapour to be analysed. For example the detector of a halothane analyser would be filled with pure halothane vapour. This arrangement helps to make the instrument selective, since the detector can only absorb those infra-red wave-lengths which can be absorbed by the sample in the sample cell. This is fitted with windows made from artificial sapphire or arsenic tri-sulphide since ordinary glass will not pass infra-red. The infra-red spectra of CO_2 and N_2O overlap, and unwanted effects in a CO_2 analyser due to the presence of N_2O can be avoided by using filter cells filled with pure N_2O. This is important when measuring expired CO_2 during nitrous oxide anaesthesia. Because of absorption in the sample cell, the beam falling on the sample side of the detector is weaker than that falling on the reference side. Hence the vapour in the reference side receives more heat than that in the sample side. As a result, the diaphragm is pushed slightly over to the sample side of the detector. The infra-red beams are interrupted at 25 Hz or more, and the alternating signal appearing across the detector is amplified with a high impedance input a.c. amplifier, rectified and displayed on a meter or recorder. A carbon dioxide infra-red gas analyser for respiratory studies is shown in *Figure 10.13*. Similar analysers to this

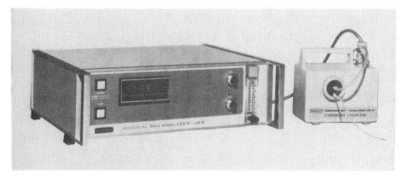

Figure 10.13. Beckman Model LB2 Medical Gas Analyser with carbon dioxide sampling head. (By courtesy of Beckman-RIIC Ltd)

are still in use for the measurement of end-tidal carbon dioxide tension values (Dohi and Gold, 1979). In some types of analyser, the whole tidal volume passes through the sample cell, but in others, such as that used by Dohi and Gold (1979) a pump draws through a steady stream of the gas mixture at a flow of the order of 500 ml min^{-1}. A comprehensive review of Luft-type infra-red gas analysers occurs in the book by Hill and Powell (1965). Hill and Stone (1964) describe a fully-transistorized infra-red gas analyser designed for anaesthetic and respiratory measurements, which can be powered from a six-volt accumulator. It uses an indium antimonide photoconductive detector and employs narrow band optical interference filters to select the appropriate wavebands for the gas and vapours of anaesthetic and respiratory interest. Recent years have seen a marked improvement in the manufacturing technology for optical interference filters and a number of gas analysers are now available based on these devices.

Infra-red gas analysers have been largely superseded by the quadrupole mass spectrometer since this is also sufficiently fast in response for a breath-by-breath analysis, but it can also measure gases such as argon, oxygen and nitrogen as well as carbon dioxide. The instrument uses a combination of d.c. and radiofrequency fields to select ions which have a specified charge-to-mass ratio. It is thus impossible with a normal mass spectrometer to resolve nitrous oxide and carbon dioxide directly since they both have a mass of 44. If carbon dioxide is measured directly, nitrous oxide can be measured indirectly by monitoring a subsidiary peak, e.g. that for nitric oxide.

The ultraviolet halothane analyser

General purpose laboratory spectrophotometers, such as the Pye Unicam SP6-550 (*Figure 10.14*) are fitted with quartz optics since ordinary glass will not pass ultraviolet and quartz can be used in both the ultraviolet and visible regions of the spectrum. A deuterium discharge lamp is used as the light source in the ultraviolet and a tungsten–halogen incandescent lamp in the visible. Wavelength selection is accomplished with a blazed holographic diffraction grating and a large digital display with an adjustable decimal point is provided for the display of concentration measurements. The wavelength range covered is 195 to 1000 nm.

Using a spectrophotometer of this type it can be easily shown that halothane exhibits a considerable absorption in the ultraviolet over the range 200–270 nm (Barrett and Nunn, 1972). Mackay and Kalow (1958) used a Beckman spectrophotometer at 228 nm to estimate the halothane concentrations produced by four different vaporizers. A quantum of ultraviolet light is more energetic than that of a quantum of infra-red radiation, and this means that a simpler means of detecting

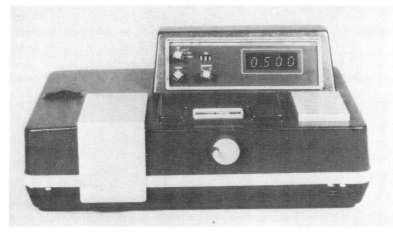

Figure 10.14. Ultraviolet spectrophotometer. (By courtesy of Pye Unicam Ltd)

ultraviolet light can be employed. This fact led to the development of the ultraviolet halothane analyser by Robinson, Denson and Summers (1962). Ultraviolet light at 253.7 nm is generated by a small mercury vapour discharge lamp and falls on to a pair of photocells. An optical absorption cell is placed between the lamp and one photocell. The output voltage from each photocell is fed to a grid of a balanced double triode cathode follower (*Figure 10.15*). The mains transformer and the

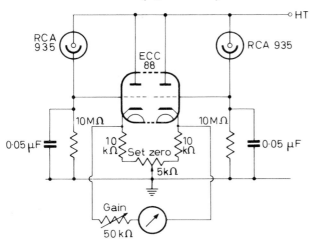

Figure 10.15. Halothane meter circuit

lamp are fed from a constant voltage transformer. The reference photocell simply monitors the output of the lamp. If there is any halothane
vapour in the absorption cell which is fitted with quartz windows, the
output of the sample photocell is diminished, and the cathode follower
measures the difference between the photocell outputs. The meter is
calibrated 0–5 per cent v/v of halothane. The lamp house carries two
V-shaped shutters. Since the reference photocell is nearer the lamp than
the sample photocell, one shutter is used to cut down the light intensity
falling on the reference photocell until it is the same as that falling on
the sample photocell. The other shutter can be switched in to provide
a signal equivalent to the absorption produced by 5 per cent halothane.

In the Research Department of Anaesthetics, the halothane analyser
has proved to be extremely useful in clinical practice. At least half an
hour must be allowed for the instrument to warm up and the zero to
stabilize. This is mainly due to the lamp. Jennings and Hersant (1965)
describe increases in the delivered halothane concentration which
occurred following the refilling of certain vaporizers. An ultraviolet
halothane analyser was employed (*Figure 10.16*). The analyser has its

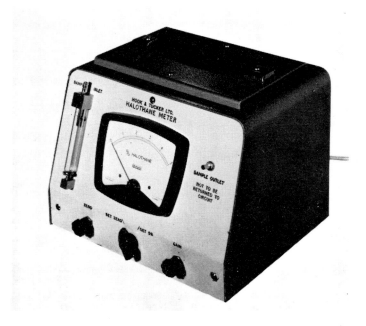

Figure 10.16. Halothane meter. (By courtesy of Hook & Tucker Ltd)

own sampling pump which draws approximately 25 ml min^{-1} of gas through the analyser from the anaesthetic circuit. The action of the ultraviolet light on the halothane gives rise to parts per million of irritant decomposition products. For this reason, it is better not to feed the effluent back into the circuit. However, if this has to be done in order for gas volume measurements to be made the effluent should be passed through a fresh soda lime canister.

The gas discharge nitrogen meter

The fact that nitrogen molecules can be excited in a low pressure electric discharge to emit visible light in the purple region forms the basis of the nitrogen meter (*Figure 10.17*). This is widely used to determine nitrogen wash-out curves in lung function testing. A fraction of the expired air is passed through the d.c. discharge tube by the action of the vacuum pump. The voltage between the electrodes is about 1500 V. Any nitrogen present is excited as a purple glow. Optical filters select the appropriate wavelengths in the violet, and the resulting light intensity is measured with a photocell and amplifier. The rotating chopping disk interrupts the light and allows the use of a stable a.c. amplifier (Lundin and Akesson, 1954).

Unfortunately, oxygen does not have suitable absorption bands in the ultraviolet, infra-red or visible and for dynamic studies it is best measured along with nitrogen and other respiratory gases by means of a quadrupole mass spectrometer. For static measurements of oxygen, a paramagnetic oxygen analyser is capable of an accuracy commensurate with that of a Haldane apparatus (Ellis and Nunn, 1968; Nunn, 1964).

Another application of the nitrogen meter occurs in the measurement of the closing volume of the lungs. The closing volume is the volume of the lungs during expiration over which emptying of the dependent (lowermost) regions of the lungs is markedly reduced or ceases. It is presumed that this action is due to closure of the small airways. Airway closure has not yet been directly demonstrated in man, but there are clinical and experimental observations which are consistent with this hypothesis. The patient having been breathing air makes a maximal inspiration of pure oxygen and then slowly exhales his vital capacity while the expired volume is required with a spirometer and the exhaled nitrogen concentration is recorded with the nitrogen meter. Using an $X-Y$ recorder, the expired volume is plotted on the

Gas discharge nitrogen meter

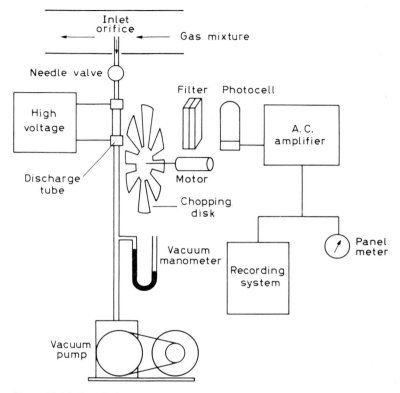

Figure 10.17. Gas discharge nitrogen meter

X-axis and the expired nitrogen concentration on the Y-axis. The graph has four phases:

(1) Dead space gas,
(2) mixed alveolar and dead space gas,
(3) an 'alveolar plateau' of alveolar gas, and
(4) a terminal and abrupt increase in the slope of the alveolar plateau.

The onset of the closure of the small airways is shown by the sharp increase in the expired nitrogen concentration when the lung volume is close to the residual volume. The closing volume is measured as the volume change from the onset of phase (4) to the end of expiration as a percentage of the vital capacity. Amaha (1979) points out that the measurement of closing volume may prove of value as a means of monitoring early signs of small airway disease. Closing volume increases linearly with age while functional residual capacity (lung volume at resting end-expiration) remains relatively constant.

Oximeters

Oximeters are used to measure the degree of oxygenation of the blood and are calibrated in terms of the percentage saturation of the blood with oxygen. Their operation depends on the fact that there is a large difference between the optical absorption coefficient of haemoglobin and oxyhaemoglobin in the red region of the spectrum around 650 nm, whilst there is an isobestic point in the near infra-red at 800 nm. At the isobesic point the molecular extinction coefficients for haemoglobin and oxyhaemoglobin are equal (*Figure 10.2*). Light from an incandescent lamp falls on the blood contained in a cuvette, and is scattered by the blood cells. In reflection oximeters, the light scattered backwards is measured, whilst in transmission oximeters the light scattered in the forward direction as well as the transmitted light is measured. Filters peaked at 650 and 800 nm select the red and infra-red wavelengths which are measured with a pair of miniature cadmium sulphide photoconductive cells. Strictly speaking, the oxygen saturation of the blood is proportional to the ratio of the optical density of the blood at the red wavelength to that at the infra-red wavelength. Cornwall, Marshall and Boyes (1963) describe an oximeter in which the output meter is a ratiometer calibrated directly in percentage saturation. Reichert (1966) shows that for practical purposes it is satisfactory to measure the difference between the absorption at the red and infra-red wavelengths. This leads him to the very simple arrangement shown in *Figure 10.18*. The cadmium sulphide photocells are used in a bridge arrangement, and give a sufficiently large output to eliminate the need for any amplifier. When resistor R_4 is placed in the diagonal of the bridge, the voltage drop appearing across it is proportional to the difference between the absorptions in the red and infra-red. The four arms of the bridge are formed by the light-sensitive resistors R_{cr} and R_{ir} together with their series resistors R, and the two fixed resistors R_3. Adjustment of the lamps is carried out with the cuvette filled with water. Since water does not produce scattering and has only a small absorption coefficient, the output meter circuits must be altered to reduce their sensitivity whilst the adjustment is made. Switched multiplier resistors allow for full-scale meter deflections of 5 and 25 V. If desired, resistor R_4 in the bridge diagonal can be short-circuited to provide two independent circuits for the red and infra-red. The ratio of these can then be calculated.

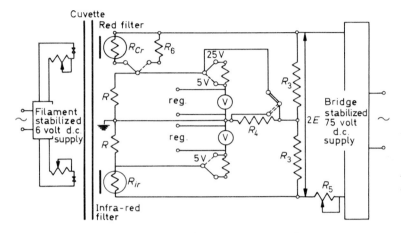

Figure 10.18. Electrical circuit of a transmission oximeter. (After Reichert, 1966)

If the red photocell is replaced with a fixed resistor, it is then possible to record dye-dilution curves for cardiac output studies using the dye cardio-green. If a blue dye is to be used, the infra-red photocell must be replaced with a fixed resistor.

Fibre optic catheter and cannula oximeters

Cuvette oximeters require the availability of a series of discrete blood samples so that they are unsuitable for following rapid changes in blood oxygenation unless the cuvette is incorporated into an extra-corporeal circulation. Cuvette densitometers for dye dilution cardiac output measurements require the use of a motor-driven syringe to draw a constant flow of blood from an artery through the cuvette. Considerable trouble can be experienced in practice with the presence of air bubbles in the line and it takes time to return the blood to the patient. An interesting development has arisen with the availability of fibre optic cardiac catheters and arterial cannulae.

A fibre optic or 'light pipe' operates on the principle of total internal reflection. The light pipe consists of a bundle of glass fibres. Each fibre is made from a central core of glass surrounded by a cladding of another glass which has a lower refractive index than that of the core. Light incident upon the interface between the two glasses at angles of incidence greater than the critical angle undergoes total internal reflection and is transmitted efficiently down the fibre, as shown in *Figure 10.19.* In fibre optic catheters and cannulae it is only required to

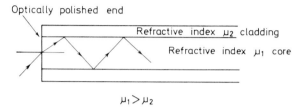

$$\mu_1 > \mu_2$$

Figure 10.19. Principle of operation of a fibre optic

transmit light intensities and not to view an image as in a gastroscope. The individual fibre diameters can be of the order of 50–100 μm and the individual fibre ends do not have to be in precise geometrical alignment at either end of the catheter. In the case of a No. 7 French gauge cardiac catheter, the fibres are mounted inside a radio-opaque sleeving. At the proximal end, they are separated to form two equal bundles. Light from a suitable wavelength source is transmitted down the length of the catheter via one bundle. With the catheter in blood, a portion of the incident light is reflected back down the other half of the fibres as a result of scattering from the erhythrocytes and is led to a suitable optical detector.

Gamble *et al.* (1965) have described an earlier version of a fibre optic catheter oximeter. Light from a tungsten filament lamp was focused by means of two lenses on to the transmitting bundle of fibres. The light reflected back from the catheter tip passed through a rotating glass disc which had alternate clear and mirror segments mounted near its periphery. This arrangement divided the reflected light into 550 pulses per second. The clear glass segments allowed the light to fall on to a 650 nm optical filter, while the reflecting segments directed the light on to an 850 nm optical filter. As a result, pulses of light alternatively of 650 and 850 nm wavelength fall on to a photomultiplier. The output signal from the photomultiplier is amplified and synchronously rectified. The reference signal for the synchronous rectifier is obtained from the phototransistor. The ratio of the reflected light intensities is then taken and displayed on a meter or recorder calibrated in percentage oxygen saturation. The response time of the oximeter was 0.1 s and it was used *in vivo* for up to 3 hours. The fast response of the instrument makes it particularly useful for exercise studies, but the need for a powerful projection lamp and a photomultiplier made the instrument and its power supplies rather bulky.

The availability of light-emitting diodes with wavelengths of 660, 805 and 930 nm has made possible the design of an elegant fibre optic oximeter/densitometer using a silicon photodetector and plastic fibre catheters. The ratio of the reflected light at 660 and 805 nm is proportional to the percentage oxygen saturation of the blood, whilst the ratio at 805 and 930 nm is proportional to the concentration of indocyanine green dye in the blood. The saturation and dye concentration values can be displayed on a digital display or on a recorder. There is no electrical risk to a cardiac patient because of the nonconducting nature of the catheter. Fibre optic catheters in the range No. 4 to No. 7 French gauge are available; the No. 6 and 7 French catheters also have a lumen for the measurement of blood pressure, the injection of dye or the withdrawal of blood. It is also possible to have an arterial cannula or a fibre optic Swan-Ganz catheter. With its inflatable balloon the Swan-Ganz catheter can easily be floated into the pulmonary artery and has two free lumina. One of these ends at the catheter tip and the other approximately 30 cm before the tip so that it can be used for the injection of cardiogreen dye. Thus with the same catheter it is possible to measure the oxygen saturation, cardiac output and blood pressure as well as inject drugs or withdraw blood. The three light-emitting diodes are located in a small box which accepts the two ends of the catheter and can be strapped to the patient's arm. The light output from the diodes is modulated at 300 Hz thus obviating the need for a rotating chopper disc. An adjustment can be made to allow for the effects of haematocrits which are substantially different from normal. The measurement accuracy is quoted as $\pm$ 1 per cent HbO_2 at 100 per cent saturation and $\pm$ 2 per cent HbO_2 at 0 per cent saturation. The accuracy with dye is $\pm$ 4 per cent of the dye concentration. A built-in integrator can be provided to measure the area under the dye dilution curve and to give a digital display of the cardiac output in litres per minute for pre-selected injectate volumes of 0.2, 0.5, 1, 2 or 5 ml of indocyanine green dye solution (2.5 mg cm^{-3}). When the dye is detected at some distance from the heart the curve will have a recirculation peak and the integrator then uses an extrapolation algorithm to find the area. If the dye is detected in the left ventricle or close to it the recirculation peak will be absent and a simple integration will be sufficient (Hugenholtz *et al.*, 1965).

The availability of a fibre optic oximeter allows the monitoring for periods of 12 hours or more of the mixed venous oxygen saturation. This has proved a valuable variable to monitor under intensive care circumstances for the detection of patients with incipient circulatory distress. Krauss *et al.* (1974) reported that in 19 patients following cardiac or lung surgery plus 12 patients with acute myocardial infarction there was a correlation coefficient of 0.85 between mixed venous oxygen saturation and the cardiac index. A mixed venous oxygen saturation of less than 65 per cent indicated a cardiac index of less than 2.5 l min^{-1} m^{-2}. In nine out of ten post-operative patients in whom the mixed venous oxygen saturation was less than 65 per cent, Krauss *et al.* (1974) found at some time during the period of monitoring serious complications such as shock, ventricular arrhythmias and renal and respiratory disturbances. A fall in the mixed venous oxygen saturation of 5 volumes per cent or a value of less than 60 per cent preceded a period of hypotension in six patients. In two of them this coincided with ventricular arrhythmias. When the mixed venous oxygen saturation rose above 65 per cent convalescence was undisturbed. Monitoring of the mixed venous oxygen saturation gave immediate warning of a respiratory failure which could occur due to endotracheal tube suctioning or discontinuous ventilatory support. It was also possible to judge easily the beneficial or deleterious effects of interventions such as rapid fluid loading, physiotherapy or the administration of inotropic agents.

The design of a fibre optic oximeter based on the use of light-emitting diodes is described by Johnson, Palm and Stewart (1971), and its use in clinical practice by Coles *et al.* (1972) and Martin *et al.* (1973). Coles *et al.* (1972) found that in six healthy subjects the mixed venous oxygen saturation was greater than 60 per cent for more than 98.4 per cent of the monitored period. However, in eight cardiac patients the mixed venous oxygen tension was less than 60 per cent for 35 per cent of the monitored period and less than 40 per cent for 45 per cent of the period.

Plastic fibre optic catheters of only 4 French gauge are now available with a lumen which can be used for blood sampling, pressure monitoring or drug/fluid/blood administration (Wilkinson, Gregory and Phibbs, 1977, 1978) and this has extended the use of the technique to measurements in sick neonates. When two catheters are available, one can be employed to monitor the arterial oxygen saturation and the other the mixed venous oxygen saturation. The difference of the saturation readings gives the A-V oxygen difference. This is being taken as a sensitive 'normalized' index of the adequacy of the cardiac output and of the prognosis of survival after an acute myocardial infarction.

References

AMAHA, K. (1979). Anesthesia and Respiration in *Advanced Health Care Technology* (Ed. by M. Saito and T. Furukawa). Tokyo; Technocrat Technical Survey Books

BARRETT, A.M. and NUNN, J.F. (1972). Absorption spectra of the common anaesthetic agents in the far ultraviolet. *Br. J. Anaesth.* **44**, 306

BROUGHTON, P.M.G. (1956). A rapid ultraviolet spectrophotometric method for the detection, estimation and identification of barbiturates in biological material. *Biochem. J.* **63**, 207

BRÜGEL, WERNER (1962). *An Introduction to Infra-red Spectroscopy.* London; Methuen

BURNS, J.J., BERGER, B.L., LIEF, P.A., WOLLACK, A., PAPPER, E.M. and BRODIE, B.B.(1955). Physiological disposition and fate of meperidine (Demerol) in man, and a method for its estimation in plasma. *J. Pharmac. exp. Ther.* **114**, 289

COLES, J.S., MARTIN, W.E., CHEUNG, P.W. and JOHNSON, C.C. (1972). Clinical studies with a solid state fibre optic oximeter. *Am. J. Cardiol.* **29**, 383

CORNWALL, J.B., MARSHALL, D.C. and BOYES, J. (1963). A cuvette oximeter and an extension to the theory of oximetry. *J. scient. instrum.* **40**, 253

COULSON, J.S. (1941). *Waves,* p. 3. Edinburgh; Oliver & Boyd

CRAWFORD, J.S. (1956). Some aspects of obstetric anaesthesia. *Br. J. Anaesth.* **28**, 146

CRUL, J.F. (1964). Lighting in operating theatres. In *Operating Theatres and Auxiliary Rooms* (Ed. by T.C. Gray and J.F. Nunn), p. 192. Altrincham; Sherratt

CURRY, A.S. (1959). Identification of barbiturates. *Nature, Lond.* **183**, 1052

DOHI, S. and GOLD, M.J. (1979). Pulmonary mechanics during general anaesthesia. *Br. J. Anaesth.* **51**, 205–214

EDMONDSON, W. (1957). Gas analysis by refractive index measurement. *Br. J. Anaesth.* **29**, 570

ELLIS, F.R. and NUNN, J.F. (1968). The measurement of gaseous oxygen tension utilizing paramagnetism: an evaluation of the Servomex OA150 analyser. *Br. J. Anaesth.* **40**, 569–578

FOX, I.J., BROOKER, L.G.S., HESELTINE, D.W., ESSEX, H.E. and WOOD, E.H. (1957). A tricarbocyanine dye for continuous recording of dilution curves in whole blood independent of variations in blood oxygen saturation. *Proc. Staff Meet. Mayo Clin.* **32**, 478

FOX, I.J., and WOOD, E.H. (1960). Indocyanine green: Physical and physiological properties. *Proc. Staff Meet. Mayo Clin.* **35**, 732

GAMBLE, W.J., HUGENHOLTZ, P.G., MONROE, R.G., POLYANI, M. and NADAS, A.S. (1965). The use of fibre optics in clinical cardiac catheterisation. *Circulation* **31**, 328

HILL, D.W. (1963). Halothane concentrations with a Dräger 'Vapor' vaporizer. *Br. J. Anaesth.* **35**, 285–289

HILL, D.W. and POWELL, T. (1965). *Non-dispersive infra-red gas analysers in science, medicine and industry.* Bristol; Adam Hilger

HILL, D.W. and STONE, R.N. (1963). A transistor-driven gas sampling pump. *J. scient. Instrum.* **40**, 421

HILL, D.W. and STONE, R.N.(1964). A versatile infra-red gas analyser using transistors. *J. scient. Instrum.* **41**, 732

HOPKINSON, R.G. (1964). The lighting of operating theatres. In *Operating Theatres and Auxiliary Rooms* (Ed. by T.C. Gray and J.F. Nunn), p. 176. Altrincham; Sherratt

HUGENHOLTZ, P.G., GAMBLE, W.J., MONROE, R.G. and POLYANI, M.L. (1965). The use of fibre optics in clinical cardiac catheterisation, 2. *In vivo* dye-dilution curves. *Circulation* **31**, 344

HULANDS, G.H. and NUNN, J.F. (1970). Portable interference refractometers in anaesthesia. *Br. J. Anaesth.* **42**, 1051–1059

KRAUSS, X.H., VERDOUW, P.D., HAGEMEIJER, F., NAUTA, J. and HUGEN-HOLTZ, P.G. (1974). Instantaneous and continuous mixed venous oxygen saturation, a leading indicator in cardiorespiratory failure. *Scient. Abstr. First World Congr. on Intensive Care*, p. 30. London

JENNINGS, A.M.C. and HERSANT, M.E. (1965). Increase in halothane concentration following refilling of certain vaporizers. *Br. J. Anaesth.* **37**, 137

JOHNSON, C.C., PALM, R.D. and STEWART, D.C. (1971). A solid state fibre optic oximeter. *J. Ass. Adv. Med. Instrum.* **5**, 77

LUDER, M.(1964). Measurement of halothane concentrations with the interferometer. *Anaesthetist* **13**, 360–364

LUFT, K.F. (1943). Uber eine neue Methode der registrierenden Gas-analyse mit Hilfe der absorption ultraroter Strahlen ohne spektrale Zerlegung. *Z. tech. Phys.* **24**, 97

LUNDIN, G. and AKESSON, L. (1954). A new nitrogen meter model. *Scand. J. clin. Lab. Invest.* **6**, 251

MACKAY, I.M. and KALOW, W. (1958). A clinical and laboratory evaluation of four fluothane vaporizers. *Can. Anaesth. Soc. J.* **5**, 248

MARTIN, W.E., CHEUNG, P.W., JOHNSON, C.C. and WONG, K.C. (1973). Continuous monitoring of mixed venous oxygen saturation in man. *Curr. Res. Anaesth. Analg.* **52**, 784

NUNN, J.F. (1964). Evaluation of the Servomex paramagnetic oxygen analyser. *Br. J. Anaesth.* **30**, 264–268

OSTER, G. and POLLISTER, A.W. (1955). *Physical Techniques in Biological Research. Vol. 1. Optical Techniques.* New York; Academic Press

PARRISH, J.A., ANDERSON, R.R., URBACH, F. and PITTS, D. (1978). *UV-A.* New York; Wiley

REICHERT, W.J. (1966). The theory and construction of oximeters. In *Oxygen Measurements in Blood and Tissues and Their Significance* (Ed. by J.P. Payne and D.W. Hill), p.81. London; Churchill

ROBINSON, A., DENSON, J.S. and SUMMERS, F.W. (1962). Halothane analyser. *Anesthesiology* **23**, 391

SALOMONSEN, R.F. (1978). A vaporizing system for programmed anaesthesia. *Br. J. Anaesth.* **50**, 425–433

SAUNDERS, K.B., HOFFMAN, J.I.E., NOBLE, M.I.M. and DOMENECH, R.J. (1970). A source of error in measuring flow with indocyanine green. *J. Appl. Physiol.* **28**, 190

WILKINSON, A.R., GREGORY, G.A. and PHIBBS, R.R. (1977). Continuous measurement of oxygen saturation in sick newborn infants. *Clinical Research* **25**, February

WILKINSON, A.R., PHIBBS, R.R. and GREGORY, G.A. (1978). *In vivo* oxygen dissociation curves in transfused and untransfused newborn infants. *Clinical Research* **26**, February

WISER, R., KNEBEL, C. and SEIFTER, J. (1960). Determination of promazine in biological materials. *Pharmacologist* **2**, 83

11 Ionizing radiations

The atomic structure of matter

For the present purpose, it is convenient to think in terms of an atomic structure comprising a relatively massive central nucleus, surrounded by one or more orbital electrons. The diameter of an atom is about 10^{-10} m, whereas that of the nucleus is some 10^{-14} m, i.e. some 10 000 times smaller. The simplest atom is that of hydrogen with one proton in its nucleus and one orbital electron. The proton is a positively charged particle of mass approximately 1840 times greater than that of an electron. Normally, an atom is electrically neutral, that is the positive charge on the nucleus is balanced by an equal negative charge due to the orbital electrons.

In addition to protons, the nuclei of elements other than hydrogen contain neutrons. A neutron is a particle of mass approximately the same as that of a proton, but uncharged.

X-radiation

The existence of X-radiation was discovered by Wilhelm Röntgen in 1895. It is always produced when high speed electrons strike matter. In a modern X-ray tube, a potential of tens of thousands of volts is generated across a pair of electrodes mounted in a highly evacuated tube (Strettan, 1965). The negative electrode or cathode contains a heated filament which acts as a source of electrons. In a fixed anode X-ray tube the positive electrode, or anode, consists of a massive copper block in which is embedded a block of tungsten. Electrons from the cathode are accelerated under the influence of the high electric field to strike the tungsten part of the anode, where X-radiation is emitted. In order to produce sharp shadows, a small area source of X-rays is required, and the beam of electrons is focused on to an area of about 3×1 mm. To prevent vaporization of the anode occurring due to the heat produced the target area of the anode is made of a high melting point material (such as tungsten). The bulk of the anode is made from a copper block which acts as a heat sink during the exposure and ensures that the heat produced is conducted away during the period between exposures. In practice, as shown in *Figure 11.1*, the radiating face of

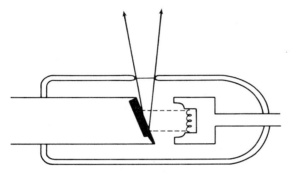

Figure 11.1. Line focus X-ray tube

the anode is cut at an angle of 19 ° with the plane perpendicular to its axis. X-rays emerging from the 'line focus' through the exit window appear to be coming from a much shorter line. If the line focus is 3 long $\times$ 1 mm wide, its length will appear to be 3 sin 19 °=0.98 mm. Its width will be unaltered and so the effective focal area is 0.98 mm $\times$ 1 mm.

From the viewpoint of the anaesthetist and surgeon, it is important to consider the precautions that are taken in the tube design to minimize stray radiation which could strike the operating team. Radiation protection is accomplished by fitting a lead shield around that part of the tube where the X-rays are produced, leaving only a small exit port (*Figure 11.2*). X-ray tube and lead shield are placed in a metal housing which is then filled with high-insulation transformer oil. The high voltage supplies are brought into it by means of heavily insulated cables. Heat generated in the X-ray tube is conducted through the oil to the outer metal casing and thence to the atmosphere. In order

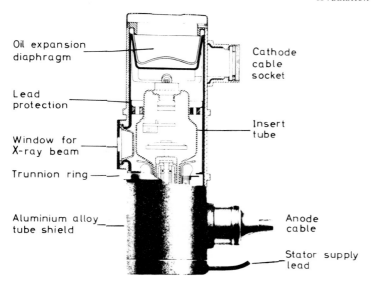

Oil expansion diaphragm

Lead protection

Window for X-ray beam

Trunnion ring

Aluminium alloy tube shield

Cathode cable socket

Insert tube

Anode cable

Stator supply lead

Figure 11.2. Section through X-ray tube housing

to guard against high pressures developing in the tube housing due to excess heating of the oil in long exposures, as in therapy, metal expansion bellows are made part of the housing. As the oil heats up, the bellows expand. When the danger limit is reached, the bellows trip a switch and cut off the mains supply to the apparatus. With this arrangement, there must be no gas inside the oil-filled metal housing, which has to be evacuated before the oil is put in. If the X-ray beam had to pass through the oil, it would be absorbed and scattered, hence an insulated cone is fitted in contact with the tube wall and through this the useful X-ray beam emerges. In all modern X-ray sets, a series of adjustable metal diaphragms is fitted in front of the tube exit window to define the size of the emergent beam. Unwanted leakage and scattered X-radiation from the tube is of concern to the surgeon and anaesthetist. Under international regulations the leakage radiation from the tube shield is limited to 0.1 mSv (100 mrem) in any one hour at 1 m, when the tube is run at its maximum rated output. This applies to tubes used in diagnostic equipment only. In practice the leakage radiation from British X-ray tubes is less than one-tenth of the permitted amount. The smaller, portable X-ray sets rated at up to 100 mA at 90 kV use a fixed anode X-ray tube, whereas for higher

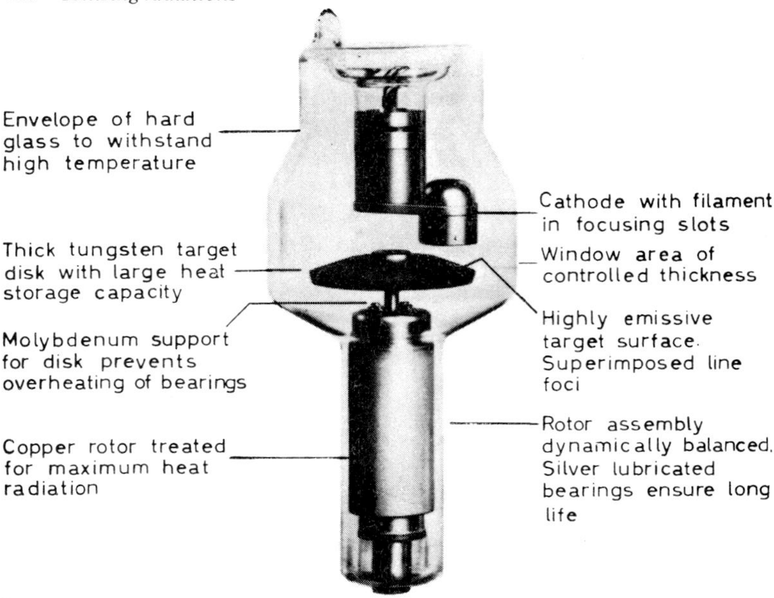

Envelope of hard
glass to withstand
high temperature

Thick tungsten target
disk with large heat
storage capacity

Molybdenum support
for disk prevents
overheating of bearings

Copper rotor treated
for maximum heat
radiation

Cathode with filament
in focusing slots

Window area of
controlled thickness

Highly emissive
target surface.
Superimposed line
foci

Rotor assembly
dynamically balanced.
Silver lubricated
bearings ensure long
life

Figure 11.3. Rotating anode X-ray tube

current ratings, rotating anode tubes (*Figure 11.3*) are usually employed. The anode is spun at about 3000 r.p.m. by means of an induction motor stator placed outside the tube. The rotating anode has a much larger effective area than a fixed anode, but all the heat dissipated must be lost by radiation. Tungsten rotating anodes are normally used, for high power pulsed operation (100 kW, 100 kV) in cardiac catheterization X-ray systems water-cooled tubes with rotating carbon anodes are encountered. Microprocessor control of the X-ray generator is common. The latest development is to use a ceramic body for the X-ray tube rather than hard glass in order to hold a better vacuum under high power operating conditions.

When the anode power dissipation is low and hence the tungsten target does not become hot enough to emit electrons by thermionic emission, the X-ray tube may be used as its own simple half-wave rectifier. However, when the target is heavily loaded, the high voltage supply to the tube must be separately rectified. *Figure 11.4* shows a portable X-ray set using a rotating anode X-ray tube with separate rectifier valves. An X-ray image intensifier is used in conjunction with a television camera and monitor. The set is capable of delivering 300 mA at up to 120 kV peak, but when used in conjunction with the image intensifer, currents of only a few milliamperes would be supplied.

The longer exposures required during fluoroscopy present the greatest risk to the surgeon and anaesthetist who are near the patient due to the presence of stray X-radiation scattered from the patient and surroundings. With an image intensifier, X-rays emerging from the

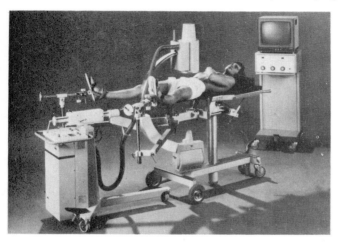

Figure 11.4. Portable X-ray set fitted with an image intensifier for use during surgery. (By courtesy of Philips Müller)

patient cause the input fluorescent screen of the intensifier to fluoresce. The resulting light releases photoelectrons from a light-sensitive cathode. The number of electrons is proportional to the brightness of each point of light forming the image on the screen. The electrons are then accelerated by a high voltage, focused with an electrostatic field and converted into a bright image on a small fluorescent screen placed at the output end of the intensifier tube (*Figure 11.5*). A gain in intensity of at least 3000 is possible with a 15 cm intensifier. The gain of an image intensifier is specified by its conversion factor, symbol Gx. This is defined as the ratio of the mean value of the luminance of the output image and the corresponding mean value of the input exposure rate measured in the entrance plane of the intensifier under specific conditions. The luminance is the amount of light emitted per unit area from a surface expressed in candelas per square metre and the exposure rate is expressed in milliröntgens per second. Gx = luminance/exposure rate and has units of Cd s m^{-2} mR. An average value of Gx for a new

15 cm image intensifier having a caesium iodide phosphor would be 150. Typical minimum values of Gx suitable for angiocardiography would be 50 and for hip pinning 35. The image can be viewed with a television camera and the resulting picture displayed on television monitors seen by the whole operating team and others in ancillary rooms. In general, the use of image intensifiers during fluoroscopy has reduced the X-ray tube current employed by about ten times. At low

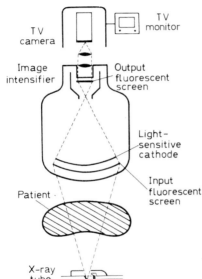

Figure 11.5. X-ray image intensifier unit and television camera. (By courtesy of Philips Müller)

tube currents, it may not be possible to see the screen well in daylight, or the noise of the intensifier amplifiers may be excessive. The use of an intensifier provides a better quality picture, and this enables the diagnosis or manoeuvre to be completed in a shorter time and the dose of radiation to the patient to be substantially reduced. It is still desirable for the surgeon and anaesthetist to wear lead-lined aprons and their radiation exposure should be monitored by film badges. Lead-lined screens may also be placed around the patient to limit scattered radiation. Rueter (1978) gives details of the radiation dose to the doctor and the patient during cardiac catheterization. A film badge service is available in the U.K. through the National Radiological Protection Board. The film badges are designed to distinguish between various qualities of radiation and to give an estimate of the dose received. Radiation hazards of interest to anaesthetists are discussed by Webster and Merrill (1957), Keen (1960), Kyle (1962), Letard and Belleau (1962) and Little and Radford (1964). Anaesthetists are some-times asked to anaesthetize patients undergoing supervoltage irradiation of tumours in conjunction with high pressure oxygen (Van Den Brenk, Madigan and Kerr, 1964; Churchill-Davidson, 1965). Anaesthetists are also called upon to anaesthetize patients for other radiotherapy procedures. Since the anaesthetist cannot remain in the room with the patient during treatment there may be a need for respiratory monitoring equipment. A good review article on linear accelerators used for radiotherapy is that of Atherton (1966).

Radioactive isotopes

Isotopes

It is possible for some elements to exist in different forms having the same atomic number but different atomic weights. These are known as isotopes. Some isotopes are stable, others are radioactive. The atomic number of an atom is equal to the number of orbital electrons in the atom, and governs the chemical properties of the atom. The atomic weight of an atom is simply its weight (relative to that of carbon whose atomic weight is taken to be 12). Since the chemical properties of isotopes of the same element are identical, their separation can be difficult by physical means, and is impossible chemically.

Atomic mass unit

This is one twelfth that of the mass of the ^{12}C atom, i.e. 1.6606×10^{-27} kg. This is the physical unit of atomic weight. It is smaller than the chemical unit which ignores the presence of the heavier isotopes of carbon.

The mass number A

It will be remembered that an atom consists of a central massive nucleus, around which moves orbital electrons. The mass number is the number of protons plus neutrons in the nucleus, and is the nearest integer to the atomic weight. The *atomic weight* of an atom no longer has the fundamental importance formerly attached to it, and is in a sense accidentally determined by the mixture of isotopes in the atom, and by their abundances. In the case of chlorine, there are two isotopes of mass 35 and 37 and having relative abundances of 3.07:1. This leads to a mean weight of 35.460 which is almost exactly the chemical atomic weight of 35.457.

Nuclide

This is the name of an atom which has a specific nuclear characteristic, e.g. phosphorus of mass number 32 and atomic number 15, and cobalt of mass number 60 and atomic number 27.

The symbolic representation of nuclides
Phosphorus-32 is represented as

A (mass number)
Z (atomic number) Chemical Symbol   i.e. $^{32}_{15}$ P

The advantage of this method is that the nuclear characteristics are kept to one side, leaving the right-hand side free for indication of valency and molecular state. Thus $^2_1$H represents an atom of heavy hydrogen (deuterium).

Stable and unstable nuclei

In a series of isotopes of the same element, the ratio of neutrons to protons varies. Some of these ratios give rise to stability, whereas other ratios lead to instability (radioactivity). Consideration of the stability of nuclei involves a study of the *binding energy* of the nucleus. This is the difference between the sum of the masses of the protons, neutrons

TABLE 11.1

Element	Atomic No.	No. of Neutrons	No. Protons	Mass No.
Hydrogen	1	0	1	1 Stable
Heavy hydrogen	1	1	1	2 Stable
Tritium	1	2	1	3 Unstable
Carbon	6	4	6	10 Unstable
"	6	5	6	11 Unstable
"	6	6	6	12 Stable
"	6	7	6	13 Unstable
"	6	8	6	14 Unstable

and electrons associated with the atom and the exact mass of the nuclide. These facts are illustrated in *Table 11.1* (Faires and Parks, 1964).

Modes of disintegration of nuclei

Beta particles

An unstable nucleus such as carbon-14 has an excess of energy. In order to achieve stability, it undergoes a random rearrangement during which energy is given out in the form of particles. Carbon-14 has too many neutrons for stability. The resulting nuclear rearrangement may be represented as the decay of an uncharged neutron into a positively charged proton and a negatively-charged electron. The maximum energy of the beta particle depends on the change in binding energy resulting from the nuclear reaction. In many cases, the nucleus still has an excess of energy after losing a beta particle. This is then dissipated in the form of gamma radiation. Gamma radiation is simply a form of electromagnetic radiation like light or X-radiation. Gamma radiation from radioactive cobalt is widely used in radiotherapy for the treatment of tumours. Since beta decay results in the formation of an extra proton, the new nuclide will have an atomic number one higher than previously. For example

$$^{14}_{6}C \longrightarrow ^{14}_{7}N + e^{-}$$

Some substances are pure beta emitters such as tritium, carbon-14, and sulphur-35, phosphorus-32 and yttrium-90. In the majority of cases, however, both beta particles and gamma radiation are emitted.

Alpha particles

The heaviest nuclides have such an excess of energy that they commonly lose larger units of mass than beta particles in the decay process. These units are known as alpha particles. They are identical to helium nuclei, having a mass of four atomic units and a positive charge of two units. The decay of radium-226 is given by:

$$^{226}_{88}Ra \longrightarrow ^{222}_{86}Rn + ^{4}_{2}He^{2+}$$

Alpha particle emitters are particularly dangerous if they are ingested, since the alpha particles cause an intense ionization in tissue. This, together with the difficulty in counting them, means that alpha particle emitters are not commonly encountered in unsealed medical practices.

Gamma radiation

In many cases the nucleus still has an excess of energy after losing an alpha or beta particle. This is then dissipated in the form of gamma radiation which is simply a form of electromagnetic radiation, like light or X-radiation. Gamma radiation is generally more penetrating than are beta particles, and is particularly useful since it can be counted from outside the body. Tantalum-182 emits both beta particles and gamma rays as does iodine-131. Powerful gamma ray sources are used to sterilize by radiation a wide range of disposable items used in anaesthesia and surgery, such as syringes, needles and scalpels.

Beta decay by positron emission

Some isotopes have too few neutrons for stability. They can become stable by changing a proton into a neutron. When this occurs it is possible for a positron (the positively-charged antiparticle of the electron) to be emitted. The positron has the same mass as an electron and loses kinetic energy in the same way as does a negative beta particle, by interaction with electrons in its path. Once it has lost all its kinetic energy it is incapable of an independent existence. It then undergoes an annihilation reaction with an ordinary negative electron to produce two 0.51 MeV gamma rays which are given off in opposite directions. By using a coincidence circuit to detect the pair of gamma rays, the positrons emitted can be counted. This technique has been used in a positron gamma camera (Yano and Anger, 1968), with positron emitting isotopes such as gallium-68 to visualize the kidneys.

Electron capture

The other process by which neutron-deficient isotopes can attain stability is by the nucleus capturing one of its orbital electrons, thus converting a proton into a neutron. As a result of this process an X-ray characteristic of the daughter element is emitted when an outer orbital electron fills the vacancy previously occupied by the captured electron. In some cases the energy, instead of being radiated, may be transferred to another orbital electron causing it to be ejected from the atom. This is called an Auger electron. Electron capture occurs, for example, in mercury-197, chromium-51 and fluorine-18.

Internal conversion

A transition can occur between two energy states of a nucleus where the energy difference is not emitted as a gamma photon, but is given to an orbital electron which is thereby ejected from the atom. An isotope in which internal conversion occurs is iodine-125.

Metastable states

In cases of normal gamma ray emission, the excited state of the nucleus only lasts about 10^{-12} s. With some isotopes the excited state may have a half-life of several hours. This is a very convenient period for isotopes which are used to visualize organs by means of a scanner or gamma camera. Examples are technetium-99m (half-life 6 hours) and indium-113m (half-life 100 minutes). (The 'm' in 'technetium-99m' conventionally indicates the metastable isotope.)

Radioactive decay and half-life

The decay of a radioactive element is governed by a simple exponential law, i.e. $N=N_0 \exp(-\lambda t)$, where N_0 is the number of atoms of the decaying substance at time $t=0$, N the number at time t, and λ is a constant for the particular element concerned, known as the decay constant. The constant $\lambda = 1/T$ where T is the time constant, i.e. the time taken for the activity to decay to $1/e$ (37 per cent) of its initial value. In considering the life of a particular radioactive substance, it is usual to express this in terms of its half-life. This is the time taken for the activity to decay to one half of its original value. In the case of radiotherapy sources, it is often desirable to have a long half-life so that the source does not need to be renewed at frequent intervals. Common sources here are caesium-137, half-life 30 years, gamma energy 0.66 MeV; cobalt-60, half-life 5.26 years, gamma energy 1.17 and 1.33 MeV; radium-226, half-life 1620 years, gamma energies of 0.19–2.43 MeV. On the other hand, for labelling drugs which have to be injected into a patient, it is desirable to work with short half-life substances. For example: iodine-131 (half-life 8.04 days), mercury-203 (half-life 47 days), mercury-197 (half-life 65 days), fluorine-18 (half-life 112 minutes).

Biological half-life

The greatest danger when working with radioactive materials occurs when they enter the body, because once they have become deposited in a tissue, they cannot readily be removed. In the body, there are two processes reducing the amount of radioactivity. These are the normal radioactive decay and excretion. The combined effect is to shorten the natural half-life of an isotope to its effective biological half-life. Hobbs (1965) states that whilst the physical half-life of iodine-125 is 60 days, its biological half-life is 3.4 hours. Ben-Porath, Case and Kaplan (1968) find a biological half-life in man of 45.5 days for selenium-75 seleno-methionine compared with the 121-day physical half-life of selenium-75. An extreme example occurs with inert gaseous isotopes such as xenon-133 which has a physical half-life of 5.27 days, but its concentration in blood is reduced by about 95 per cent in the first pass through the lungs.

The effective half-life (T_{eff}) for the elimination of a radioactive nuclide from an organ can be calculated from a knowledge of the half-life for the physiological elimination of the particular compound (T_b) and the half-life $(T_{1/2})$ for the decay of radioactivity with which the compound has been labelled. The time constants T_b and $T_{1/2}$ act in parallel so that

$$T_{eff} = \frac{(T_b T_{1/2})}{(T_b + T_{1/2})}$$

The compound chlormerodrin labelled with mercury-197 can be used to obtain gamma camera pictures of the kidney. It is removed from the kidney with a physiological half-life of 5.6 hours (0.23 days). The half-life for the decay of mercury-197 is 2.7 days, so that the effective half-life for the clearance of mercury-197 chlormerodrin is

$$T_{eff} = \frac{0.23 \times 2.7}{0.23 + 2.7} = 0.21 \text{ days}$$

Taking into account the nature and energy of the radiation emitted, and the radiosensitivity of the tissue concerned, the International

Committee on Radiological Protection has laid down a maximum permissible body burden for each radioisotope.

The unit of energy of radioactivity

In the SI system, the basic unit of energy is the joule and one electron volt is approximately equal to 1.6×10^{-19} J. Since 1 femtojoule = 10^{-15} J, 1 keV = 0.16 fJ and 1 MeV = 160 fJ. Thus the 35 keV radiation from iodine-125 has an energy of 5.6 fJ and the 0.51 MeV radiation from fluorine-18 has an energy of 81.6 fJ.

For any electromagnetic radiation the following relationship holds:

$$E = h\upsilon$$

where E is the photon energy in joules, h is Planck's constant (6.6×10^{-34} J s), and υ is the frequency.

For the fluorine-18 radiation, $E = 81.6 \times 10^{-15}$ J, so the frequency of the radiation is

$$(81.6 \times 10^{-15})/(6.6 \times 10^{-34}) = 12.36 \times 10^{-19} \text{ Hz}$$

The wavelength of the radiation can be determined from the relationship

velocity of light = wavelength $\times$ frequency

Since the velocity of light is 3×10^{8} m s^{-1}, the wavelength of the fluorine-18 radiation is

$$(3 \times 10^{8})/(12.36 \times 10^{19}) = 2.34 \times 10^{-12} \text{ m}$$

Units of activity

The pre-SI unit of radioactivity is the curie (symbol Ci). This was originally defined as the activity of one gram of radium, but it is now also applied to alpha and beta emitters. The value of the curie is taken as 3.7×10^{10} disintegrations per second. In nuclear medicine the mCi (10^{-3} Ci) and the μCi (10^{-6} Ci) are commonly encountered. Thus 1 μCi of phosphorus-32 will decay at a rate of 3.7×10^{-4} disintegrations per second corresponding with the emission of 3.7×10^{-4} beta particles per second. It does not automatically follow that, because a beta emitter is decaying at a certain rate, it must be emitting beta particles at that rate. Thus, iodine-126 decays with a negative beta particle in

44 per cent of the transitions: it produces a positive beta particle (positron) in 1 per cent of the transitions and the characteristic X-ray of electron capture in 55 per cent of the transitions. In this case 1 μCi of iodine-126 will emit only $0.44 \times 3.7 \times 10^{10}$ negative beta particles per second.

The SI unit of activity is the becquerel (symbol Bq), equal to one nuclear transformation per second; 3.7×10^{10} becquerels equal 1 curie exactly. 1 μCi = 3.7×10^4 Bq = 37 kBq; 1 mCi = 37 MBq.

Radiological protection

It is now widely known that the action of radiation on tissue can be dangerous, and the dose limits are carefully laid down in the United Kingdom by codes of practice. Practical problems arise when handling radioisotopes, since radiation by itself is invisible. Further, harmful effects arising from exposure to it may not be evident until many years after the exposure. In order to specify dose levels, it is first necessary to lay down units by means of which the dose can be defined (Boag, 1963).

Units of exposure

The pre-SI unit of radiation exposure is the röntgen (R). The röntgen is defined as the quantity of X- or gamma radiation that the associated corpuscular emission per 0.001293 g of air, produces ions carrying one electrostatic unit of electricity (0.001293 g is the mass of 1 ml of air at STP). The röntgen can be regarded as the total energy given to 1 ml of air. It is not used to measure alpha or beta particle radiation because of practical difficulties in its application. It is not a unit of body exposure dose, since it does not necessarily give an indication of the energy absorbed by tissue but is a unit of exposure.

The SI unit of exposure is the coulomb per kilogram (symbol C kg^{-1}). No special name has been adopted for this unit as its use is expected to decrease. 1 coulomb per kilogram equals 3876 röntgens. One röntgen equals 258 μC kg^{-1}.

The intensity of a beam of X or gamma rays is measured by its exposure rate expressed in C kg^{-1} s^{-1} or röntgens per second.

Units of absorbed dose

When a beam of gamma or X-rays passes through air ionization occurs due to the primary radiation or secondary electrons. A quantity known as exposure which is a measure of the intensity of the radiation has now been defined in terms of the amount of the ionization produced in air. When X-rays or gamma rays are incident on tissue, damaging effects occur due to the ionization produced in the tissue. Ionization within a living cell may cause its death or give rise to changes in its nucleus which may lead to malignancy.

The biological effects of radiation depend not only on the intensity but more particularly on the amount of the radiation energy which is absorbed in the tissue. One röntgen gives 258 microcoulombs of energy to one kilogram of air, but 289 microcoulombs to one kilogram of water. Since tissue is radiologically equivalent to water, one röntgen will give 289 microcuries to one kilogram of tissue. The fact that one röntgen gives different amounts of energy to the same mass of air and tissue led to the introduction of the rad (from *R*öntgen *a*bsorbed *d*ose). It is defined as that quantity of ionizing radiation which produces an energy absorption of 100 ergs per gram and it applies to all types of radiation. For soft tissue the röntgen and the rad are approximately equal.

The SI unit of absorbed dose is the gray (symbol Gy) and equals one joule per kilogram. $1 \text{ Gy} = 1 \text{ J kg}^{-1} = 10\,000 \text{ erg g}^{-1} = 100 \text{ rad}$.

Relative biological effectiveness (r.b.e.)

This is defined as

$$\frac{\text{Amount of 200 keV X-rays required to produce a given effect}}{\text{Amount of the radiation in question required to produce the same effect}}$$

For 200 keV X-rays the r.b.e. is by definition unity, while for the usual range of gamma radiation or beta particles the r.b.e. varies between 1.2 and 0.8. However, for fast neutrons, protons and naturally occurring alpha particles it has values of up to 100. For example, two rads of alpha particles produce the same biological damage as 20 rads of 100 keV X-rays. That is, alpha particles have an r.b.e. of 10. Alpha particles can be stopped by a single layer of paper and have a range of a few centimetres in air. In this short path, however, they give rise to intense ionization and heavy damage to tissues. It is for this reason that alpha particle emitters constitute a real hazard if they become ingested. A 3 MeV alpha particle has a range in air of 16 mm and is stopped by an aluminium foil about 0.015 mm, whereas a 3 MeV beta particle would require about 6.5 mm thickness of aluminium. In 1959 the International Commission on Radiological Units recommended that the term r.b.e. should be used in radiobiology work, and the term quality factor in radiation protection work (Neary, 1963).

Units of dose equivalent

The rem is a unit of radiation dose which relates the radiation effect of different types of irradiation per rad of the radiation. 1 rem is taken as the effect of 1 rad of 200 keV X-rays in man.

The SI unit of dose equivalent is the joule/kilogram. It is proposed by the International Commission on Radiological Protection that this unit be named the sievert (symbol Sv). 1 sievert equals 100 rems exactly.

As an example, 1 gray of alpha particles is equal in effect to 10 sieverts. The advantage of a unit of dose equivalent is that the effect of various types of radiation in man can be summed and expressed in terms of a single unit. Thus if tissue is subjected to 0.01 Gy of alpha particles and 0.02 Gy of 200 keV X-rays the total dose can be expressed as $(0.01 \times 10 + 0.02 \times 1) = 0.12$ Sv. In more detail, the dose equivalent (Sv) = absorbed dose (Gy) $\times$ various factors. These factors include the distribution factor and the quality factor (Neary, 1963). When the risk is of late effects from a low dose as in tracer studies, the distribution factor is unity. The quality factor takes into account the relative effects of different types of radiation. It is 1.0 for X-rays and gamma rays and beta particles of maximum energy more than 0.03 MeV, 10 for neutrons and protons up to 10 MeV and 20 for alpha particles. This reflects the fact that heavy particles do more damage to tissue because they lose all their energy in a short distance.

For all X-rays, gamma rays and beta particles at the energies and dose rates normally found in nuclear medicine studies, the modifying factors may be taken as unity so that dose equivalent and absorbed dose are numerically equal, thus 1 gray is approximately equal to 1 sievert and 1 rad is approximately equal to 1 rem.

Maximum permissible doses

In the United Kingdom, the maximum permissible doses have been laid down by Codes of Practice. The *Code of Practice for the Protection of Persons Exposed to Ionizing Radiations in Research and Teaching* (H.M.S.O., 1968) applied to Medical Schools and Research Laboratories. In U.K. hospitals, the *Code of Practice for the Protection of Persons Against Ionizing Radiations Arising from Medical and Dental Use* (H.M.S.O., 1972) applied.

However, the Commission of the European Community has proposed to the Council of Ministers that the Euratom Directive (76/579 Euratom) should be implemented from July 1980. For members of the general public the Directive lays down that in the case of whole body irradiation the dose limit shall be 5 mSv (0.5 rem) per year. For designated 'exposed workers' the dose limit for whole body irradiation shall be 50 mSv (5 rem) per year. Exposed workers are defined as persons subjected, as a result of their work, to an exposure liable to result in an annual dose greater than one tenth of the limits of the annual dose laid down for workers.

For the purposes of monitoring and surveillance, a distinction shall be made between two categories of exposed workers: Category A — those who are liable to receive a dose greater than three tenths of a limit of annual dose; Category B — those who are not liable to receive this dose.

For women of reproductive capacity (in the U.K. under 50 years of age) the dose to the abdomen shall not exceed 13 mSv (1.3 rem) in a quarter. As soon as pregnancy is declared, measures shall be taken to ensure that exposure of the woman concerned in the context of her employment is such that the dose to the fetus, accumulated over the period of time between declaration of pregnancy and the date of delivery, remains as small as is reasonably practicable and in no case exceeds 10 mSv (1 rem). In general, this limitation can be achieved by employing the woman in working conditions appropriate to category B workers.

Workers under 18 years of age may not carry out *any* activity which would result in their being exposed workers.

Subject to certain conditions, and with their permission, Category A workers can be subjected to planned special exposures each of which must be the subject of an appropriate permit. The doses received as a result of planned special exposures must not in any year exceed twice the limits of the appropriate annual dose, or in a lifetime, five times those dose limits.

In the case of partial body irradiation, the dose limit for the effective dose shall be 50 mSv (5 rem) per year; the average dose in each of the organs or tissues involved shall not exceed 500 mSv (50 rem) per year. The dose limit for the lens of the eye is 300 mSv (30 rem) per year, for the skin 500 mSv (50 rem) per year and applies to the dose average over any area of 100 cm^2. The dose limit for the hands, forearms, feet and ankles is 500 mSv (50 rem) per year.

Radiation protection

Users of radioactive substances are required to register with the Department of the Environment, and the amounts of material which can be

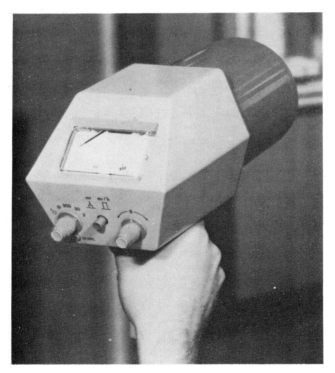

Figure 11.6. Ionization chamber radiation monitor. (By courtesy of Philips Ltd Medical Systems Division)

kept on the premises and the routes of its disposal are carefully controlled. The accomodation for the storage of the material and the safety precautions taken during its use are the concern of the Inspectors of the Health and Safety Executive. The safety aspects of work with radioactive materials or equipment producing X-rays or gamma rays must be overseen by a Radiological Protection Adviser.

Users must also have a calibrated monitor available to check the dose or dose rates. For quantitative work an ionization chamber type of monitor is needed (*Figure 11.6*) but a simple transistorized Geiger counter monitor (*Figure 11.7*) is very convenient for locating lost

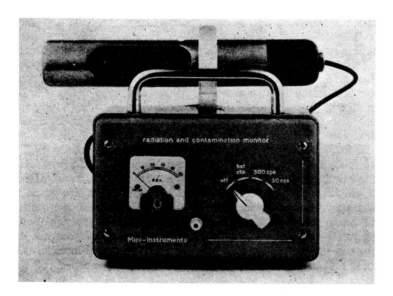

Figure 11.7. Transistorized Geiger counter radiation monitor

sources or checking on spillages. For low energy gamma emitting isotopes, such as iodine-125, a version with a scintillation counter probe should be employed. Dosimetry techniques are described by Aglintsev *et al.* (1965) and the principles of radiation protection by Eaves (1964). Hendee (1973) gives examples of the calculation of the internal absorbed dose when typical doses of radionuclides are administered to patients, while Shapiro (1972) gives a practical guide for scientists and clinicians to the principles of radiation protection.

From June 1980 medical practitioners in the United Kingdom

wishing to administer radioisotopes to persons will have to be licensed to do so by the Department of Health and Social Security.

Under the Euratom Directive the assessment of the individual doses must be systematic for Category A workers.

In order to restrict exposure, it will be necessary to classify and demarcate areas. No special arrangements need be made for areas of work where the exposure is not liable to exceed one tenth of the limits of the annual dose for exposed workers. Controlled areas must be established where the doses are liable to exceed three tenths of the limits of the annual dose for exposed workers. Controlled areas must be demarcated, radiological environmental surveillance must be organized; activities, doses and dose rates as the case may be shall be monitored and results recorded; the hazards inherent in the sources shall be indicated, signs indicating sources shall be displayed and qualified experts must be concerned in the discharge of these duties.

In the United Kingdom, radiation protection services are provided for hospitals in various ways. Some Regional Health Authorities provide a comprehensive advisory and monitoring service from Regional Centres with routine personal dosimetry by film badges and thermoluminescent dosimeters while others may make use of the film badge and thermo-luminescent dosimeter (TLD) services offered by the National Radio-logical Protection Board. The Board also offers a specialist advisory service in radiological protection.

The introduction in the United Kingdom of the Health and Safety at Work Act and the activities in hospitals of the Health and Safety Executive Inspectors has undoubtedly focussed attention on the need to maintain strict safety precautions when dealing with potential health hazards such as radioactivity and ionizing radiations.

Clinical applications of radioisotopes

Hobbs (1965) describes the use of human serum albumin labelled with iodine-131 and 125 to replace dye in the indicator dilution method for determining cardiac output. The method offers the advantage that water may be used for the preparation of standard solutions for calibration purposes. Methods for analysing the 'radiocardiogram' curves are discussed by Hill *et al.* (1973). Hobbs also discusses an adaptation of the method to enable blood volume to be measured. Regional blood-flow studies can be undertaken with the use of the radioactive gas xenon-133 (half-life 5.27 days). Dollery, Hugh-Jones and Matthews (1962) discuss the use of radioactive xenon for studies of regional lung function. When xenon-133 is rapidly injected into a suitable arm vein, nearly all the injected dose is evolved into the alveolae on the first passage through the pulmonary circulation, giving a counting rate for each zone of the lung which is proportional to its blood supply. Bentivoglio *et al.* (1963a) have used xenon-133 to study regional ventilation and perfusion in pulmonary emphysema, and in bronchial asthma (1963b). Holzman *et al.* (1964) used xenon-133 to study the muscle blood flow in the human forearm. The blood flow in skeletal muscle was studied by Lassen, Lindbjerg and Munck (1964) using xenon-133. Radioactive methods of estimating hepatic blood flow are discussed by Sherlock (1964) and isotope renograms as a test of renal function by Tauxe, Maher and Hunt (1964).

Harper, Jacobson and McDowall (1965) used krypton-85 to determine the effect of hyperbaric oxygen on the blood flow through the cerebral cortex. Veall and Vetter (1958) describe the application of many isotopes to clinical studies including the measurement of blood volume using chromium-51 and red-cell survival studies with chromium-51.

Van Dyke, Chenoweth and Van Poznak (1964) describe the use of carbon-14 and chlorine-36 to label cyclopropane, methoxyflurane and ether in studies on the metabolism of volatile anaesthetics. The metabolism of carbon-14 labelled halothane is described by Van Dyke, Chenoweth and Larson (1965).

Daniel (1963) used chlorine-36 labelling to study the metabolism of trichloroethylene and tetrachloroethylene in the rat. Dal Santo (1964) investigated the distribution of dimethyl-*d*-tubocurarine by labelling it with carbon-14. By labelling succinylcholine with carbon-14, Dal Santo (1968) showed in dogs that under pentobarbitone anaesthesia, after five minutes 80 per cent of the activity had disappeared into the plasma and 10 per cent into the urine. The fate, distribution and excretion of promazine has been studied by Walkenstein and Seifter (1959) with the aid of sulphur-35 labelled promazine.

The monograph by Lajth (1961) gives a concise account of the use of iodine-131 labelled serum albumin for the estimation of blood volume and the use of chromium-51 to estimate red-cell survival time. The book by Parker, Smith and Taylor (1978) deals in a most clear manner with the basic science of nuclear medicine including basic physics, counting techniques and radiopharmaceuticals.

References

AGLINTSEV, K.K., KODYUKOV, V.M., LYZKOV, A.P. and SIVINTSOV, Y.V. (1965). *Applied Dosimetry.* London; Iliffe

ATHERTON, L. (1966). Design evolution of an advanced linear accelerator for supervoltage therapy. *Wld med. Electron. Instrum., Lond.* **4**, 66

BEN-PORATH, M., CASE, L. and KAPLAN, E. (1968). The biological half-life of Se-75 selenomethionine in man. *J. nucl. Med.* **9**, 168

BENTIVOGLIO, L.G., BEEREL, F., BYRAN, A.C., STEWART, P.B., ROSE, B. and BATES, D.V. (1963a). Regional pulmonary function studied with xenon-133 in patients with bronchial asthma. *J. clin. Invest.* **42**, 1193

BENTIVOGLIO, L.G., BEEREL, F., STEWART, P.B., BYRAN, A.C., BALL, W.C. and BATES, D.V. (1963b). Studies of regional ventilation and perfusion in pulmonary emphysema using xenon-133. *Am. Rev. Resp. Dis.* **68**, 315

BOAG, J.W. (1963). Radiological quantities and units, their inter-relationships and conditions of use. *Physics Med. Biol.* **7**, 409

CHURCHILL-DAVIDSON, I. (1965). The use and effects of high-pressure oxygen in radio-therapy. In *Clinical Application of Hyperbaric Oxygen* (Ed. by I. Boerema, W.H. Brummelkamp, and N.G. Meijne) p. 14. Amsterdam; Elsevier

DAL SANTO, G. (1964). Kinetics of distribution of radioactive-labelled muscle relaxants. I. Investigation with C14 dimethyl-*d*-tubocurarine. *Anesthesiology* **25**, 788

DAL SANTO, G. (1968). Kinetics of distribution of radioactive labelled muscle relaxants. *Anesthesiology* **29**, 435

DANIEL, J.W. (1963). The metabolism of [36]Cl-labelled trichloroethylene and tetra-chlorethylene in the rat. *Biochem. Pharmac.* **12**, 795

DOLLERY, C.T., HUGH-JONES, P. and MATTHEWS, C.M.E. (1962). Use of radioactive xenon for studies of regional lung function. *Br. med. J.* **2**, 1006

EAVES, G. (1964). *Principles of Radiation Protection.* London; Iliffe

FAIRES, R.A. and PARKS, B.H. (1964). *Radioisotope Laboratory Techniques.* 2nd edn, p. 6. London; Newnes

HARPER, A.M., JACOBSON, I. and McDOWALL, D.G. (1965). In *Hyperbaric Oxygenation* (Ed. by I. McA. Ledingham), p. 184. Edinburgh; Livingstone

HENDEE, W.R. (1973). *Radioactive Isotopes in Biological Research.* New York; Wiley

HILL, D.W., THOMPSON, D., VALENTINUZZI, M.E. and PATE, T.D. (1973). The use of a compartmental hypothesis for the estimation of cardiac output from dye dilution curves and the analysis of radiocardio-grams. *Med. Biol. Engng* **11**, 43

HOBBS, J.T. (1965). Semi-automatic instruments to measure cardiac output and blood volume. *Wld. med. Electron. Instrum., Lond.* **3**, 324

HOLZMAN, G.B., WAGNER, H.N., ILO, M., RABONWITZ, D. and ZIERLER, K. L. (1964). Measurement of muscle blood flow in the human forearm with radioactive krypton and xenon. *Circulation* **30**, 27

KEEN, R.I. (1960). The radiation hazard to anaesthetists. *Br. J. Anaesth.* **32**, 224

KYLE, W.D. (1962). Radiation exposure of anaesthetists. *Can. Anaesth. Soc. J.* **9**, 161

LAJTH, L.G. (1961). *The Use of Isotopes in Haematology.* Oxford; Blackwell

LASSEN, N. A., LINDBJERG, J. and MUNCK, O. (1964). Measurement of blood flow through skeletal muscle by intramuscular injection of xenon-133. *Lancet* **1**, 686

LETARD, R. and BELLEAU, C.D.(1962). Radiation exposure. *Anesthesiology* **23**, 267

LITTLE, J.B. and RADFORD, E.P. (1964). Effects of ionising radiation and their importance in anesthesiology. *Anesthesiology* **25**, 479

NEARY, G.J. (1963). The significance of the rem and parameters on which it depends. *Physics Med. Biol.* **7**, 419

PARKER, R.P., SMITH, P.H.S. and TAYLOR, D.M. (1978). *Basic Science of Nuclear Medicine.* Edinburgh; Churchill Livingstone

RUETER, F.G. (1978). Physician and patient exposure during cardiac catheterization. *Circulation* **58**, 134–139

SHAPIRO, J. (1972). *Radiation Protection.* Cambridge, Mass; Harvard University Press

SHERLOCK, S. (1964). Measurement of hepatic blood flow. In *Dynamic clinical studies with radioactive isotopes. TID-7678*, p. 359. United States Atomic Energy Commission Report

STRETTAN, J.S. (1965). *Ionizing Radiations.* Oxford; Pergamon

TAUXE, W.N., MAHER, F.T. and HUNT, J.C. (1964). The isotope renogram as a test of renal function. In *Dynamic clinical studies with radioactive isotopes. TID-7678*, p. 383. United States Atomic Energy Commission Report

VAN DEN BRENK, H.A.S., MADIGAN, J.P. and KERR, R.C. (1964). Experience with megavoltage irradiation of advanced malignant disease using high pressure oxygen. In *Clinical Application of High Pressure Oxygen* (Ed. by I Boerema, W.H. Brummelkamp and N.G. Meijne), p. 140. Amsterdam; Elsevier

VAN DYKE, R.A., CHENOWETH, M.B. and VAN POZNAK, A. (1964). Metabolism of volatile anaesthetics: Conversion *in vivo* of several anaesthetics to $^{14}CO_2$ and chloride. *Biochem. Pharmac.* **13**, 1239

VAN DYKE, R.A., CHENOWETH, M.B. and LARSON, E.R. (1965). Synthesis and metabolism of halothane 1-14C. *Nature, Lond.* **204**, 471

VEALL, N. and VETTER, H. (1958). *Radioisotope Techniques in Clinical Research and Diagnosis.* London; Butterworths

WALKENSTEIN, S.S. and SEIFTER, J. (1959). Fate, distribution and excretion of S 35 promazine. *J. Pharmac. exp. Ther.* **125**, 283

WEBSTER, E.W. and MERRILL, O.F. (1957). Radiation hazards: Measurement of gonadal dose in radiographic examinations. *New Engl. J. Med.* **257**, 811

YANO, Y. and ANGER, H.O. (1968). Visualization of heart and kidneys in animals with ultra-short-lived Rb-82 and the positron scintillation camera. *J. nucl. Med.* **9**, 412

12 Anaesthesia machines

Anaesthetic machines are designed to provide known flow rates of gases which may contain the vapour of a volatile anaesthetic agent in various forms of anaesthetic circuit such as an open circuit or circle arrangement. A typical arrangement is that shown in *Figure 12.1* which is the well known Boyle M anaesthetic apparatus by the British Oxygen Company. The trolley is constructed from square section stainless steel and runs on four large-diameter castors fitted with antistatic rubber castors. A top frame carries all the gas circuit components, i.e. cylinder yokes and pressure regulators or pipeline connectors or both. Above the stainless steel working surface a backbar carries the flowmeter unit which has up to four rotameter tubes and their associated needle valves, a choice of up to three vaporizers including one Boyle ether bottle as standard together with a combined non-return valve and pressure relief safety valve. The swivel-type fresh gas outlet incorporating an emergency oxygen control valve and a manoeuvring handle is fitted at the front right-hand corner of the table. The gas circuit layout is shown in *Figure 12.2*. A maximum of six non-interchangeable pin index cylinders can be carried. Various combinations are possible such as three oxygen, two nitrous oxide and one carbon dioxide or two oxygen, two nitrous oxide, one carbon dioxide and one cyclopropane. The individual cylinder capacities are 700 litres (24 cubic feet size) oxygen, 2000 litres (400 gallon size) nitrous oxide, 400 litres (80 gallon size) cyclopropane and 500 litres (2 lb size) carbon dioxide. Non-return valves fitted in the cylinder yokes facilitate changing an empty cylinder whilst a second cylinder is in use. Cylinder contents pressure gauges are fitted as standard on the oxygen cylinder

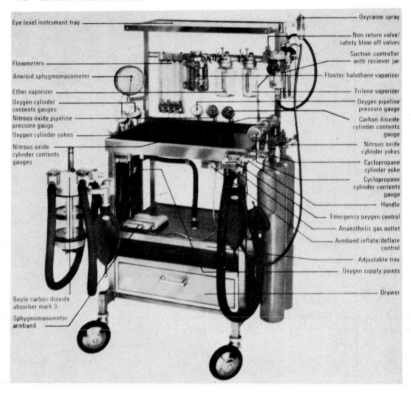

Figure 12.1. The Boyle anaesthetic apparatus Model M. (By courtesy of the British Oxygen Co. Ltd)

yokes and they are available as optional extras on the yokes for the other gases. Each cylinder yoke is provided with a Bodok washer to make a gas-tight joint.

All the gas lines of the Boyle M are made from chromium-plated copper tubing with threaded connections throughout. Each cylinder yoke (except cyclopropane) is fitted with a pressure reducing regulator to give an output pressure of 60 lbf in^{-2}g (414 kN m^{-2}) so that each yoke can be used independently of the others. No pressure regulators are required for the pipeline connections since these operate at 60 lbf in^{-2}g (414 kN m^{-2}). A regulator safety valve is provided so that the regulator output pressure cannot exceed 85 lbf in^{-2}g (586 kN m^{-2}). The maximum cylinder pressure which can be handled is 3000 lbf in^{-2}g (20.69 MN m^{-2}). The maximum individual flow rates possible as

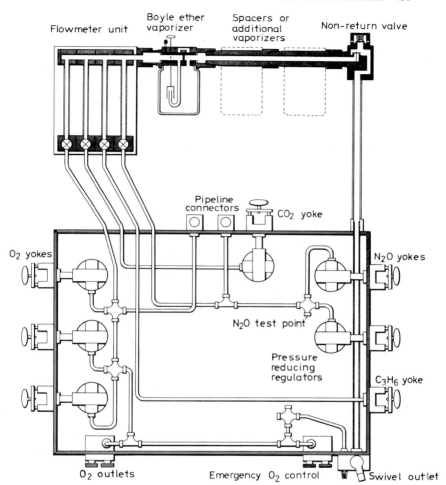

Figure 12.2. The gas circuit arrangement of the Boyle anaesthetic apparatus Model M. (By courtesy of the British Oxygen Co. Ltd)

measured by the flowmeters are: oxygen 0–8 litres per minute; nitrous oxide 0–12 litres per minute; cyclopropane 0–1 litres per minute, carbon dioxide 0–2 litres per minute. The maximum pressure of the fresh gas is limited to 5 lbf in^{-2}g (34.5 kN m^{-2}). By depressing the emergency oxygen control level the oxygen flowmeter and vaporizers are bypassed and a flow of 35–40 litres per minute of oxygen is available to the anaesthetic circuit.

A built-in manifold panel on the front of the apparatus carries four self-sealing oxygen supply points for ancillary equipment. The supply pressure is 60 lbf in^{-2} g (414 kN m^{-2}). Provision is made for fitting an oxygen inflate/deflate valve for pressurizing a blood pressure sphygmo-manometer cuff. Either a diaphragm aneroid-type manometer scaled 0–300 mmHg or a mercury manometer scaled 0–260 mmHg can be mounted on one of the upright pillars of the anaesthetic machine to measure blood pressure. A spray for the administration of local anaes-thetic agents can be powered from one of the oxygen supply points.

One or more of the following vaporizers are mounted on the back bar of the trolley: the Boyle ether vaporizer; the Boyle trichloro-ethylene vaporizer; the Fluotec Mark 2 or Mark 3 vaporizer; the Halox vaporizer or the Goldman vaporizer. The Goldman dental vaporizer can be used for either halothane in concentrations up to 3 per cent v/v or for trichloroethylene in low concentrations. In the Penlon SM anaesthesia apparatus, vaporizers can be mounted on individual off-line mounting blocks which are permanently mounted as part of the machine's manifold. Vaporizers can then be quickly disconnected from the machine without disturbing the joints of the manifold. The use of the mounting blocks is claimed to minimize contamination of com-ponents such as the flowmeters with anaesthetic vapours since the vaporizers can be removed from the machine at the end of the anaes-thetic.

Epstein and Hunter (1968) have provided a pictorial review of the development of the modern anaesthetic machine and Komesaroff (1974) has developed an anaesthetic machine for developing countries. Adams (1969) has given a good account of the various components of anaesthetic machines and Mayer (1974) has given a guide for the maintenance of anaesthetic machines. Eger and Epstein (1964) have pointed out a number of possible hazards which can arise with routine anaesthetic apparatus and Ditzler (1970) discusses the checking of anaesthetic machines, whilst Nainby-Luxmoore (1967) discusses the hazards which can arise with dental anaesthetic gas machines.

All the major manufacturers of anaesthetic machines pride themselves on their service organization. It is essential that anaesthetic machines and their ancillary equipment, which may be required for use at any time of day or night, are regularly serviced. This will ensure that gas leaks, sticking valves, rotating parts jammed with soda lime particles, sticking flowmeters and faulty vaporizers are detected and repaired.

Microprocessor controlled anaesthesia machine

As was mentioned in the chapter Computer Techniques, microcomputers based on the use of integrated circuit microprocessors are finding increased applications in scientific instruments. It was a logical development to find this approach being adopted for a new generation of anaesthesia machines. Cooper *et al.* (1978) describe a new type of anaesthesia machine whose flow diagram is given in *Figure 12.3*. The

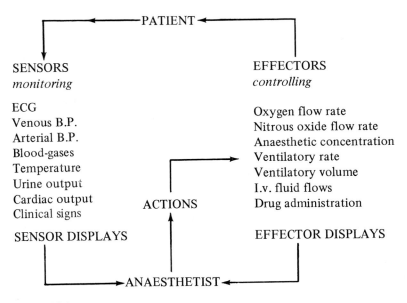

Figure 12.3

desired mixture of oxygen and nitrous oxide is generated by means of special valves. Liquid anaesthetic agent is added directly into this gas mixture in pulses by an injector. All the liquid vaporizes in a passive evaporator coil. All the active devices are under the control of a microprocessor which receives instructions from the control panel and scans a number of machine sensors. The processor continuously monitors the system functions and either corrects or alarms when the machine or the operator acts in an unsafe or inappropriate manner. The processor itself is monitored repeatedly to ensure appropriate warning or corrective action in the event of a functional problem. A rechargeable battery provides back-up power in the event of a mains power failure. A description of the vaporizer used is given in the chapter on Anaesthetic Vaporizers.

Anaesthetic circuits

Anaesthetic circuits in this context consist of an assembly of hoses and components through which the patient breathes. The circuit concerned is supplied with fresh gas and anaesthetic vapour from the anaesthetic machine or fresh gas alone. If the fresh gas flow supplied to the circuit is less than the patient's minute volume, rebreathing occurs. It is possible to classify circuits on the basis of the amount of rebreathing which takes place:

(1) Non-rebreathing circuits (open circuits)
(2) Partial rebreathing circuits without carbon dioxide absorption (semi-open circuits)
(3) Partial rebreathing circuits with carbon dioxide absorption (semi-closed circuits)
(4) Complete rebreathing circuits (closed circuits)

The five common circuit configurations are:

(1) Circuits with non-rebreathing valves
(2) T-piece systems
(3) Magill circuits
(4) To-and-fro circuits
(5) Circle systems

When assembling the components for an anaesthetic circuit care must be taken to see that the total resistance to gas flow will not impose an undue burden in terms of the work cost of breathing on a spontaneously breathing patient. The measurement of the resistance to gas flow of breathing apparatus is discussed in Chapter 2.

Circuits with non-rebreathing valves

Non-rebreathing anaesthetic circuits may be used in conjunction with a draw-over vaporizer and the entrainment of air or oxygen-enriched air

or they may be fed with an anaesthetic gas mixture from an anaesthetic machine. In the latter case there must be an interposed reservoir
bag or tube so that the patient can draw from this during inspiration.
Figure 12.4 illustrates the Penlon Quantitative Apparatus Mark 2.
A suitable mixture of oxygen and nitrous oxide is fed from the two
rotameters into a corrugated reservoir tube and then into an EMO ether
inhaler. At the outlet of the EMO is mounted a Penlon bellows unit.

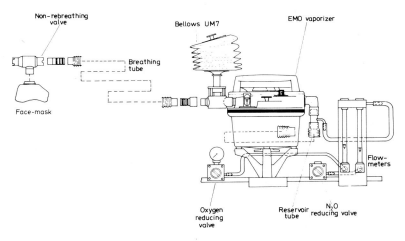

Figure 12.4. Schematic diagram of the Penlon Quantitative
Anaesthetic Apparatus Mark 2. (By courtesy of Penlon Ltd)

The bellows are fitted with a disc non-return valve. A corrugated hose
leads from the T-piece of the bellows unit to a non-rebreathing valve
and a facemask. During inspiration, the patient inspires an anaesthetic
gas and vapour mixture via the inspiratory porting of the non-rebreathing
valve. During expiration he expires directly to the atmosphere via the
expiratory porting of the valve.

There are a number of suitable non-rebreathing valves. *Figure 12.5*
is a sectional view of the Ambu E valve. During spontaneous inspiration
or the inflation of the patient by the bellows the fresh gas flow from
the right opens the labial side of the elastic shutter. The shutter then
swells outwards and occludes the expiratory port at seating B. The side
port to the patient is left open. As soon as the inspiration or inflation is
finished, the labial openings close the opening to A. The elastic shutter
returns to its original position allowing the patient to exhale through
valve C. Upon the completion of expiration, the labial valve C in the

expiratory port closes and the re-entry of air into the valve through the outlet is prohibited. Grogono and Porterfield (1970) point out the danger which can occur if an Ambu valve is wrongly assembled. If an Ambu E valve has been dismantled, it is important to be sure that on re-assembly both shutters face the same way and are fitted to points A and C in *Figure 12.5*. A shutter must never be fitted at point B as it

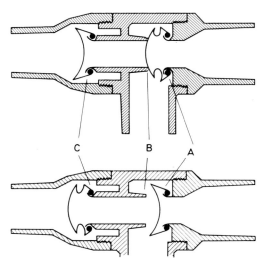

Figure 12.5. Sectional view of an Ambu E non-rebreathing valve. (By courtesy of Penlon Ltd)

would completely occlude expiration. In the well known Ruben valve the operating principle is the same, but plastic discs connected to form a shuttle are used (Ruben, 1955). Sykes (1968) has reviewed various types of non-rebreathing valves. For the accurate measurement of inspiratory and expiratory tidal volumes it is essential that at any given time the inspiratory and the expiratory valves are not open together. Hill and Hook (1958) have described an electrically operated valve for this purpose.

Magill system

This is the standard open circuit breathing attachment supplied with the Boyle apparatus, and is illustrated in *Figure 12.6*. A two-litre volume rebreathing bag is attached to a bag mount which connects with

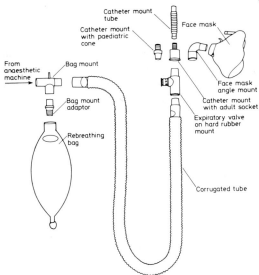

Figure 12.6. A Magill anaesthetic circuit. (By courtesy of the British Oxygen Co. Ltd)

the anaesthetic gas outlet of the anaesthetic machine. At the other end of the 1 metre long corrugated rubber hose is an expiratory valve on an antistatic mount. This can lead to a facemask or an endotracheal tube. No carbon dioxide absorber is used so that there is always the possibility of some carbon dioxide being present in the inspired gas mixture. Whether any rebreathing occurs, and if so how much, depends upon a number of variables such as the ratio of the fresh gas flow to the patient's minute volume, the patient's anatomical dead space, the respiratory flow pattern and the duration of the expiratory pause (Suwa and Yamamura, 1970).

The action of a Magill system with a spontaneously breathing patient can be seen in *Figure 12.7*. During the first part of the expiratory phase, expired gas returns to the corrugated hose and to the partially empty bag. It comes mainly from the apparatus and anatomical dead spaces and contains little carbon dioxide. The next portion of the expirate will normally contain up to about 6 per cent CO_2 and will also enter the tube and bag, but some will be vented out though the relief valve as the bag fills with the incoming fresh gas. When inspiration commences, some portion of the previous expirate can be rebreathed. Mapleson (1954) predicted that the rebreathing would be prevented by making the fresh gas flow equal to the patient's alveolar ventilation.

Then, at the moment of commencing an inspiration the circuit will only contain fresh gas and dead space gas of the same composition. Mapleson recommended that in practice the fresh gas flow should be made equal to the patient's minute volume. Kain and Nunn (1968) showed that in lightly-anaesthetized patients the fresh gas flow could be reduced to 71 per cent of the minute volume before rebreathing commenced.

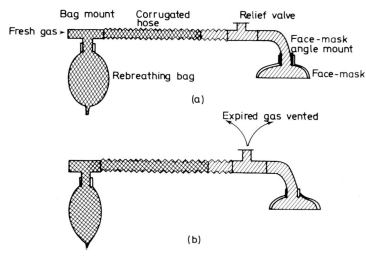

Figure 12.7. The movement of fresh gas (cross-hatched) and gas containing CO_2 (shaded) in the Magill circuit during spontaneous respiration with a medium flow of fresh gas. (a) During expiration; the bag is taut and the relief valve is about to open; (b) Start of next inspiration

Intermittent positive pressure respiration can be performed by manually squeezing the rebreathing bag. The relief valve opens at a predetermined inflation pressure and vents excess gas from the circuit to the atmosphere. During expiration, the patient expires passively into the hose and bag. The degree of rebreathing will depend upon the fresh gas flow, tidal volume, respiratory rate and the rate of rise of pressure during inspiration. It can be reduced by having a high fresh gas flow, increasing the tidal volume, reducing the respiratory rate and having a high pressure early in inspiration to vent a greater amount of alveolar gas from the circuit. Norman, Adams and Sykes (1968) discuss re-breathing with a Magill attachment.

T-piece systems

From the viewpoint of the components, T-piece systems (Ayre, 1937; 1956) represent the simplest configuration. This makes for reliability, but T-piece systems have the disadvantage of being uneconomical in their use of fresh gas. Under favourable conditions the fresh gas flow can be 2 to 2½ times the patient's minute volume without the occurrence of rebreathing. The particular feature of the T-piece is that the fresh gas is introduced between the connection to the patient and the gas outlet. Depending on the amount of the fresh gas flow the system can function as a non-rebreathing system or as a partial rebreathing system without carbon dioxide elimination. Referring to *Figure 12.8*, in the original design the volume of the corrugated hose on

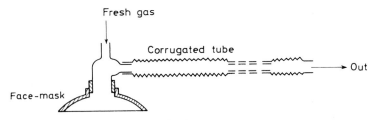

Figure 12.8. T-piece anaesthetic circuit

the expiratory limb of the T-piece was greater in volume than the patient's tidal volume in order to avoid diluting the fresh gas with room air. During expiration both expired and fresh gas flow down the expiratory limb. Since the peak expiratory flow rate occurs early in expiration, as expiration proceeds the proportion of fresh gas in the expiratory limb increases. During the expiratory pause fresh gas will accumulate at the patient end of the limb. During inspiration both fresh gas and gas from the expiratory limb will be inspired. When the fresh gas flow rate is greater than the peak inspiratory flow rate then only fresh gas will be inspired. This requires that the fresh gas flow is about three times the patient's minute volume. For lower fresh gas flows, gas will be inspired from the expiratory limb. At first this will be the accumulated fresh gas but after this it will contain an increasing proportion of carbon dioxide. The effect of rebreathing should be greatest at the end of inspiration, but then the gas containing carbon dioxide will occupy the patient's dead space and will take part in gas exchange. Intermittent positive-pressure respiration can be obtained by an intermittent occlusion of the expiratory limb. The inspirate will consist entirely of fresh gas. During expiration both fresh gas and expired gas will be discharged from the expiratory limb. Since the circuit does not have a reservoir bag the fresh gas flow and the ratio of inspiration-to-expiration time must be adjusted to produce the desired minute volume. In practice this amounts to a fresh gas flow of about three times the minute volume. For this reason T-piece arrangements have been used for the ventilation of neonates and infants. It is interesting to note that T-piece systems have been in use for more than 25 years. In Jackson-Rees's (1950) modification, an open-tailed bag is added to the expiratory limb. Analyses of the behaviour of T-piece systems have been given by Mapleson (1954), Inkester (1956) and Nightingale, Richards and Glass (1965). Bush (1971) makes the point that whereas with spontaneous respiration the fresh gas flow should be three times the patient's minute volume in order to prevent rebreathing, with intermittent positive-pressure ventilation the gas mixing makes it possible to have a fresh gas flow of only 220 ml kg^{-1} body weight. Bush suggests that in order to allow for the inaccuracies of the gas flow-meters, a flow of 2 $1 min^{-1}$ is recommended during neonatal anaesthesia. A comprehensive account of the use of a T-piece with a ventilator for the ventilation of neonates is given by Urban and Weitzner (1974).

The Waters' to-and-fro systems

This is shown in *Figure 12.9*. Fresh gas from the anaesthetic machine is run in to the circuit close to the face-mask or endotracheal tube. The

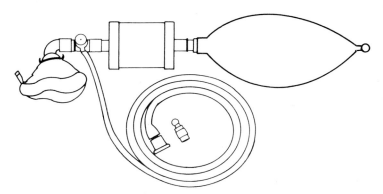

Figure 12.9. The Waters' to-and-fro absorber. (By courtesy of the British Oxygen Co. Ltd)

relief valve is also situated where the fresh gas enters. The main portion of the circuit is from the patient via a carbon dioxide absorber to a rebreathing bag. According to the relationship between the fresh gas input to the system and the patient's minute volume, a to-and-fro circuit can function either as a non-rebreathing system, a partial re-breathing system or a complete rebreathing system. Although a carbon dioxide absorber is present, rebreathing of CO_2 is not completely prevented. In the illustration the absorber is made of transparent acrylic material so that indicating soda lime may be used. A 30 cm length of corrugated tubing can be inserted between either the canister and the expiratory valve mount or between the canister and the rebreathing bag when intermittent positive-pressure respiration is to be used by squeezing the bag.

The to-and-fro arrangement provides an inspired gas mixture with a relatively high humidity when low fresh gas flows are used. This arises from the release of water vapour from the soda lime and the rise in temperature of the gases due to heat generated in the absorbent. Channelling of gas through the absorbent may occur because of the horizontal position of the absorber. The dead space extends out to the proximal boundary of the carbon dioxide absorber. The gradual exhaustion of the absorber leads to a steady increase in the dead space and a loss of circuit efficiency. Because the circuit is compact and the absorber is close to the patient, there is a risk of the patient inhaling soda lime dust. Robsen and Pask (1954) investigated the performance of Waters' canisters and discuss a more effective method for packing the canister with soda lime. Ten Pas, Brown and Elam (1958) have compared circle and to-and-fro absorption systems.

Circle systems

Circle systems came into prominence with the introduction of expensive and flammable agents such as cyclopropane. The agent is contained within the circle except for the relatively small amount which is vented from the relief valve, and the rebreathing of the agent conserves the amount which must be supplied. The components of a typical circle system are shown diagrammatically in *Figure 12.10*. If there are no leaks present, the fresh gas flow rate need only be sufficient to supply the oxygen uptake requirements of the patient, no gas being vented from the circuit. This is then a *closed circuit* arrangement. Because of leaks, a flow rate of about 500 cm^{-3} min^{-1} into the circle may be

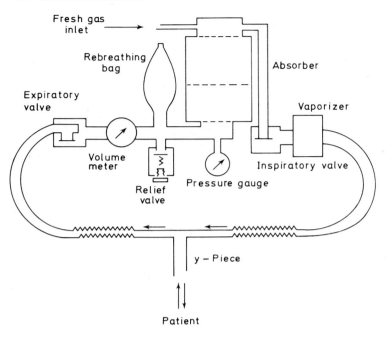

Figure 12.10. The components of a typical circle anaesthetic circuit

required to prevent the rebreathing bag from collapsing. At low fresh gas flows, the circle may require a regular readjustment of the fresh gas input in order to balance the circuit flows. It is common practice in the United Kingdom to work with fresh gas flows of the order of 4 1 min^{-1}, i.e. less than the patient's minute volume but more than the uptake per minute of the patient and the absorber. Excess gas is vented from the relief valve and rebreathing of carbon dioxide is prevented by the soda lime absorber. When the fresh gas inflow is equal to or greater than the patient's minute volume, the circle is said to be open and no rebreathing occurs. Under these conditions a carbon dioxide absorber is not required. Fitton (1958) has investigated oxygen consumption in semi-closed circuits.

Components of the circle system

The uni-directional flow of gas round a circle system is normally achieved by the use of a pair of valves, the inspiratory valve and the expiratory valve. In order to minimize the apparatus dead space the valves may be mounted in a valve block forming part of the Y-piece to which is connected a face-mask, tracheostomy connection or endotracheal tube. In many circle anaesthetic systems the pair of valves is mounted on the circle absorber housing. The valves usually operate in a fixed position with the valve disc being returned by gravity. The valve disc is often made of mica and works in conjunction with a metal seat. The sideways movement of the disc is restrained by a cage fixed to the edge of the seating. A transparent plastic dome is fitted above each valve so that the motion of the disc can be observed. Each disc may also carry a visible mark such as a white spot. Guides are also required to limit the travel of the disc in a vertical direction. The expiratory valve, in particular, becomes very wet from the condensation of breath moisture. The design must prevent valves from sticking under these circumstances and they should be cleaned at regular intervals. A number of types of gas circulator have been described to provide an efficient circulation of gas in a circle system. They also minimize the mechanical dead space especially that existing under a face-mask (Revell, 1958; Roffey, Revell and Morris, 1961; Neff, Burke and Thompson, 1968).

The carbon dioxide absorber

The Boyle circle-type carbon dioxide absorber Mark 3, *Figure 12.11,* is representative of current absorber design practice. It consists of a double chamber, reversible, soda lime canister holding 1.8 kg (4 lb) of soda lime and is fitted to a control head by means of a central tube. It is screwed into the central tube with a large plastic hand nut. The canister is made from a transparent acrylic material in order that any change in colour of the indicating soda lime may be easily observed. A condensation trap fitted to the base of the central tube prevents any accumulation of condensed water vapour in the soda lime. Unidirectional inspiratory and expiratory valves are mounted in the control head as well as an adjustable pressure relief valve and a lever which can shut off the canister from the circle when it is not required or when it is being refilled. A pressure gauge can be screwed into the control head as an optional extra. All the internal gas passages are treated to protect against corrosion by moist halothane vapour. The transparent canister is divided centrally by a perforated metal baffle which reduces channelling through the soda lime. When the absorber is in use, the gases are

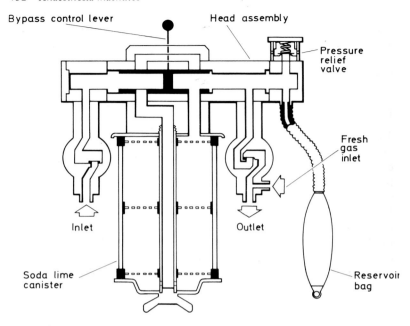

Figure 12.11. Cross-section of the Boyle Mark 3 carbon dioxide absorber. (By courtesy of the British Oxygen Co. Ltd)

routed down through the central tube and up through the soda lime; hence the soda lime in the lower chamber becomes exhausted first. When all the colour has changed in the lower chamber, the soda lime in that chamber can be replaced and the canister refitted with the freshly filled chamber uppermost. When used with the Boyle anaesthetic apparatus, the absorber is mounted on a support bracket fitted to either front leg of the table frame. The fresh gas supply tube for the circle is plugged into the anaesthetic gas outlet on the manifold panel. The makers claim that the soda lime used in the Mark 3 absorber will last approximately twice as long as it would if used in a conventional single chamber canister. Elam (1958) worked on the basis of servicing the absorber after eight hours of intermittent use. With tidal volumes in the range 0.5–1 litre the patient produced 12–18 litres of carbon dioxide per hour. Assuming that 100 g of soda lime absorbs 15 litres of carbon dioxide before the exit gas contains one per cent of carbon dioxide, Elam calculated that 870 g of soda lime would be needed per eight hour period. About 47 per cent of the soda lime would be void space which would accommodate one average tidal volume and it would increase by 60 ml per hour as absorption proceeded, hence the need for a second chamber. Other papers dealing with the design of absorbers are those of Brown, Seniff and Elam (1964) and Bracken and Cox (1968).

Relief valve

The relief valve is also known as a pop-off valve (U.S.A.), exhaust valve or pressure limiting valve. It is best located downstream from the expiratory valve but upstream from the absorber. In this way gas vented from the circle dow not have to pass through the absorber. The relief valve is often mounted on the housing of the absorber unit, but in the Boyle circle absorber, *Figure 12.11,* it is located on the outlet side of the absorber. The relief valve is usually a simple spring-loaded check valve with provision for the screw adjustment of the opening pressure. One-way valves of the Heidbrink pattern, *Figure 12.12,* are frequently

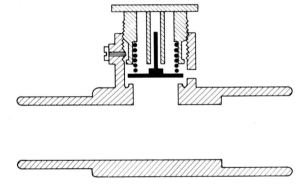

Figure 12.12

encountered in circle systems, semi-closed anaesthetic circuits and in the 'manual' circuits attached to automatic lung ventilators. Adjustment of the spring resistance allows the venting of gas to be controlled by the anaesthetist. When a greater accuracy of the opening is required, a dead weight valve is used. Apart from limiting the pressure in the circle, the relief valve serves to vent excess fresh gas to the atmosphere. When the patient is breathing spontaneously, the relief valve is set to a low opening pressure, typically 1 cmH_2O so that it opens towards the end of expiration. When intermittent positive-pressure respiration is in use, the valve is adjusted to give the maximum required inflation pressure and opens towards the end of inflation when the pressure in the circuit overcomes the spring tension. By screwing the valve adjustment knob hard down it is possible to close the valve completely. Linker, Holaday and Waltuck (1970) have described a simply constructed automatic pressure relief valve and Rusz and Duncalf (1970) have described a controlled pop-off valve. Eger and Ethans (1968) investigated several arrangements of inspiratory and expiratory valves and relief valve locations in a circle absorber system to determine which arrangement best conserved fresh gas and preferentially eliminated alveolar gas. During spontaneous ventilation the greatest economy of fresh gas occurred with the relief valve situated close to the patient. However, with one exception, when the ventilation was controlled, the worst conditions for economy were found with the relief valve near the patient. The exception was the arrangement with the inspiratory and expiratory valves close to the patient and the relief valve immediately downstream from the expiratory valve. This was the most economical arrangement.

Nott and Norman (1978) have measured the resistance of Heidbrink-type expiratory valves at a flow rate of 30 litres per minute. The average resistance of 70 valves currently in clinical use was 318 Pa and of these about 44 per cent had resistances in excess of 294 Pa which was the limit suggested by Nunn (1977). Mushin and Mapleson (1954) suggested that during spontaneous respiration Heidbrink-type valves should be set so that the pressure in the circuit was of the order of 50 Pa.

The scavenging of anaesthetic gases from circuits may produce a risk for the patient if it gives rise to subatmospheric pressures in the circuit. This can arise if there is an imbalance between the fresh gas flow and the gas evacuation rate. The use of a negative pressure relief valve will prevent this by opening at a small negative pressure and permitting a high rate of gas inflow (Brinløv, Andersen and Jørgensen, 1978).

Corrugated hoses

Corrugated hoses or breathing tubes are normally available in standard lengths of 20, 30, 80 and 107 cm (7½, 12, 32 and 42 in) and are usually made of antistatic rubber. The internal diameter should be at least 20 mm, and the hoses should be flexible but resist kinking. Hoses are also available made in various types of plastic such as neoprene, poly-vinyl chloride, polyethylene, polyurethane or polyolefin. Rubber hoses, breathing bags, face-masks, etc. should be stored in a dark, cool, location and not exposed for lengthy periods to sunlight or ultraviolet light which can affect the composition of the rubber. They should not be over-stretched and should be cleansed with warm water and a suitable detergent. They should be kept clear of grease, oil and solvents. As was mentioned in Chapter 5, rubber components of anaesthetic circuits can absorb substantial amounts of agents such as halothane and methoxyflurane. This fact must be taken into consideration when a quantitative approach is adopted to the uptake and elimination of volatile anaesthetic agents. Corrugated hoses are relatively compliant and their expansion during the inflation phase of ventilation can significantly alter the waveform generated by a ventilator. Non-distensible tubing should be used with modern, low compliance, ventilators (Bushman and Collis, 1967).

Rebreathing bags

Rebreathing bags are made from antistatic rubber and typically have volumes of 1, 2, 3, 4 and 6 litres. The shape and compliance of the bag used should be such that it will expand comfortably during expiration without causing an undue amount of gas to be lost via the relief valve. The neck of the bag is reinforced often with a separate short rubber connection piece which is inserted into the neck of the bag and makes contact with the metal bag mount.

The disposal of effluent gases and vapours from anaesthetic circuits

Studies such as those of Linde and Bruce (1969) and Cohen, Belville and Brown (1971) have led to an awareness of the harmful effects of the chronic exposure of operating room staff to low concentrations of anaesthetic gas and vapour mixtures which are discharged into the operating room and have led to many investigations such as those of Davenport *et al.* (1976, 1977) and the recommendations of Vickers (1975). By means of a gas chromatograph it is readily possible to measure gas and vapour concentrations in the parts per million range. Yanagida *et al.* (1973) measured an average concentration of 880 parts per million after three hours at 0.5 m from the circuit relief valve in an operating room with 15 changes of air per hour. Saloojee and Cole (1978) describe a gas chromatographic technique for the measurement of trace levels of nitrous oxide in whole blood. Trace levels of halothane can be measured with a gas chromatograph fitted with an electron capture detector.

Bruce (1974) replaced the relief valve with a venting valve which connected with a length of tubing to duct the effluent to the outside atmosphere. Enderby, Booth and Churchill-Davidson (1978) use a T-piece connected to the expiratory valve, the second limb of the T being open to the room atmosphere and the third limb connecting to the hospital's wall suction unit. They confirm that this arrangement does not harm the vacuum pump.

Halliday and Carter (1978) have described a chemical absorption system for sampling gaseous organic pollutants in operating room atmospheres and over 19 sessions found mean concentrations of 13.3 parts per million of ethanol with figures of 3.6 for isopropanol and 2.6 for halothane. Corbett (1969) has also described a gas trap.

Low oxygen pressure warning devices

The risk of cerebral damage consequent upon anoxia is still a real hazard for patients undergoing anaesthesia. The transposition of oxygen and nitrous oxide cylinders on the anaesthetic machine has been rendered impossible when pin index cylinders are used, but cases do occur where nitrous oxide is put into an oxygen pipeline. Another well known hazard occurs with the emptying of the oxygen cylinder passing unnoticed by the anaesthetist. The situation is aggravated if the anaesthetic machine is not carrying a spare oxygen cylinder. One possible warning device for this situation is the Ritchie whistle, shown in *Figure 12.13*. It sounds an audible warning of a reduction in the oxygen pressure below normal when connected into the oxygen line of an anaesthetic machine. It is powered solely by the oxygen pressure in the system and is not dependent upon a battery. When correctly adjusted, it starts to whistle when the oxygen pressure has fallen to 50–60 per cent of the normal value. The whistle is connected into the oxygen line between the outlet of the reducing valve and the inlet to the flowmeter. The maximum working pressure is 690 kPa (100 lbf in^{-1}) and the unit is normally supplied to sound an alarm at a pressure of 207 kPa (30 lbf in^{-1}), the normal supply pressure lying in the range

275–415 kPa (40–60 lbf in^{-1}). The whistle will continue to sound until the oxygen pressure has fallen to 70 kPa (10 lbf in^{-1}). Devices for warning of a low oxygen pressure have been described by Adler and Burn (1967), Ward (1968) and Rosen and Hillard (1971). A nitrous oxide cut-off valve can also be fitted to cut-off the nitrous oxide supply should the oxygen pressure fall below 207 kPa (30 lbf in^{-2}).

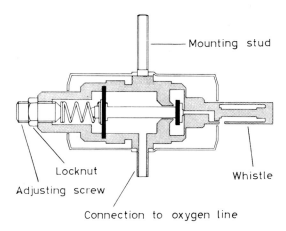

Figure 12.13. The Ritchie whistle low oxygen pressure warning device. (By courtesy of Penlon Ltd)

Hypoxic conditions can arise in anaesthetic circuits, particularly circle systems, due to an insufficient fresh gas flow of oxygen. The availability of compact oxygen concentration monitors has led to their increasing use with anaesthetic machines. One type is based on the use of a galvanic cell with a gold cathode and a lead anode in a potassium hydroxide electrolyte (Weil, Sodal and Speck, 1967; Torda and Collis, 1967). Gaseous oxygen from the circuit in which the sensor is placed diffuses into the cell via a polytetrafluoroethylene membrane and initiates redox reactions which generate a very small electric current which is proportional to the oxygen partial pressure. After amplification the current is caused to actuate a meter scaled 0–50 per cent and 0–100 per cent oxygen. The calibration is claimed to be linear within ±1 per cent of full-scale at a constant ambient temperature and the accuracy is claimed to be ±1 per cent of full-scale deflection. The 90 per cent response time is less than 20 seconds. The entire sensing element is encapsulated in an inert plastic and can withstand a maximum pressure of 500 lbf in^{-2} g (3.45 MN m^{-2}). A recorder and remote alarms can be fitted. The sensor is claimed to have a life under warranty of 180 000 per cent-hours or one year, and to be insensitive to carbon dioxide, nitrous oxide and humidity up to 100 per cent. It is temperature compensated between 0 and 40 °C. Other forms of compact oxygen monitor work on the polarographic Clark oxygen electrode principle much used in blood-gas analysers. For a range of 0–100 per cent oxygen a polarographic monitor would have a typical response time of 20 seconds to 95 per cent response. The accuracy is quoted as ±1 per cent oxygen when calibrated on room air. The device can be powered from 3.0–4.05 V mercury batteries and is fitted with high and low oxygen concentration alarm settings. The electrode membrane is changeable. This should normally be performed at three-monthly intervals and is said to take less than 30 seconds.

The British Oxygen Medishield oxygen failure warning device comprises two audible warning systems: one operated by a falling oxygen pressure, the other by patient-inspired air. When the oxygen powered whistle sounds, there is a short delay before anaesthetic gases are cut off. When the inspiratory whistle sounds the anaesthetic gases cut-off valve prevents the patient from breathing a hypoxic mixture. The oxygen failure warning section of the device is powered entirely by residual oxygen.

Figure 12.14 illustrates the operation of the British Oxygen Medishield oxygen failure warning device. Driving oxygen enters the inlet valve and pressurizes the rolling diaphragm, opening the anaesthetic gases cut-off valve and closing the air inspiratory valve and the port to the oxygen failure whistle. Anaesthetic gases flow freely to the breathing circuit. When the driving gas pressure falls to 262 kPa (38 lbf in^{-2}), the anaesthetic gases cut-off valve commences to close and the oxygen failure whistle valve starts to open, permitting a flow of oxygen, via the restrictor, to operate the oxygen failure whistle. The whistle sounds continuously until the pressure has fallen to approximately 35.4 kPa (6 lbf in^{-2}). At a pressure of 165–179 kPa (28–30 lbf in^{-2}), the force of the magnet keeper return spring and magnet causes the anaesthetic gases cut-off valve to be snapped shut, cutting off the supply of the anaesthetic gases. At the same time, the spring load on the air inspiratory valve is released, allowing the patient to inspire room air. Whenever the patient inspires, the inspiratory air whistle sounds. With the anaesthetic gases cut-off valve closed, fresh gases vent through the pressure relief valve on the Boyle apparatus, preventing gas pressure

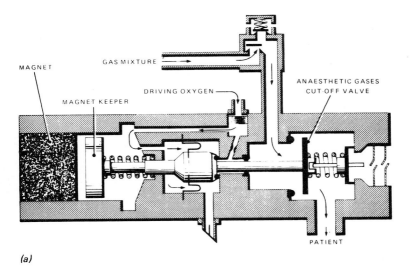

(a)

(b)

Figure 12.14. British Oxygen Medishield oxygen failure warning
device. (a) Normal operation; (b) oxygen failure. (Courtesy of the
Medishield Corporation)

in this part of the circuit from rising above 250–300 mmHg. Sounding of the air inspiratory whistle indicates:

(1) The oxygen supply has failed.
(2) When commencing anaesthesia, the oxygen supply is not connected
(3) The oxygen supply, if connected, has not been turned ON.

References

ADAMS, P. (1969). Anaesthetic machines. *Br. J. Hosp. Med.* April Equipment Supplement 35

ADLER, L. and BURN, N. (1967). A warning device for failure of the oxygen supply. *Anaesthesia* **22**, 156

ADRIANI, J. and ROWENSTINE, E.A. (1941). Experimental studies on carbon dioxide absorbers for anaethesia. *Anesthesiology* **2**, 1

AYRE, P. (1937). Endotracheal anaesthesia for babies: with special reference to hare lip and cleft palate operations. *Curr. Res. Anesth. Analg.* **16**, 330

AYRE, P. (1956). The T-piece technique. *Br. J. Anaesth.* **28**, 550

BENSON, D.W., GRAFF, T.D. and HURT, H.H. (1968). The circle semi-closed system control of $PACO_2$ by inflow rates of anaesthetic gases and hyperventilation. *Anesthesiology* **29**, 174

BRACKEN, A. and COX, L.A. (1968). Apparatus for carbon dioxide adsorption. *Br. J. Anaesth.* **40**, 660

BRINKLØV, M.M., ANDERSEN, P.K. and JØRGENSEN, S. (1978). The negative pressure relief valve: Pressure-flow relationships. *Br. J. Anaesth.* **50**, 1025–1029

BROWN, E.S., SENIFF, A.M. and ELAM, J.O. (1964). Carbon dioxide elimination in semiclosed systems. *Anesthesiology* **25**, 31

BRUCE, D.L. (1974). A simple way to vent anaesthetic gases. *Curr. Res. Anesth. Analg.* **52**, 595

BRUCE, D.L. and LINDE, H.W. (1972). Halothane content in recovery room air. *Anesthesiology* **36**, 517

BUSH, G.H. (1971). Neonatal anaesthesia. In *General Anaesthesia* (Ed. by I.C. Gray and J.F. Nunn), p. 410–427. London; Butterworths

BUSHMAN, J.A. and COLLIS, J.M. (1967). The estimation of gas losses in ventilator tubing. *Anaesthesia* **22**, 664

COHEN, E.N., BELVILLE, J.W. and BROWN, B.W. (1971). Anesthesia–pregnancy and miscarriage. A study in operating room nurses and anesthetists. *Anesthesiology* **35**, 343

COOPER, J.B., NEWBOWER, R.S., MOORE, J.W. and TRAUTMAN, E.D. (1978). A new anesthesia delivery system. *Anesthesiology* **49**, 310–318

CORBETT, T.H. (1969). The gas trap: a device to minimize chronic exposure. *Anesthesiology* **31**, 464

DAVENPORT, H.T., HALSEY, M.J., WARDLEY-SMITH, B. and WRIGHT, B.M. (1976). Measurement and reduction of occupational exposure to inhaled anaesthetics. *Br. med. J.* **2**, 1219–1221

DAVENPORT, H.T., HALSEY, M.J., WARDLEY-SMITH, B. and WRIGHT, B.M. (1977). Occupational exposure to inhaled anaesthetics. *Br. med. J.* **1**, 506–507

DITZLER, J.W. (1970). Checking anaesthesia machines. *Anesthesiology* **32**, 87

EGER, E.I. II and EPSTEIN, R.M. (1964). Hazards of anaesthetic equipment. *Anesthesiology* **25**, 490

EGER, E.I. II and ETHANS, C.T. (1968). The effects of inflow, overflow and valve placement on economy of the circle system. *Anesthesiology* **29**, 93–100

ENDERBY, D.H., BOOTH, A.M. and CHURCHILL-DAVIDSON, H.C. (1978). Removal of anaesthetic waste gases. *Anaesthesia* **33**, 820–826

ELAM, J.O. (1958). The design of circle absorbers. *Anesthesiology* **19**, 99

EPSTEIN, H.G. and HUNTER, A.R. (1968). A pictorial review of the development of the modern anaesthetic machine. *Br. J. Anaesth.* **40**, 636

FITTON, E.P. (1958). A theoretical investigation of oxygen concentrations in gases inspired from various semi-closed anaesthetic systems. *Br. J. Anaesth.* **30**, 269

GROGONO, A.W. and PORTERFIELD, J. (1970). Ambu valve: danger of wrong assembly. *Br. J. Anaesth.* **42**, 978

HALLIDAY, M.M. and CARTER, K.B. (1978). A chemical adsorption system for the sampling of gaseous organic pollutants in operating theatre atmospheres. *Br. J. Anaesth.* **50**, 1013–1018

HILL, D.W. and HOOK, J.R. (1958). A solenoid-operated inspiratory - expiratory valve. *J. Physiol. (Lond.)* **145**, 1P

INKESTER, J.S. (1956). The T-piece technique in anaesthesia. *Br. J. Anaesth.* **28**, 512

KAIN, M.L. and NUNN, J.F. (1968). Fresh gas economics of the Magill circuit. *Anesthesiology* **29**, 964

KOMESAROFF, D. (1974). A new anaesthetic machine and technique with particular application to developing countries. *Curr. Res. Anesth. Anal.* **52**, 605

LEE, S. (1964). A new pop-off valve. *Anesthesiology* **25**, 240

LINDE, H.W. and BRUCE, D.L. (1969). Occupational exposure of anesthetists to halothane, nitrous oxide and radiation. *Anesthesiology* **30**, 363

LINKER, S.G., HOLADAY, D.A. and WALTUCK, B. (1970). A simply constructed automatic pressure-relief valve. *Anesthesiology* **32**, 563

MAPLESON, W.W. (1954). The elimination of rebreathing in various semi-closed anaesthetic systems. *Br. J. Anaesth.* **26**, 323

MARSHALL, M. and HENDERSON, G.A. (1968). Positive pressure ventilation using a semiclosed system: a reassessment. *Br. J. Anaesth.* **40**, 265

MAYER, A. (1974). Malfunction of anaesthesia machines: a guide for maintenance. *Curr. Res. Analg. Anesth.* **52**, 376

MUSHIN, W.W. and MAPLESON, W.W. (1954). Pressure—flowrate characteristics of expiratory valves. *Br. J. Anaesth.* **26**, 3—10

NAINBY-LUXMOORE, R.C. (1967). Some hazards of dental gas machines. *Anaesthesia* **22**, 545

NEFF, W.B., BURKE, S.F. and THOMPSON, R.(1968). A venturi circulator for anesthetic systems. *Anesthesiology* **29**, 838

NIGHTINGALE, D.A., RICHARDS, C.C. and GLASS, A. (1965). An evaluation of rebreathing in a modified T-piece system during controlled ventilation of anaesthetized children. *Br. J. Anaesth.* **37**, 762

NORMAN, J., ADAMS, A.P. and SYKES, M.K. (1968). Rebreathing with a Magill attachment. *Anaesthesia* **23**, 75

NOTT, M.R. and NORMAN, J. (1978). Resistance of Heidbrink-type expiratory valves. *Br. J. Anaesth.* **50**, 477—480

NUNN, J.F. (1977). *Applied Respiratory Physiology.* 2nd edn, p. 103 London; Butterworths

REES, G.J. (1950). Anaesthesia in the newborn. *Br. Med. J.* **2**, 1419

REVELL, D.G. (1958). An improved circulator for closed circle anaesthesia. *Can. Anaesth. Soc. J.* **6**, 104

ROBSEN, J.G. and PASK, E.A. (1954). Some data on the performance of Water's canister. *Br. J. Anaesth.* **26**, 333

ROFFEY, P.J., REVELL, D.G. and MORRIS, L.E. (1961). Assessment of the Revell circulator. *Anesthesiology* **22**, 583

ROSEN, M. and HILLARD, E.K. (1971). Oxygen-fail-safe device for an anaesthetic apparatus. *Br. J. Anaesth.* **43**, 103

RUBEN, H. (1955). A new non-rebreathing valve. *Anesthesiology* **16**, 643

RUTLEDGE, R.R. (1973). A safe pressure-relief valve and scavenging system. *Curr. Res. Anesth. Analg.* **52**, 870

RUSZ, Th. and DUNCALF, D. (1970). A safe controlled pop-off valve. *Anesthesiology* **33**, 459

SALOOJEE, Y. and COLE, P. (1978). Estimation of nitrous oxide in blood. Gas chromatographic analysis of trace or analgesic levels. *Anaesthesia* **33**, 779—783

SUWA, K. and YAMAMURA, H. (1970). The effect of gas inflow on the regulation of CO_2 levels with hyperventilation during anesthesia. *Anesthesiology* **33**, 440

SYKES, M.K. (1968). Rebreathing circuits: A review. *Br. J. Anaesth.* **40**, 666

TEN PAS, R.H., BROWN, E.S. and ELAM, J.O. (1958). Carbon dioxide absorption, the circle versus the to-and-fro. *Anesthesiology* **19**, 231

TORDA, T.A. and COLLIS, J.M. (1967). The estimation of gas losses in ventilator tubing. *Anaesthesia* **22**, 664

URBAN, B.J. and WEITZNER, S.W. (1974). The Amsterdam infant ventilator and the Ayre T-piece in mechanical ventilation. *Anesthesiology* **40**, 423

VICKERS, M.D. (1975). Pollution of the atmosphere of operating theatres: Advice to members from the Council of the Association of Anaesthetists of Great Britain and Ireland. *Anaesthesia* **30**, 697–699

WARD, C.S. (1968). Oxygen warning device. *Br. J. Anaesth.* **40**, 907

WEIL, J.W., SODAL, I.E. and SPECK, R.P. (1967). A modified fuel cell for the analysis of oxygen concentration of gases. *J. Appl. Physiol.* **23**, 419

YANAGIDA, H., KEMI, C., SUWA, K. and YAMAMURA, H. (1973). Nitrous oxide content in the operating suite. *Curr. Res. Anesth. Analg.* **53**, 347

Index